Cutaneous Oncology and Dermatologic Surgery

Editors

RAJIV I. NIJHAWAN

DIVYA SRIVASTAVA

DERMATOLOGIC CLINICS

www.derm.theclinics.com

Consulting Editor
BRUCE H. THIERS

July 2019 • Volume 37 • Number 3

ELSEVIER

1600 John F. Kennedy Boulevard • Suite 1800 • Philadelphia, Pennsylvania, 19103-2899

http://www.theclinics.com

DERMATOLOGIC CLINICS Volume 37, Number 3
July 2019 ISSN 0733-8635, ISBN-13: 978-0-323-68237-4

Editor: Jessica McCool
Developmental Editor: Laura Kavanaugh

Dermatologic Clinics (ISSN 0733-8635) is published quarterly by Elsevier Inc., 360 Park Avenue South, New York, NY 10010-1710. Months of publication are January, April, July, and October. Business and editorial offices: 1600 John F. Kennedy Blvd., Suite 1800, Philadelphia, PA 19103-2899. Customer service office: 11830 Westline Drive, St. Louis, MO 63146. Periodicals postage paid at New York, NY, and additional mailing offices. Subscription prices are USD 404.00 per year for US individuals, USD 736.00 per year for US institutions, USD 456.00 per year for Canadian individuals, USD 898.00 per year for Canadian institutions, USD 510.00 per year for international individuals, USD 898.00 per year for international institutions, USD 100.00 per year for US students/residents, and USD 240.00 per year for Canadian and international students/residents. International air speed delivery is included in all *Clinics* subscription prices. All prices are subject to change without notice. **POSTMASTER:** Send address changes to *Dermatologic Clinics*, Elsevier Health Sciences Division, Subscription Customer Service, 3251 Riverport Lane, Maryland Heights, MO 63043. **Customer Service: 1-800-654-2452 (U.S. and Canada); 314-447-8871 (outside U.S. and Canada). Fax: 314-447-8029. E-mail: journalscustomerservice-usa@elsevier.com (for print support); journalsonlinesupport-usa@elsevier.com (for online support).**

Reprints. For copies of 100 or more, of articles in this publication, please contact the Commercial Reprints Department, Elsevier Inc., 360 Park Avenue South, New York, New York 10010-1710. Tel.: 212-633-3874; Fax: 212-633-3820; Email: reprints@elsevier.com.

The *Dermatologic Clinics* is covered in *MEDLINE/PubMed (Index Medicus), Current Contents/Clinical Medicine, Excerpta Medica, Chemical Abstracts,* and *ISI/BIOMED.*

Contributors

CONSULTING EDITOR

BRUCE H. THIERS, MD
Professor and Chairman Emeritus, Department of Dermatology and Dermatologic Surgery, Medical University of South Carolina, Charleston, South Carolina

EDITORS

RAJIV I. NIJHAWAN, MD
Assistant Professor, Department of Dermatology, The University of Texas Southwestern Medical Center, Dallas, Texas

DIVYA SRIVASTAVA, MD
Assistant Professor, Department of Dermatology, The University of Texas Southwestern Medical Center, Dallas, Texas

AUTHORS

SUMAIRA Z. AASI, MD
Director, Mohs and Dermatologic Surgery, Clinical Professor, Surgery – Plastic and Reconstructive Surgery, Clinical Professor, Department of Dermatology, Stanford University School of Medicine, Redwood City, California

NNENNA G. AGIM, MD
Associate Professor of Dermatology, Pediatric Dermatology, The University of Texas Southwestern Medical Center, Dallas, Texas

NEHA AGRAWAL, BA
Medical Student, University of Nevada, Reno, Nevada

SARAH T. ARRON, MD, PhD
Associate Professor, Department of Dermatology, University of California, San Francisco, San Francisco, California

EILEEN AXIBAL, MD
Fellow, Mohs Micrographic Surgery and Dermatologic Oncology, Department of Dermatology, University of Colorado Hospital and School of Medicine, University of Colorado, Aurora, Colorado

THOMAS S. BANDER, MD
Micrographic Surgery and Dermatologic Oncology Fellow, Memorial Sloan Kettering Cancer Center, Weill Cornell Medical College, New York, New York

DAVID G. BRODLAND, MD
Assistant Professor, Zitelli and Brodland PC, Departments of Dermatology, Otolaryngology, and Plastic Surgery, University of Pittsburgh Medical Center, Pittsburgh, Pennsylvania

MARIAH BROWN, MD
Director of Mohs Surgery and Cutaneous Oncology, Associate Professor, Department of Dermatology, University of Colorado Hospital and School of Medicine, University of Colorado, Aurora, Colorado

CHRISTINE CORNEJO, MD
Department of Dermatology, University of Pennsylvania, Philadelphia, Pennsylvania

M. LAURIN COUNCIL, MD
Associate Professor, Division of Dermatology, Department of Medicine, Washington University School of Medicine, St Louis, Missouri

LAUREN D. CROW, MD, MPH
Postdoctoral Clinical Research Fellow, Department of Dermatology, University of California, San Francisco, San Francisco, California

ASHLEY DECKER, MD
Dermatologic Surgery Attending, Cooper University Hospital, Marlton, New Jersey; Assistant Professor of Medicine, Cooper Medical School of Rowan University, Camden, New Jersey

CATHERINE A. DEGESYS, MD
Fellow, Mohs Micrographic Surgery and Dermatologic Oncology, Department of Dermatology, The University of North Carolina at Chapel Hill, Chapel Hill, North Carolina

DANIEL B. EISEN, MD
Director of Dermatologic Surgery and Head of the Micrographic and Dermatologic Oncology Fellowship, Department of Dermatology, University of California, Davis Medical System, Sacramento, California

JEREMY R. ETZKORN, MD
Assistant Professor, Department of Dermatology, University of Pennsylvania, Philadelphia, Pennsylvania

NICHOLAS GOLDA, MD
Medical Director of Dermatology Clinics, Director of Dermatologic Surgery, Fellowship Program Director for Micrographic Surgery and Dermatologic Oncology, Associate Professor, Department of Dermatology, University of Missouri, Columbia, Missouri

S. TYLER HOLLMIG, MD
Director, Laser and Aesthetic Dermatology, Clinical Associate Professor, Department of Dermatology, Stanford University School of Medicine, Redwood City, California

HILLARY JOHNSON-JAHANGIR, MD, PhD, MHCDS
Clinical Associate Professor, Dermatology, University of Iowa, Iowa City, Iowa

HAILEY M. JUSZCZAK, BA
Medical Student, University of California, San Francisco, San Francisco, California

KATHERINE A. KAIZER-SALK, BA
Research Assistant, Department of Dermatology, University of California, San Francisco, San Francisco, California

NAOMI LAWRENCE, MD
Head, Division of Dermatology, Cooper University Hospital, Marlton, New Jersey; Professor of Medicine, Cooper Medical School of Rowan University, Camden, New Jersey

ERICA H. LEE, MD
Assistant Attending Physician, Memorial Sloan Kettering Cancer Center, Assistant Professor of Dermatology, Weill Cornell Medical College, New York, New York

MICHAEL P. LEE, BS
Clinical Research Fellow, Department of Dermatology, University of Pennsylvania, Philadelphia, Pennsylvania

JEFFREY N. LI, BS, BBA
Department of Dermatology, The University of Texas Southwestern Medical Center, Dallas, Texas

BRADLEY G. MERRITT, MD
Associate Professor, Department of Dermatology, The University of North Carolina at Chapel Hill, Chapel Hill, North Carolina

CHRISTOPHER J. MILLER, MD
Associate Professor of Dermatology, Director of Penn Dermatology Oncology Center, Department of Dermatology, Perelman Center for Advanced Medicine, University of Pennsylvania, Philadelphia, Pennsylvania

KISHWER S. NEHAL, MD
Attending Physician, Memorial Sloan Kettering Cancer Center, Professor of Dermatology, Weill Cornell Medical College, New York, New York

KATHLEEN M. NEMER, MD
Micrographic Surgery and Dermatologic Oncology Fellow, Division of Dermatology, Department of Medicine, Washington University School of Medicine, St Louis, Missouri

RAJIV I. NIJHAWAN, MD
Assistant Professor, Department of
Dermatology, The University of Texas
Southwestern Medical Center, Dallas,
Texas

ROBERTO NOVOA, MD
Clinical Assistant Professor, Department
of Dermatology, Clinical Associate Professor,
Department of Pathology, Associate
Program Director, Division of
Dermatopathology, Stanford University
School of Medicine, Redwood City,
California

MICHAEL RENZI Jr, MD
PGY-2 Resident, Division of Dermatology,
Cooper University Hospital, Camden, New
Jersey

MICHAEL SACO, MD
Micrographic Surgery and Dermatologic
Oncology Fellow, Department of
Dermatology, University of Missouri,
Columbia, Missouri

JOSH SCHIMMEL, BS
Cooper Medical School of Rowan University,
Camden, New Jersey

KISHAN M. SHAH, BA
Indiana University School of Medicine,
Indianapolis, Indiana

LINDSAY R. SKLAR, MD
Mohs Fellow, Department of Dermatology,
University of California, Davis Medical System,
Sacramento, California

CORY SMITH, BS
Medical Student, The University of Texas
Southwestern Medical Center, Dallas, Texas

JOSEPH F. SOBANKO, MD
Assistant Professor, Department of
Dermatology, University of Pennsylvania,
Philadelphia, Pennsylvania

TEO SOLEYMANI, MD
Resident, Department of Dermatology,
Stanford University School of Medicine,
Redwood City, California

DIVYA SRIVASTAVA, MD
Assistant Professor, Department of
Dermatology, The University of Texas
Southwestern Medical Center, Dallas, Texas

RACHEL E. WARD, MD
Chief Resident, Department of Dermatology,
Wayne State University School of Medicine,
Detroit, Michigan

SHANNON W. ZULLO, MS
Clinical Research Fellow, Department of
Dermatology, University of Pennsylvania,
Philadelphia, Pennsylvania

Contents

Cutaneous squamous cell carcinoma (cSCC) is one of the most common cancers in the United States. Outcomes are generally favorable, but a subset of cSCC is biologically distinct and requires a different approach because of its higher risk of local recurrence, metastasis, and death. This article focuses on the recent literature regarding identification of this high-risk subset, efforts to validate and improve the prognostic ability of staging systems, and updates in management.

Atypical fibroxanthoma and undifferentiated pleomorphic sarcoma, or pleomorphic dermal sarcoma, are rare malignant cutaneous neoplasms existing along a clinicopathologic spectrum. Although these tumors share many similarities, recognition of distinguishing characteristics may predict differences in clinical behavior and outcomes. Salient features defining atypical fibroxanthoma include superficial tumors with minimal high-risk histologic features. Deeper tumors with high-risk histologic features are often clinically aggressive and should be appropriately designated as pleomorphic dermal sarcoma. Surgery remains gold standard in management; tumor extirpation with complete margin control is critical. In the high-risk tumor cohort, comprehensive evaluation and multidisciplinary management is paramount for optimal outcomes.

Extramammary Paget disease is an intraepidermal adenocarcinoma, most often limited to the epidermis, with typical cases affecting genital skin. When limited to the epidermis, primary extramammary Paget disease is not life-threatening, but invasive disease may portend a poor prognosis. Surgical excision remains the mainstay of treatment of extramammary Paget disease, and Mohs micrographic surgery is the surgical treatment of choice. Alternative treatments include topical 5-fluorouracil and imiquimod, photodynamic therapy, laser vaporization, chemotherapy, and radiation therapy but data are limited. Implementation of cytokeratin 7 immunostain has increased the ability to detect extramammary Paget disease on frozen section.

Merkel cell carcinoma is an aggressive neuroendocrine carcinoma with increasing incidence over the past few decades. The TNM Staging System used for Merkel cell carcinoma was updated by the American Joint Committee on Cancer in 2017. Clinical practice guidelines were updated by the National Comprehensive Cancer Network on August 31, 2018. This article reviews the most recent evidence-based updates on staging and management.

Over the next 30 years, dermatologists face a rising population of elderly patients, causing a marked increase in the incidence of cutaneous malignancies. For this reason, it is important to review the approach to the management of skin cancer in the elderly. In the current medical environment, there has been debate as to how cutaneous malignancy should be treated in elderly patients, especially those with multiple comorbid conditions. Clinicians should use a comprehensive approach that accounts for functional status, impact on quality of life, cost, and potential adverse outcomes when managing high- and low-morbidity skin cancers in the elderly.

Chemoprevention of nonmelanoma skin cancer should be considered in patients likely to develop numerous, invasive, or metastatic nonmelanoma skin cancers. This article reviews the various topical and systemic substances studied as chemopreventive agents.

A number of medications for short-term and long-term use have been linked to an increased risk for keratinocyte carcinoma (KC). Immunosuppressive medications are associated with an increased risk for KC and melanoma due to reduction of antitumor immune surveillance, and some immunosuppressive agents directly impact DNA replication and repair. Clinical and epidemiologic studies have shown an increased risk for KC in users of photosensitizing medications. Additional mechanisms include drug-induced modulation of DNA damage repair, enhancement of keratinocyte proliferation, and direct carcinogenic effect. Alternatively, some medications potentially decrease KC risk. This article reviews the literature on medications associated with KC risk.

Dermatologic surgery in pregnant/postpartum patients requires deliberate consideration. Although surgery can be safely performed during any trimester, the second trimester and immediate postpartum period is optimal. Surgery should not be delayed for melanoma/high-risk skin cancers. Perioperative positioning, analgesic, antiseptic, and antibiotic selection should be deliberate to avoid risk to the patient/fetus/infant. The left lateral tilt position reduces aortocaval compression syndrome. Lidocaine and epinephrine can be used safely. Alcohol and chlorhexidine are considered safe. Antibiotics commonly used in skin surgery are safe in pregnancy and lactation. Acetaminophen is first line for pain management. Nonsteroidal antiinflammatory drugs should be avoided.

Overall, dermatologic surgery performed in the outpatient setting is very low risk to patients and safer than similar procedures performed under general anesthesia, and is also more cost-effective. There are several approaches to mitigating the risk of complications while optimizing patient outcomes. Strict oversight of the dermatology clinic helps to ensure team members all adhere to standards of care. Vial safety, strict hand hygiene, limiting the use of topical antibiotics, generally continuing all blood thinners perioperatively, and prebiopsy photographs are all examples of approaches to help maximize patient safety.

Oral antibiotic prophylaxis is overly prescribed for procedures involving the integumentary system (skin, hair, nails, and related subcutaneous tissue) and mucosa. Preoperative antibiotic prophylaxis preventing infective endocarditis or hematogenous prosthetic joint infection is recommended only when operating on infected or mucosal sites of select, high-risk patients. There are limited data supporting oral antibiotic use to prevent surgical site infections, and antibiotics are not recommended for routine use. Alternatives to oral antibiotics that may reduce infection risk, such as wound antisepsis, are sought. Altogether, risk stratification and antibiotic stewardship are both necessary for appropriate perioperative oral antibiotic use for dermatologic surgery.

Given the opposing pressures placed on dermatologists and dermatologic surgeons by the need for adequate postoperative analgesia and the current US opioid epidemic, a systematic review was performed to analyze postoperative pain management in outpatient dermatologic surgery. Dermatologic procedures are generally associated with minor postoperative pain of short duration. Anxiety reduction may lead to less postoperative pain. Studies vary on which anatomic locations and repair types are more or less associated with pain. Evidence supports the use of acetaminophen and ibuprofen for first-line postoperative analgesia in dermatologic surgery. Opioids, if given, should only be prescribed in small quantities.

Dressings are integrally tied to wound outcomes in dermatologic surgery. Due to the wide range of wound types and dressing options available, dressing selection can be a formidable task. An understanding of dressing materials and their unique properties allows for a tailored approach to postoperative wound care. Conventional layered dressings often are suitable for uncomplicated dermatologic surgery wounds. Occlusive dressings and tissue-engineered skin substitutes may be warranted in more complex cases. This review is intended to equip the reader with the knowledge and confidence to successfully manage surgical wounds in dermatology.

Patient-centered care in dermatologic surgery emphasizes addressing the preferences, values, and concerns of the surgical patient in an effort to improve the overall experience. Impediments affecting the delivery of Mohs micrographic surgical treatment of skin cancers are present throughout the perioperative period. Defining actionable strategies to improve outcomes can be challenging due to sparse literature and minimal high-quality scientific studies. This review focuses on the current evidence supporting practical recommendations in each surgical setting to improve the patient experience and increase visit satisfaction.

Scar revision is of premier importance to the dermatologic surgeon. Some of the least invasive modalities include use of silicone gel sheets, resurfacing with electrosurgical instruments, dermabrasion, chemical peels, and subcision. Laser technology also has been implemented to selectively target and ablate fibrous scar tissue via selective thermolysis. Other lasers have been used to target dyschromia associated with scar formation. Lastly, invasive modalities of scar revision include excisional modalities and/or rearrangement of skin to enhance cosmesis of unsightly or morbid scars. Herein is a discussion of the multiple modalities of scar revision as well as advantages and disadvantages of each.

To achieve successful dermatologic surgery in a pediatric patient, several factors should be considered, including recognizing a child's inherent anxiety, ability to understand/comply with instructions, engaging their caregiver, and minimizing pain. Distraction techniques, including use of smart devices or classic play, have been shown to reduce anxiety, perception of pain, and increase overall satisfaction with the needed procedure. Customizing the child's need based on their stage of development and family preferences further improves how effectively the techniques are deployed. Because children are naturally playful, suturing techniques and dressing of surgical wounds may also require modification for best possible outcome.

DERMATOLOGIC CLINICS

SERIES OF RELATED INTEREST

Facial Plastic Surgery Clinics
Available at: http://www.facialplastic.theclinics.com/
Surgical Oncology Clinics
Available at: https://www.surgonc.theclinics.com/

THE CLINICS ARE AVAILABLE ONLINE!
Access your subscription at:
www.theclinics.com

Erratum

An error was made in the article on "Atopic Dermatitis: New Developments" appearing in the January 2019 issue of *Dermatologic Clinics* (Volume 37, Issue 1). The sentence, "However, these trials were notable for their strong vehicle effect—with 40.6% in the vehicle control group achieving clear/almost clear with a 2 or more grade improvement in the AD-301 study, leading to questions about the true efficacy of the active ingredient." should read "However, these trials were notable for their strong vehicle effect—with 40.6% and 29.7% in the vehicle control groups achieving clear/almost clear in the AD-301 and 302 studies." The online version of this article has been corrected.

Dermatol Clin 37 (2019) xiii
https://doi.org/10.1016/j.det.2019.04.002
0733-8635/19/© 2019 Published by Elsevier Inc.

Preface

Practical Updates in Cutaneous Oncology and Dermatologic Surgery

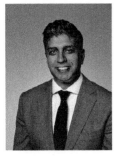 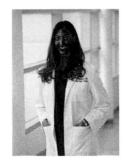

Rajiv I. Nijhawan, MD   Divya Srivastava, MD

Editors

In 1984, Ervin Epstein, MD edited the first special issue on dermatologic surgery in *Dermatologic Clinics*. Over the last three and a half decades, the fields of cutaneous oncology and dermatologic surgery have exploded with evidence-based advances in treating high-risk and rare skin cancers as well as in innovative approaches to dermatologic surgery. The landscape of health care has also evolved, giving dermatologic surgeons the opportunity to reflect on topics ranging from health care delivery for the elderly to optimizing patient satisfaction to serving as stewards for appropriate antibiotic and pain medication use.

Our goal was to identify the challenges and potential knowledge gaps that face the dermatologic surgeon on a daily basis. We tasked the authors with the mission to provide comprehensive and practical updates on these topics. Each article has real-world strategies and solutions to conundrums that we hope can be implemented in practice. We believe that whether read by a resident or seasoned dermatologic surgeon, the information conveyed by the authors will enhance the ability to provide optimal patient care.

It has been an absolute honor to be invited to edit this issue on Cutaneous Oncology and Dermatologic Surgery for *Dermatologic Clinics*. We are grateful to our patients, who continuously motivate us to learn and who stimulate many of the tough questions that we hope are addressed in these articles. The opportunity to invite respected colleagues and mentors alike to contribute to this special issue has been inspirational. We cannot thank the authors enough for their invaluable contributions of time and wisdom. We have learned an incredible amount from these experts and believe anyone who reads this issue will similarly find it to be not only informative but also clinically relevant.

We must also sincerely thank Dr Bruce Thiers for giving us this unique opportunity as well as Ms Sara Watkins and Ms Laura Kavanaugh at Elsevier for all of their assistance. Finally, we would like to thank our families for their endless love and support.

Rajiv I. Nijhawan, MD
Department of Dermatology
University of Texas
Southwestern Medical Center
5939 Harry Hines Boulevard
Suite 400
Dallas, TX 75390-9191, USA

Divya Srivastava, MD
Department of Dermatology
University of Texas
Southwestern Medical Center
5939 Harry Hines Boulevard
Suite 400
Dallas, TX 75390-9191, USA

E-mail addresses:
Rajiv.Nijhawan@utsouthwestern.edu
(R.I. Nijhawan)
Divya.Srivastava@utsouthwestern.edu
(D. Srivastava)

Dermatol Clin 37 (2019) xv
https://doi.org/10.1016/j.det.2019.04.001
0733-8635/19/© 2019 Published by Elsevier Inc.

Cutaneous Squamous Cell Carcinoma
Updates in Staging and Management

Thomas S. Bander, MD, Kishwer S. Nehal, MD,
Erica H. Lee, MD*

KEYWORDS

- Cutaneous squamous cell carcinoma • High-risk skin cancer • AJCC staging
- Squamous cell carcinoma staging • Skin cancer radiologic imaging • Sentinel lymph node biopsy
- PD-1 inhibitor • EGFR inhibitor

KEY POINTS

- Outcomes for cutaneous squamous cell carcinoma (cSCC) are generally favorable, but a subset of cSCC is biologically distinct and requires a different approach because of its higher risk of local recurrence, metastasis, and death.
- Updates to staging systems have improved their prognostic ability, but further study is needed to identify and include the most important risk factors.
- Uniform reporting of clinical and pathologic characteristics is important for clinical risk assessment and future population-based study.
- Although surgical resection with negative margins remains the goal of treatment, radiation and new systemic therapies have shown promise for advanced disease.

INTRODUCTION

Cutaneous squamous cell carcinoma (cSCC) is one of the most common cancers in the United States. Together with basal cell carcinoma (BCC), these cancers of epidermal keratinocyte lineage are often referred to as nonmelanoma skin cancer, or more specifically, keratinocyte carcinoma to differentiate their origins from melanoma and other skin cancers, such as Merkel cell carcinoma, adnexal carcinoma, and dermatofibrosarcoma protuberans.[1] Although cSCC and BCC have many similarities, a subset of cSCC is biologically distinct and requires a different approach because of its higher risk of local recurrence, metastasis, and death. This article focuses on the recent literature regarding identification of this high-risk subset, efforts to improve the prognostic ability of staging systems, and updates in management. Much of these data and expert opinion are incorporated in recent cSCC guidelines.

Incidence

Approximately 5.4 million cases of BCC and cSCC occur annually in the United States, with increasing incidence over time.[2] Although cSCC was previously estimated to represent about 20% of keratinocyte carcinomas, recent data suggest a 1:1 ratio of cSCC to BCC.[2–4] Because cSCC development is associated with older age and greater cumulative ultraviolet (UV) radiation exposure, these numbers are expected to increase as the population ages.

Disease-related Outcomes

Outcomes for cSCC are generally favorable, with low rates of local recurrence (LR; 3%–5.2%), NM

Disclosure: The authors have nothing to disclose.
Memorial Sloan Kettering Cancer Center, 16 East 60th Street, New York, NY 10022, USA
* Corresponding author.
E-mail address: leee@mskcc.org

Dermatol Clin 37 (2019) 241–251
https://doi.org/10.1016/j.det.2019.03.009

(NM; 1.5%–4%), and disease-specific death (DSD; 1.5%–2.8%).[5–11] Poor outcomes typically occur in elderly patients with multiple comorbidities but may be underreported because cSCC is not always identified as the official cause of death. In 2012, an estimated 3932 to 8791 deaths could be attributed to cSCC, with the highest mortality rates in the southern and central United States rivalling renal and oropharyngeal cancer and melanoma.[5] However, cSCC is not included in national cancer registries, limiting understanding of its true impact. In this context, increased focus has been placed on identifying high-risk patients that may benefit from a more intensive diagnostic and therapeutic approach.

Risk Factors

Over the past 80 years, numerous studies have identified risk factors for poor outcomes. Rowe and colleagues[12] reviewed all studies of cSCC outcomes from 1940 to 1992 and identified the following risk factors for LR and metastasis: treatment modality, prior treatment, location, size, depth, histologic differentiation, perineural involvement, host immunosuppression, and precipitating factors other than UV light. Recent studies have built on this work by further examining the following risk factors:

- Increased tumor size[6,7,12–16]
- Location on ear, lip, or genitals[7,12,15,17]
- Poorly differentiated, desmoplastic, or acantholytic histologic subtype[6–10,12,13,15,18,19]
- Perineural involvement[7,12,16,18,20–24]
- Lymphovascular involvement[10,18]
- Increased depth of invasion[6–8,12,14–16,18,25]
- Immunocompromised status[8,12,26–28]

These studies vary in the definition and reported magnitude of each risk factor, making a standard definition of high risk elusive (Fig. 1). For instance, some studies report tumor depth as Breslow thickness (measured from the granular layer to deepest point of invasion), whereas others consider anatomic depth to subcutaneous fat, muscle, bone, or cartilage. Perineural invasion may be reported as a binary variable (present or absent) or a continuous variable based on nerve diameter. Risk factors such as tumor depth and perineural or lymphovascular invasion tend to co-occur, potentially minimizing their individual contribution in multivariate analyses. Despite the heterogeneity in current data, great strides have been made in assessing the risk of poor outcomes.

STAGING SYSTEMS

Standardized staging systems help physicians provide prognostic information to patients, design treatment plans based on tumor risk, communicate with other physicians, and study new treatment paradigms through clinical trials. These staging systems help physicians reassure patients with favorable prognoses and better evaluate, manage, and monitor those at risk for adverse outcomes.

The ideal staging system is easily applicable to daily clinical practice and shows distinctiveness, homogeneity, and monotonicity. Distinctiveness means that disease-related outcomes should differ between stages, homogeneity refers to similar outcomes in patients within the same stage, and monotonicity implies worsening outcomes with increasing stage.[29]

Tumor Staging

At present, there are 2 major cSCC staging systems in the United States: the American Joint Committee on Cancer (AJCC) system and the Brigham and Women's Hospital (BWH) system (Table 1). The International Union Against Cancer (UICC) also has a staging system for cSCC that has been consistent with the AJCC system and is not discussed further in this article. Before 2010, the first 6 editions of the AJCC manual grouped cSCC in a chapter with all nonmelanoma skin cancers and included only tumor size and bony invasion as high-risk features.[29] The seventh edition added more risk factors but was criticized for its complexity and poor prognostic ability.[25,30,31] Retrospective cohorts showed that the bulk of poor outcomes occurred in tumor (T) stage T2 (69% of LRs, 83% of NM, and 92% of DSDs) and that T3 and T4 were too rare to be useful.[16,22]

The eighth edition was published in 2017 and reclassified cSCC in the head and neck chapter.[32,33] There are separate AJCC tumor classifications for cSCC on the eyelid, vulva, penis, and perianal region but none for tumors on other sites of the body. Changes from AJCC 7 include expansion of T3 and removal of poorly differentiated histology as a risk factor (see Table 1).

Validation of AJCC 8 with population-level data in the United States is challenging because national registries exclude cSCC. Karia and colleagues[34] attempted to validate the AJCC 8 T classification with a 10-year retrospective cohort of 680 primary head and neck cSCCs treated at BWH from 2000 to 2009. AJCC 8 showed a significant improvement in homogeneity and monotonicity compared with AJCC 7 based on expansion of the T3 and T4 categories, which together accounted for 17.8% of total cases

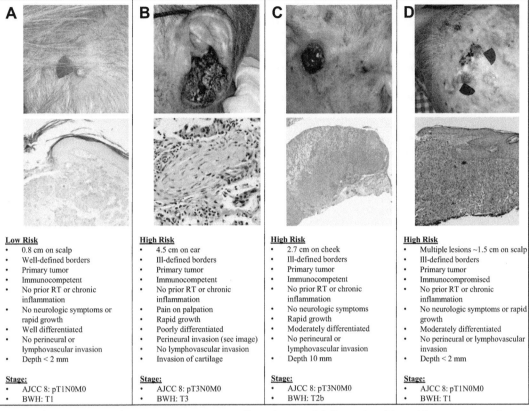

Fig. 1. Risk assessment of cutaneous squamous cell carcinoma. (*A*) Example of low-risk squamous cell carcinoma with well-differentiated pathology (H&E, original magnification ×4). (*B–D*) Examples of squamous cell carcinoma with a variety of high-risk features. Pathology images stained with hematoxylin and eosin (H&E, original magnification [B] ×10; [C] ×1.25; [D] ×2). AJCC, American Joint Committee on Cancer staging; BWH, Brigham and Women's Hospital staging; RT, radiation therapy. See Table 1 for AJCC and BWH criteria.

and 70.4% of disease-related poor outcomes compared with only 0.7% and 16.9%, respectively, in AJCC 7. Furthermore, T2, T3, and T4 cases together included 85.9% of poor outcomes. Despite these improvements, several weaknesses were identified, including similar risk of disease-related outcomes between AJCC 8 T2 and T3, making these categories indistinct. The investigators suggest that some T2 tumors may still warrant adjuvant therapy or nodal staging. Of note, most of the poor outcomes in AJCC 8 T1 and T2 were cases of poorly differentiated tumors, but this parameter was thought to be too inconsistently defined in clinical practice to be included by the AJCC 8 committee. Consistently reporting clinical tumor size and reproducibly grading histologic differentiation and depth will be critical for future population-based validation.

An alternative tumor staging system was proposed by Jambusaria-Pahlajani and colleagues[22] based on retrospective analysis of 256 tumors at BWH. Their multivariate analysis determined the strongest independent predictors of the following poor outcomes: LR, NM, DSD, or all-cause death. The resulting high-risk features determine staging (see Table 1). The model eliminates the rare T4 category and better stratifies stage T2 such that T2b tumors have a statistically significantly increased risk of NM, DSD, and all-cause death. The 4 selected risk factors were confirmed on multivariate analysis of a larger cohort of 1818 tumors from the same center.[16]

Their group also compared the BWH system with AJCC 7 and UICC 7, showing better homogeneity with only 40% of poor outcomes in T1 and T2a compared with 86% in AJCC 7 T1/T2 and 70% in UICC 7 T1/T2. BWH staging also showed better monotonicity with 60% of poor outcomes in T2b and T3 compared with only 14% in AJCC 7 T3/T4 and 30% in UICC 7 T3/T4. Of note, their model does not include N or M criteria because

Table 1
Overview of United States staging systems for cutaneous squamous cell carcinoma

	AJCC 7	AJCC 8 (Head and Neck Only)	BWH
T1	Tumor diameter ≤2 cm with <2 high-risk features	Tumor diameter <2 cm	0 high-risk features
T2	Tumor diameter >2 cm or tumor any size with ≥2 high-risk features	Tumor diameter ≥2 cm but <4 cm	T2a: 1 high-risk feature T2b: 2–3 high-risk features
T3	Tumor with invasion of maxilla, mandible, orbit, or temporal bone	Tumor diameter ≥4 cm or tumor any size with any 1 high-risk feature	All 4 high-risk features
T4	Tumor with invasion of skeleton (axial or appendicular) or perineural invasion of skull base	T4a: gross cortical bone or marrow invasion T4b: skull base invasion or skull base foramen involvement	Not applicable

High-risk features	• Tumor depth >2 mm (or Clark level IV or higher)
	• Perineural invasion of any size
	• Location (ear or nonglabrous lip)
	• Histologic differentiation (poorly differentiated or undifferentiated)
		• Deep invasion (beyond subcutaneous fat or >6 mm)
		• Minor bone erosion
		• Perineural invasion: tumor cells within the nerve sheath of a nerve
		  ○ Deeper than the dermis, or
		  ○ Measuring ≥0.1 mm, or
		  ○ Clinical or radiographic involvement of named nerves without skull base invasion
			• Poorly differentiated histology
			• Tumor diameter ≥2 cm
			• Perineural invasion
			• Deep tumor invasion (beyond subcutaneous fat but excluding bone invasion, which qualifies as T3)

Abbreviation: T, tumor staging.
Data from Refs.[22,30,32]

of the rarity of these events. The investigators assert that their system provides greater separation of high-risk and low-risk tumors, although it may not have had the power to detect other important factors that are not uniformly reported on pathology reports, such as immunosuppression or depth of invasion.

A recent population-based study in Norway[11] attempted to validate AJCC 7, AJCC 8, BWH, and a proposed staging model by Breuninger and colleagues[25] based on tumor diameter, thickness, and other risk factors. They found a lower metastatic rate compared with previous studies (1.5% of 6721 patients), possibly reflecting a more generalizable population than cohorts from tertiary referral systems. In their analysis, the Breuninger system was best able to discriminate between patients who developed metastasis and those who did not. AJCC 8 was an improvement over AJCC 7, but both showed worse discrimination than Breuninger and BWH. The investigators also commented on the simplicity of the BWH and Breuninger systems, which is an important

determinant of adoption in daily clinical practice. Continued refinement of T staging is vital for improved prognosis because most cSCCs (about 96%) do not metastasize.

Nodal Staging

Nodal (N) and distant metastasis is rare in cSCC but significantly affects prognosis when it occurs. This article highlights 4 nodal staging systems: AJCC 8, the parotid system by O'Brien and colleagues,[35] the N1S3 system, and the ITEM (immunosuppression, treatment, extranodal spread, and margin status) system. These systems stratify patients into higher stages based on increasing number of affected nodes and node size. AJCC 8 recently added extranodal extension (ENE) as an adverse risk factor, resulting in 7 nodal categories compared with 6 in AJCC 7. A recent retrospective cohort of 382 patients with metastatic cSCC in Australia showed AJCC 8 had poor prognostic ability, because there was no significant difference in disease-specific survival or overall survival between N1 and N2a, N2b, N2c, or N3b.[36] The investigators note that although studies support ENE as an independent risk factor, it is too common in metastatic cSCC (78% of cases) to make it appropriately discriminatory. Another weakness of AJCC 8 is its joint consideration of both cutaneous and mucosal squamous cell carcinoma (SCC) of the head and neck. Moeckleman and colleagues[37] found that AJCC 8 better stratified patients with mucosal SCC than those with cSCC.

The O'Brien staging system proposes separation of parotid and neck metastasis based on a retrospective cohort showing significantly worse survival with parotid and neck disease compared with parotid involvement alone.[35] Further analysis with larger cohorts is needed to validate the system and determine whether the added complexity is worthwhile.

The N1S3 system is a simpler alternative developed by Forest and colleagues[38] in 2010 from a cohort of 215 patients in Australia and then later validated with a separate group of 250 patients. Multivariate analysis revealed number and size of nodes as independent predictors of disease-specific survival (DSS), yielding 3 distinct prognostic groups:

- I: single lymph node less than or equal to 3 cm with 90% DSS
- II: single lymph node greater than 3 cm or multiple nodes less than or equal to 3 cm with 75% DSS
- III: multiple nodes greater than 3 cm with 42% DSS

In addition, the ITEM prognostic score stratifies patients with metastatic cSCC into low-risk, moderate-risk, and high-risk groups based on a weighted ranking system (1.8 for immunosuppression, negative 1.8 for treatment with surgery and radiation therapy [RT] compared with surgery alone, 4.8 for ENE, and 1.0 for involved surgical margins).[39] In this model, number and size of lymph nodes were not independent predictors of survival. The 5-year risk of death from disease for the low-risk, moderate-risk, and high-risk patients was 6%, 24%, and 56%, respectively.

Note that the most widely used staging systems do not account for patient characteristics known to increase risk of poor outcomes, such as immunosuppression, tumors associated with chronic scars or inflammatory disease, and treatment history (primary vs recurrent).[40] Future studies may lead to their incorporation into staging systems.

MANAGEMENT
Diagnosis

National Comprehensive Cancer Network (NCCN) guidelines recommend that skin biopsies include deep reticular dermis to enable complete histologic evaluation.[41] American Academy of Dermatology (AAD) guidelines recommend that important clinical information be conveyed to pathologists, including age, sex, anatomic location, recurrent versus primary lesion, size of lesion, immunosuppression, and relevant history (especially radiation, burn, or organ transplant).[42] Similarly, to ensure optimal identification of high-risk features, pathology reporting should uniformly include degree of differentiation; presence of aggressive histologic subtypes; depth of invasion (in millimeters); Clark level of invasion; perineural invasion (PNI); lymphovascular invasion (LVI); invasion of fascia, muscle, or bone; number of high-risk features; margin status; and AJCC TNM stage. Some clinicians argue that it is impractical to report all of these features in routine clinical practice, but standardized reporting would significantly improve the ability to evaluate the impact of high-risk features. Future study is needed to determine the frequency of standardized clinical histories and pathology reports and barriers to their completion.

Risk Stratification

On diagnosis of cSCC, clinical evaluation should include inspection and palpation of the involved site and regional draining lymph node basins. According to NCCN guidelines, patients should be stratified based on the presence of clinical or radiographic lymph node involvement. In the absence of nodal disease, local cSCC is divided into low-risk and high-risk tumors based on location, size, treatment history, presence of rapid growth or neurologic symptoms, patient characteristics (immunocompromised status, site of prior RT, or chronic inflammatory process), histologic differentiation, depth of invasion, and presence of PNI or LVI. These factors were selected based on available evidence and expert opinion and are intended to provide guidance on treatment rather than accurate prognostic information.

Local Control for Low-risk Tumors

Low-risk tumors may be treated with curettage and electrodessication (except in terminal hair-bearing regions or when adipose tissue is reached) or standard excision with 4-mm to 6-mm clinical margins and postoperative margin assessment. These recommendations are based primarily on expert consensus and retrospective and observational studies showing 95% to 96% cure rates.[12,43,44] RT as primary treatment may be considered only for nonsurgical candidates older than 60 years because of the risk of long-term secondary malignancy. Superficial therapies, such as topical fluorouracil, topical imiquimod, photodynamic therapy, and cryotherapy, should be reserved for cSCC in situ.[41]

Local Control for High-risk Tumors

Standard excision with wider margins, Mohs micrographic surgery (MMS), and RT are treatment options for high-risk tumors. There is no specific recommendation for margins on standard excision given the heterogeneity of the high-risk group, and few prospective studies have compared standard excision with MMS. One meta-analysis showed lower recurrence rates with MMS compared with standard excision, with 3.1% versus 8.1% for primary tumors and 10% versus 23.3% for locally recurrent tumors.[12] The improved cure rates of MMS were amplified with higher-risk tumors, because those with perineural involvement had LR of 0% with MMS compared with 47.2% with standard excision. Even in the context of newer adjuvant treatments (discussed later), surgical clearance with negative margins remains the primary goal.

Adjuvant Treatment for Local Control

NCCN guidelines recommend consideration of adjuvant therapy if postoperative margins are positive and further surgery is contraindicated, or if margins are negative and there is extensive perineural involvement. In these situations, RT or multidisciplinary tumor board consultation should be considered. Data have been mixed about the benefits of adjuvant RT, but retrospective studies are limited by selection bias because only the highest-risk patients are considered for adjuvant therapy.[45,46]

Regional Control

Regional nodal disease is associated with increased risk of LR and mortality.[15,19] Haisma and colleagues[15] reported a 5-year DSS rate of 37.3% and overall survival rate of 22.5% in patients with NM compared with 98.8% and 71.4%, respectively, in patients without NM. On clinical or radiologic identification of nodal involvement and confirmation with fine-needle aspiration (FNA) or core biopsy, NCCN guidelines recommend regional lymph node dissection for operable disease, which has shown excellent 5-year DSS of 97% in patients with low nodal tumor burden.[47] RT or systemic therapy may be considered for inoperable NM.

Increased nodal disease burden with multiple involved nodes or ENE may warrant adjuvant RT to the nodal basin. A retrospective study of 167 metastatic head and neck SCCs from Australia showed that patients undergoing lymph node dissection and adjuvant nodal basin RT had a trend toward a lower rate of locoregional recurrence (20% vs 43%) and significantly better 5-year disease-free survival rate (73% vs 54%) than surgery alone.[48] In contrast, Forest and colleagues[38] found no improvement in overall survival with adjuvant nodal RT. More data are needed, because current studies are limited by retrospective design, patient heterogeneity, and treatment selection bias.

Role of Radiologic Imaging

Because the overall risk of cSCC metastasis is low, routine radiologic imaging is not recommended. Imaging should be considered to evaluate locoregional and distant disease, bony or soft tissue invasion, perineural spread, or postoperative recurrence.[49] Ruiz and colleagues[50] retrospectively studied the use of radiologic imaging in high-risk cSCCs (BWH stage T2b or T3) over a 13-year period.[50] In their cohort, imaging was performed in 46% of patients.

Computed tomography (CT), MRI, ultrasonography, and PET/CT have all been used in the work-up of mucosal and cutaneous SCC, with CT identified as the most commonly used modality in retrospective cohorts (79%–83% of cases).[50,51] The best imaging modality depends on the clinical question and available resources (Table 2).[49,50,52,53] For evaluation of NM, a 2012 meta-analysis compared CT, MRI, PET/CT, and ultrasonography. CT was superior to ultrasonography in specificity, but there were no other differences in sensitivity or specificity.[53] A 2007 meta-analysis of head and neck mucosal SCC showed higher sensitivity and specificity for ultrasonography with FNA (87% and 98%, respectively) compared with CT and MRI.[54] A retrospective cohort study of 31 patients found that addition of PET/CT resulted in no change in management in 77% despite improved sensitivity for NM.[55] Its high cost may also limit its utility.

Ruiz and colleagues[50] found that imaging in high-risk cSCC cases (defined as BWH stage T2b or T3) resulted in treatment changes in 33%. Furthermore, 5-year disease-free survival rate was higher in patients that were imaged (78%) compared with those that were

Table 2
Comparison of imaging modalities for evaluation of cutaneous squamous cell carcinoma

Imaging Modality	CT	MRI	Ultrasonography	PET/CT
Optimal Use in cSCC	Bone or lymph node disease	Perineural, CNS, deep soft tissue, bone marrow, or lymph node disease	Superficial lymph node disease and image-guided FNA	Distant metastasis
Advantages	Less expensive, more widely available, and faster image acquisition than MRI	No exposure to ionizing radiation	Least expensive, no exposure to contrast dye or ionizing radiation, rapid image acquisition	Functional and anatomic information, distinguish postoperative scar tissue from recurrence
Disadvantages	Exposure to contrast dye and ionizing radiation	Less widely available, longer acquisition time, more expensive than CT	Operator and technique dependent, limited visualization of deep structures	Most expensive
Sensitivity for Head and Neck Nodal Disease (%)[a]	52	65	66	66
Specificity for Head and Neck Nodal Disease (%)[a]	93	81	78	87

Abbreviation: CNS, central nervous system.
[a] Only statistically significant difference is CT with superior specificity compared with ultrasonography.
Data from Refs.[49,50,53]

not (51%), raising the possibility that earlier detection of nodal disease may improve outcomes.

Although there are no specific guidelines for imaging in cSCC, some groups have proposed criteria:

- Que and colleagues[40] recommend CT imaging of draining lymph node basins for BWH stage T2b or T3 tumors and AJCC 8 stage T4 tumors because these patients have 20% risk of NM.
- Breuninger and colleagues[25] recommend ultrasonography for tumors greater than 2 mm in thickness or CT or MRI for infiltrative or destructive tumors.
- NCCN guidelines recommend consideration of CT with contrast and/or ultrasonography in those with significant risk of NM.[41]
- In Europe, ultrasonography is recommended as the initial imaging modality for regional nodal basins in high-risk cSCC, especially for superficial basins such as parotid and cervical nodes.[25,56]

Imaging is not a substitute for clinical palpation of regional nodal basins. Compared with clinical palpation, MRI showed no advantage in a prospective study of 60 patients in Taiwan who later underwent lymphadenectomy.[57] Clinical palpation and MRI had similar sensitivity, specificity, and rate of occult cervical metastasis, underscoring the importance of clinical evaluation.

Sentinel Lymph Node Biopsy

The potential benefit of early detection has led to increased interest in sentinel lymph node biopsy (SLNB) for cSCC. Retrospective studies and meta-analyses have shown the feasibility of SLNB in this patient population along with low false-negative rates (2.6%–7.1%).[58–62] In their review of 173 patients, Allen and Stolle[60] found a sensitivity of 79%, specificity of 100%, and negative predictive value of 96%. Fukushima and colleagues[63] showed that 7% of 41 patients with negative PET/CT or ultrasonography had occult micrometastases on SLNB. Sensitivity of SLNB is improved with use of combined radioisotope and blue dye for identification of the sentinel node (SN) and serial sections with immunohistochemistry to identify microscopic foci of disease. SN positivity rates varied in these studies between 11.3% and 24%, possibly reflecting varying definitions of high-risk tumors selected for this procedure.[58–62,64] These rates are in keeping with the 10% risk threshold generally thought to warrant SLNB for melanoma. Furthermore, complications from SLNB are rare and mild, including dye allergy, lymphedema, infection, hematoma, seroma, or wound dehiscence. A meta-analysis by Schmitt and colleagues[61] determined that there was a statistically higher rate of SLNB positivity in BWH T2b tumors than T2a tumors (29.4% vs 7.1%). They propose that high-risk lesions T2b or higher be considered for SLNB. They found no such clear cutoff by AJCC 7 criteria, but their review was published before AJCC 8.

One difficulty in applying SLNB to cSCC is that many tumors are staged intraoperatively or postoperatively. In these situations, SLNB may still be considered based on extrapolation from data in melanoma management.[65] At our institution, previous surgery at the melanoma primary site is not a contraindication for SLNB; however, the accuracy and utility of SLNB likely decreases with complex reconstruction or location on head, neck, or trunk where multiple lymph node basins could be involved. Delayed repair or reconstruction that minimizes lymphatic disruption may be considered in these high-risk cases. Microstaging saucerization or excisional biopsies may also be helpful to evaluate high-risk pathologic features before definitive surgical intervention. Prospective studies are needed to determine optimal patient selection and evaluate the effect of SLNB on patient outcomes.

Systemic Treatment

New systemic therapies may help the subset of patients with poor outcomes from cSCC. Historically, combinations of 5-fluorouracil (5-FU)/cisplatin, 5-FU/carboplatin, and paclitaxel/carboplatin showed 80% remission in observational studies. However, responses are short lived, and side effects are often intolerable for the elderly population affected by cSCC. Epidermal growth factor receptor (EGFR) inhibitors target the Ras-Raf mitogen-activated protein kinase (MAPK) pathway, which controls cell cycle progression and proliferation. Cetuximab is now Food and Drug Administration (FDA) approved for locally or regionally advanced mucosal SCC of the head and neck and is used off label for cSCC. Phase II trials of cetuximab monotherapy and phase III trials for gefitinib monotherapy have shown some

benefit for unresectable cSCC.[66,67] The addition of cetuximab to traditional platinum/fluorouracil chemotherapy or RT has also shown promise.[68–70]

Immunotherapy with anti–programmed cell death protein 1 (PD-1) inhibitors has also shown efficacy for cSCC, leading to FDA approval of cemiplimab in September 2018. Improved immune surveillance with PD-1 blockade seems to be particularly beneficial in solid tumors with high mutational burden and PD-L1 expression, such as melanoma, non-small cell lung cancer, and cSCC. Phase I data for cemiplimab showed a 52% response rate for unresectable locally advanced or metastatic cSCC,[71] and early data for the phase II cohort with metastatic cSCC showed objective response in 47% over a median of 7.9 months.[72] Data for the phase II trial in locally advanced disease have not yet reached the time point for primary analysis. These treatments have been well tolerated, with fatigue, diarrhea, and rash being the most common adverse effects. Caution in transplant patients has been recommended given the risk of allograft rejection.[73,74]

Further study is needed to determine which patients will benefit from systemic therapy and the role of adjuvant or neoadjuvant therapy.

Immunocompromised Patients

Immunocompromised patients require special mention. Although immunosuppression is not generally included in staging systems, numerous studies have shown higher risk of cSCC development and worse outcomes for cSCC in immunocompromised individuals.[8,12,26–28,75] NCCN guidelines discuss several strategies for treatment of SCC in such high-risk patients that rapidly develop multiple cSCCs. First, destructive techniques that allow treatment of multiple lesions at a single visit may be beneficial. Similarly, field treatment of precancers with 5-FU, imiquimod, or photodynamic therapy may be helpful. In addition, dose reduction of immunosuppression therapy or use of mammalian target of rapamycin (mTOR) inhibitors have shown benefit.[76,77]

Follow-up Monitoring

Patients with cSCC are more likely than the general population to develop another cSCC and are also at higher risk of developing BCC and melanoma. Long-term surveillance and education about sun protection are important in these patients. Furthermore, because most LR occurs within 2 years of treatment, frequent follow-up is recommended during this time.[7,12,75] NCCN recommends physical examination every 3 to

12 months during the first 2 years, every 6 to 12 months for another 3 years, then annually for life. Patients with metastatic disease may be monitored with CT scans, with frequency every 3 to 6 months depending on individual patient risk factors. Importantly, these recommendations should be adjusted depending on individual patient risk.

SUMMARY

The increasing incidence of cSCC in the United States and a renewed focus on high-risk tumors have resulted in exciting new staging and treatment paradigms. Although significant strides have been made, further study is needed to identify, evaluate, and manage the subset of patients at risk for poor outcomes.

REFERENCES

1. Nehal KS, Bichakjian CK. Update on keratinocyte carcinomas. N Engl J Med 2018;379(4):363–74.
2. Rogers HW, Weinstock MA, Feldman SR, et al. Incidence estimate of nonmelanoma skin cancer (keratinocyte carcinomas) in the US population, 2012. JAMA Dermatol 2015;151(10):1081–6.
3. Kaldor J, Shugg D, Young B, et al. Non-melanoma skin cancer: ten years of cancer-registry-based surveillance. Int J Cancer 1993;53:886–91.
4. Miller DL, Weinstock MA. Nonmelanoma skin cancer in the United States: incidence. J Am Acad Dermatol 1994;30(5):774–8.
5. Karia PS, Han J, Schmults CD. Cutaneous squamous cell carcinoma: Estimated incidence of disease, NM, and deaths from disease in the United States, 2012. J Am Acad Dermatol 2013;68(6):957–66.
6. Brantsch KD, Meisner C, Schönfisch B, et al. Analysis of risk factors determining prognosis of cutaneous squamous-cell carcinoma: a prospective study. Lancet Oncol 2008;9(8):713–20.
7. Schmults CD, Karia PS, Carter JB, et al. Factors predictive of recurrence and death from cutaneous squamous cell carcinoma. JAMA Dermatol 2013;149(5):541.
8. Eigentler TK, Leiter U, Häfner HM, et al. Survival of patients with cutaneous squamous cell carcinoma: results of a prospective cohort study. J Invest Dermatol 2017;137(11):2309–15.
9. Mourouzis C, Boynton A, Grant J, et al. Cutaneous head and neck SCCs and risk of NM - UK experience. J Craniomaxillofac Surg 2009;37(8):443–7.
10. Brougham ND, Dennett ER, Cameron R, et al. The incidence of metastasis from cutaneous squamous cell carcinoma and the impact of its risk factors. J Surg Oncol 2012;106(7):811–5.
11. Roscher I, Falk RS, Vos L, et al. Validating 4 staging systems for cutaneous squamous cell carcinoma using population-based data. JAMA Dermatol 2018;154(4):428–34.
12. Rowe DE, Carroll RJ, Day CL. Prognostic factors for local recurrence, metastasis, and survival rates in squamous cell carcinoma of the skin, ear, and lip. Implications for treatment modality selection. J Am Acad Dermatol 1992;26(6):976–90.
13. Krediet JT, Beyer M, Lenz K, et al. Sentinel lymph node biopsy and risk factors for predicting metastasis in cutaneous squamous cell carcinoma. Br J Dermatol 2015;172(4):1029–36.
14. Thompson AK, Kelley BF, Prokop LJ, et al. Risk factors for cutaneous squamous cell carcinoma recurrence, metastasis, and disease-specific death. JAMA Dermatol 2016;152(4):419.
15. Haisma MS, Plaat BEC, Bijl HP, et al. Multivariate analysis of potential risk factors for lymph node metastasis in patients with cutaneous squamous cell carcinoma of the head and neck. J Am Acad Dermatol 2016;75(4):722–30.
16. Karia PS, Jambusaria-Pahlajani A, Harrington DP, et al. Evaluation of American Joint Committee on Cancer, International Union Against Cancer, and Brigham and Women's Hospital tumor staging for cutaneous squamous cell carcinoma. J Clin Oncol 2014;32(4):327–34.
17. Wang DM, Kraft S, Rohani P, et al. Association of nodal metastasis and mortality with vermilion vs cutaneous lip location in cutaneous squamous cell carcinoma of the lip. JAMA Dermatol 2018;154(6):701–7.
18. Moore BA, Weber RS, Prieto V, et al. Lymph node metastases from cutaneous squamous cell carcinoma of the head and neck. Laryngoscope 2005;115(9):1561–7.
19. Mullen JT, Feng L, Xing Y, et al. Invasive squamous cell carcinoma of the skin: defining a high-risk group. Ann Surg Oncol 2006;13(7):902–9.
20. Carter JB, Johnson MM, Chua TL, et al. Outcomes of primary cutaneous squamous cell carcinoma with perineural invasion. JAMA Dermatol 2013;149(1):35.
21. Goepfert H, Dichtel WJ, Medina JE, et al. Perineural invasion in squamous cell skin carcinoma of the head and neck. Am J Surg 1984;148(4):542–7.
22. Jambusaria-Pahlajani A, Kanetsky PA, Karia PS, et al. Evaluation of AJCC tumor staging for cutaneous squamous cell carcinoma and a proposed alternative tumor staging system. JAMA Dermatol 2013;149(4):402–10.
23. Leibovitch I, Huilgol SC, Selva D, et al. Cutaneous squamous cell carcinoma treated with Mohs micrographic surgery in Australia II. Perineural invasion. J Am Acad Dermatol 2005;53(2):261–6.
24. Ross AS, Miller Whalen F, Elenitsas R, et al. Diameter of involved nerves predicts outcomes in cutaneous

squamous cell carcinoma with perineural invasion: an investigator-blinded retrospective cohort study. Dermatol Surg 2009;35(12):1859–66.

25. Breuninger H, Brantsch K, Eigentler T, et al. Comparison and evaluation of the current staging of cutaneous carcinomas. J Dtsch Dermatol Ges 2012; 10(8):579–86.

26. Manyam BV, Gastman B, Zhang AY, et al. Inferior outcomes in immunosuppressed patients with high-risk cutaneous squamous cell carcinoma of the head and neck treated with surgery and radiation therapy. J Am Acad Dermatol 2015;73(2):221–7.

27. Martinez JC, Otley CC, Stasko T, et al. Defining the clinical course of metastatic skin cancer in organ transplant recipients. Arch Dermatol 2003;139: 301–6.

28. Winkelhorst JT, Brokelman WJ, Tiggeler RG, et al. Incidence and clinical course of de-novo malignancies in renal allograft recipients. Eur J Surg Oncol 2001;27(4):409–13.

29. Greene F, Page D, Fleming I, et al. AJCC cancer staging manual. 6th edition. New York: Springer International Publishing; 2002.

30. Edge S, Byred D, Compton C, et al. AJCC cancer staging manual. 7th edition. New York: Springer International Publishing; 2010.

31. Farasat S, Yu SS, Neel VA, et al. A new American Joint Committee on Cancer staging system for cutaneous squamous cell carcinoma: creation and rationale for inclusion of tumor (T) characteristics. J Am Acad Dermatol 2011;64(6):1051–9.

32. Califano J, Lydiatt W, Nehal K, et al. Cutaneous squamous cell carcinoma of the head and neck. In: AJCC cancer staging manual. 8th edition. New York: Springer International Publishing; 2017. p. 171–81.

33. Lydiatt W, Patel S, O'Sullivan B, et al. Head and neck cancers-major changes in the American Joint Committee on Cancer Eighth Edition Cancer Staging Manual. CA Cancer J Clin 2017;67(2):122–37.

34. Karia PS, Morgan FC, Califano JA, et al. Comparison of tumor classifications for cutaneous squamous cell carcinoma of the head and neck in the 7th vs 8th edition of the AJCC cancer staging manual. JAMA Dermatol 2018;154(2):175–81.

35. O'Brien CJ, McNeil EB, McMahon JD, et al. Significance of clinical stage, extent of surgery, and pathologic findings in metastatic cutaneous squamous carcinoma of the parotid gland. Head Neck 2002; 24(5):417–22.

36. Liu J, Ebrahimi A, Low THH, et al. Predictive value of the 8th edition American Joint Commission Cancer (AJCC) nodal staging system for patients with cutaneous squamous cell carcinoma of the head and neck. J Surg Oncol 2018;117(4):765–72.

37. Moeckelmann N, Ebrahimi A, Dirven R, et al. Analysis and comparison of the 8th Edition American Joint Committee on Cancer (AJCC) nodal staging system in cutaneous and oral squamous cell cancer of the head and neck. Ann Surg Oncol 2018;25(6): 1730–6.

38. Forest VI, Clark JJ, Veness MJ, et al. N1S3: a revised staging system for head and neck cutaneous squamous cell carcinoma with lymph node metastases - Results of 2 Australian cancer centers. Cancer 2010;116(5):1298–304.

39. Oddone N, Morgan GJ, Palme CE, et al. Metastatic cutaneous squamous cell carcinoma of the head and neck. Cancer 2009;115(9):1883–91.

40. Que SKT, Zwald FO, Schmults CD. Cutaneous squamous cell carcinoma: management of advanced and high-stage tumors. J Am Acad Dermatol 2018; 78(2):249–61.

41. Bichakjian CK, Olencki T, et al. NCCN clinical practice guidelines in oncology (NCCN guidelines) squamous cell skin cancer 2 2018.

42. Alam M, Armstrong A, Baum C, et al. Guidelines of care for the management of cutaneous squamous cell carcinoma. J Am Acad Dermatol 2018;78(3): 560–78.

43. Chren MM, Linos E, Torres JS, et al. Tumor recurrence 5 years after treatment of cutaneous basal cell carcinoma and squamous cell carcinoma. J Invest Dermatol 2013;133(5):1188–96.

44. Louise L, Jo LB, William P, et al. Interventions for non-metastatic squamous cell carcinoma of the skin. Cochrane Database Syst Rev 2010;4.

45. Jambusaria-Pahlajani A, Miller CJ, Quon H, et al. Surgical monotherapy versus surgery plus adjuvant radiotherapy in high-risk cutaneous squamous cell carcinoma: a systematic review of outcomes. Dermatol Surg 2009;35(4):574–85.

46. Babington S, Veness MJ, Cakir B, et al. Squamous cell carcinoma of the lip: is there a role for adjuvant radiotherapy in improving local control following incomplete or inadequate excision? ANZ J Surg 2003;73(8):621–5.

47. Ebrahimi A, Clark JR, Lorincz BB. Metastatic head and neck cutaneous squamous cell carcinoma: defining a low-risk patient. Head Neck 2012;34:365–70.

48. Veness MJ, Morgan GJ, Palme CE, et al. Surgery and adjuvant radiotherapy in patients with cutaneous head and neck squamous cell carcinoma metastatic to lymph nodes: combined treatment should be considered best practice. Laryngoscope 2005;115(5):870–5.

49. Humphreys TR, Shah K, Wysong A, et al. The role of imaging in the management of patients with nonmelanoma skin cancer: When is imaging necessary? J Am Acad Dermatol 2017;76(4):591–607.

50. Ruiz ES, Karia PS, Morgan FC, et al. The positive impact of radiologic imaging on high-stage cutaneous squamous cell carcinoma management. J Am Acad Dermatol 2017;76(2):217–25.

51. Marrazzo G, Thorpe R, Condie D, et al. Clinical and pathologic factors predictive of positive radiologic findings in high-risk cutaneous squamous cell carcinoma. Dermatol Surg 2015;41(12):1405–10.

52. Macfarlane D, Shah K, Wysong A, et al. The role of imaging in the management of patients with nonmelanoma skin cancer: diagnostic modalities and applications. J Am Acad Dermatol 2017;76(4):579–88.

53. Liao LJ, Lo WC, Hsu WL, et al. Detection of cervical lymph node metastasis in head and neck cancer patients with clinically N0 neck—a meta-analysis comparing different imaging modalities. BMC Cancer 2012;12(1):236.

54. de Bondt RBJ, Nelemans PJ, Hofman PAM, et al. Detection of lymph node metastases in head and neck cancer: a meta-analysis comparing US, USgFNAC, CT and MR imaging. Eur J Radiol 2007;64(2):266–72.

55. Supriya M, Suat-Chin N, Sizeland A. Use of positron emission tomography scanning in metastatic head and neck cutaneous squamous cell cancer: does it add to patient management? Am J Otolaryngol 2014;35:347–52.

56. Bonerandi JJ, Beauvillain C, Caquant L, et al. Guidelines for the diagnosis and treatment of cutaneous squamous cell carcinoma and precursor lesions. J Eur Acad Dermatol Venereol 2011;25(Suppl. 5):1–51.

57. Hao SP, Ng SH. Magnetic resonance imaging versus clinical palpation in evaluating cervical metastasis from head and neck cancer. Otolaryngol Head Neck Surg 2000;123(3):324–7.

58. Durham AB, Lowe L, Malloy KM, et al. Sentinel lymph node biopsy for cutaneous squamous cell carcinoma on the head and neck. JAMA Otolaryngol Head Neck Surg 2016;142(12):1171.

59. Ross AS, Schmults CD. Sentinel lymph node biopsy in cutaneous squamous cell carcinoma: a systematic review of the English literature. Dermatol Surg 2006;32(11):1309–21.

60. Allen JE, Stolle LB. Utility of sentinel node biopsy in patients with high-risk cutaneous squamous cell carcinoma. Eur J Surg Oncol 2015;41(2):197–200.

61. Schmitt AR, Brewer JD, Bordeaux JS, et al. Staging for cutaneous squamous cell carcinoma as a predictor of sentinel lymph node biopsy results: meta-analysis of American Joint Committee on Cancer criteria and a proposed alternative system. JAMA Dermatol 2014;150(1):19–24.

62. Navarrete-Dechent C, Veness MJ, Droppelmann N, et al. High-risk cutaneous squamous cell carcinoma and the emerging role of sentinel lymph node biopsy: a literature review. J Am Acad Dermatol 2015;73(1):127–37.

63. Fukushima S, Masuguchi S, Igata T, et al. Evaluation of sentinel node biopsy for cutaneous squamous cell carcinoma. J Dermatol 2014;41(6):539–41.

64. Takahashi A, Imafuku S, Nakayama J, et al. Sentinel node biopsy for high-risk cutaneous squamous cell carcinoma. Eur J Surg Oncol 2014;40(10):1256–62.

65. Gannon CJ, Rousseau DL, Ross MI, et al. Accuracy of lymphatic mapping and sentinel lymph node biopsy after previous wide local excision in patients with primary melanoma. Cancer 2006;107(11):2647–52.

66. Stewart JSW, Cohen EEW, Licitra L, et al. Phase III study of gefitinib 250 compared with intravenous methotrexate for recurrent squamous cell carcinoma of the head and neck. J Clin Oncol 2009;27(11):1864–71.

67. Maubec E, Petrow P, Avril M, et al. Phase II study of cetuximab as first-line single-drug therapy in patients with unresectable squamous cell carcinoma of the skin. J Clin Oncol 2011;29:3419–26.

68. Vermorken J, Remenar E, Kawecki A, et al. Platinum-based chemotherapy plus cetuximab in head and neck cancer. N Engl J Med 2008;359:1116–27.

69. Bonner JA, Harari PM, Giralt J, et al. Radiotherapy plus cetuximab for squamous-cell carcinoma of the head and neck. N Engl J Med 2006;354:567–78.

70. O'Bryan K, Sherman W, Niedt GW, et al. An evolving paradigm for the workup and management of high-risk cutaneous squamous cell carcinoma. J Am Acad Dermatol 2013;69(4):595–603.

71. Papadopoulos K, Owonikoko T, Homsi J, et al. REGN2810: a fully human anti-PD-1 monoclonal antibody, for patients with unresectable locally advanced or metastatic cutaneous squamous cell carcinoma (CSCC)- initial safety and efficacy from expansion cohorts (ECs) of phase I study. J Clin Oncol 2017;35:9503.

72. Migden MR, Rischin D, Schmults CD, et al. PD-1 blockade with cemiplimab in advanced cutaneous squamous-cell carcinoma. N Engl J Med 2018;379(4):341–51.

73. Spain L, Higgins R, Larkin J, et al. Acute renal allograft rejection after immune checkpoint inhibitor therapy for metastatic melanoma. Ann Oncol 2016;27:1135–7.

74. Alhamad T, Venkatachalam K, Brennan D, et al. Checkpoint inhibitors in kidney transplant recipients and the potential risk of rejection. Am J Transplant 2016;16:1332–3.

75. Johnson TM, Rowe DE, Nelson BR, et al. Squamous cell carcinoma of the skin (excluding lip and oral mucosa). J Am Acad Dermatol 1992;26(3):467–84.

76. Euvrard S, Morelon E, Rostaing L, et al. Sirolimus and secondary skin-cancer prevention in kidney transplantation. N Engl J Med 2012;367:329–39.

77. Salgo R, Gossmann J, Schofer H, et al. Switch to a sirolimus-based immunosuppression in long-term renal transplant recipients: reduced rate of (pre-)malignancies and nonmelanoma skin cancer in a prospective, randomized, assessor-blinded, controlled clinical trial. Am J Transplant 2010;10:1385–93.

Atypical Fibroxanthoma and Pleomorphic Dermal Sarcoma
Updates on Classification and Management

Teo Soleymani, MD*, Sumaira Z. Aasi, MD,
Roberto Novoa, MD, S. Tyler Hollmig, MD

KEYWORDS

- Atypical fibroxanthoma • Pleomorphic dermal sarcoma • Malignant fibrous histiocytoma
- Undifferentiated pleomorphic sarcoma • Cancer • Sarcoma • Mohs • Micrographic surgery

KEY POINTS

- AFX and UPS/PDS tumors are rare malignant cutaneous neoplasms that exist along a clinicopathologic spectrum.
- AFX tumors are generally more superficial without high-risk histologic features; they tend to display minimal metastatic potential in their clinical course.
- PDS, rather than MFH or UPS, is the preferred term for cutaneous tumors that are deeper with more extensive subcutaneous involvement than AFX, and demonstrate high-risk features on histopathology; these tumors have a higher propensity for local recurrence, distant metastases, and death.
- Surgical tumor extirpation with comprehensive tumor margin control is paramount and remains gold standard in management.
- In high-risk tumors, multidisciplinary management with comprehensive evaluation using imaging and possible adjuvant chemoradiation is prudent for optimal outcomes.

INTRODUCTION AND DEFINITION

Atypical fibroxanthoma (AFX) is a distinctive cutaneous neoplasm of fibrohistiocytic mesenchymal origin.[1–6] Atypical fibroxanthoma tumors typically develop on sun-damaged skin of the elderly, with a greater predilection for developing in highly sun-damaged or previously radiated sites and in men greater than women.[6–8] Clinically, presentation is most commonly as a superficial rapidly growing tumor that may ulcerate and bleed (**Fig. 1**A). Historically, a subset of these tumors demonstrated deeper cutaneous involvement and a more aggressive course, with higher rates of local recurrence, distant metastases, and death. This presented challenges not only in terminology and diagnosis, but more importantly in risk stratification and management paradigms. Since its initial introduction in the literature in 1961, the entire spectrum of AFX and related neoplasms has been a topic of extensive controversy; the terminology and precise diagnostic criteria of these tumors continue to be a topic of ongoing debate. Historically, the terms AFX and superficial malignant fibrous histiocytoma (MFH) were used interchangeably or as a continuum for many years, with more superficial tumors termed AFX and

Disclosure Statement: The authors have nothing to disclose.
Department of Dermatology, Stanford University School of Medicine, 450 Broadway Street, Pavilion C, 2nd Floor–MC5334, Redwood City, CA 94063, USA
* Corresponding author.
E-mail address: teo.soleymani@gmail.com

Dermatol Clin 37 (2019) 253–259
https://doi.org/10.1016/j.det.2019.02.001
0733-8635/19/

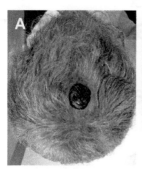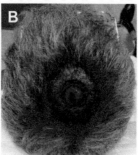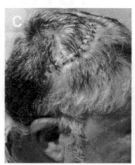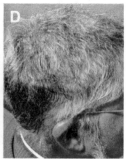

Fig. 1. AFX clinical photos. (*A*) Initial preoperative clinical photo of an AFX presenting as a relatively superficial, rapidly growing, ulcerated, friable tumor on the scalp. (*B*) Intraoperative photograph demonstrating the surgical defect after tumor extirpation using Mohs micrographic technique. (*C*) Immediate postoperative repair using a rotation flap to reconstruct the surgical defect. (*D*) Postoperative photograph at 3 months.

deeper tumors MFH; notably, consequences of such an imprecise approach continue to reverberate in the literature.[1–4,8–11] With the advent of contemporary histologic techniques and advances in basic science research, many tumors previously deemed "MFH" were more appropriately recategorized as other tumor types entirely. As a result, the term MFH has become somewhat antiquated—as well as imprecise—and has been supplanted by the term "undifferentiated pleomorphic sarcoma" (UPS).[1–4,6,9–11] Alternatively, the term "pleomorphic dermal sarcoma" (PDS) has been proposed to better encapsulate tumors specifically of cutaneous origin, because the term UPS also represents a diverse heterogeneous cohort of malignant soft tissue neoplasms, including tumors of internal organ, retroperitoneal, and osteoid origin.[4,6,11–14] In this review we will thus refer to these deeper but cutaneous neoplasms as PDS.

The diagnosis of AFX and PDS tumors remains a challenge and one of exclusion, because these tumors show no reliable discriminatory morphologic or immunohistochemical (IHC) features.[2–4,6,11,12] However, careful differentiation and correct categorization is critical in risk stratification and management for optimal outcomes. An evolving consensus has developed in the literature to better aid in the appropriate categorization and nomenclature of these tumors: more superficial tumors limited to the dermis or associated with minimal subcutaneous involvement have demonstrated minimal metastatic potential and may be termed AFX, whereas deeper cutaneous subtypes with clinical and histologic features similar to AFX but with more extensive subcutaneous invasion, tumor necrosis, or high-grade histologic features including abundant atypical mitoses, lymphovascular and/or perineural invasion, are designated as PDS (**Fig. 2**A–C).[1–4,6,9,11,12]

ETIOLOGY AND ONCOGENETICS

Until recently, very little was known about the oncogenetic background of AFX and PDS. There was, and to a certain degree still is, considerable debate as to whether or not these tumors are related neoplasms arising from a common mesenchymal progenitor cell and represent either end of a "spectrum," or whether they are 2 distinct, separate, and malignant entities. Contemporary studies support a fibrohistiocytic mesenchymal origin.[1–5,11,12,15]

Most AFX and PDS tumors demonstrate C->T mutations in dipyrimidines in the P53 and TERT promoter genes, suggesting that tumorigenesis is, at least in part, driven by UV-induced mutations.[5,15–18] AFX tumors have demonstrated a markedly increased gene expression profile in pathways involved in epithelial to mesenchymal transition, indicated by an upregulation of mesenchymal markers with a downregulation of epithelial markers, and can be activated and promote tumor progression through a variety of different pathways, including the AKT-PI3K, RAS, ERK, MAPK, and FGF pathways.[5,15,17] Atypical fibroxanthoma and PDS tumors demonstrate shared gene alteration profiles commonly seen in FAT1, NOTCH1/2, CDKN2A, COL11A1, PDGFR, TP53, and the TERT promoter genes, indicating that AFX and PDS tumors are in fact genetically related, potentially representing 2 ends of a common tumor spectrum.[5,15–19] Of note, several recent studies have identified that activating RAS gene mutations are commonly seen in PDS tumors, but only rarely if at all in AFX tumors, suggesting that this gene mutation may be unique to the development of PDS tumors and may play a pivotal role in the divergence of these 2 tumors, with activating RAS gene mutations being a poor prognosticator.[15,16,18,19] Importantly, this also suggests

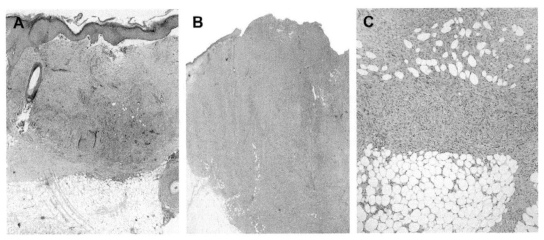

Fig. 2. AFX and PDS. (*A*) Low-power view of AFX architecture demonstrating proximity of tumor to the epidermis minimal depth of invasion. The tumor is composed of pleomorphic, atypical spindle-shaped cells arranged in a storiform pattern. Note the relatively superficial depth in comparison with (*B*) and (*C*). (*B*) Low-power view of PDS demonstrating a markedly dense, pleomorphic, hypercellular tumor composed of atypical spindle-shaped cells arranged infiltrating throughout the dermis and into the subcutaneous fat. Note the sheet-like appearance of the atypical cells and the extensive subcuticular infiltration in comparison with the AFX noted in (*A*). (*C*) Higher-power magnification demonstrating a densely cellular tumor composed of large, pleomorphic, mixed epithelioid, and spindle-shaped cells haphazardly arranged in a storiform pattern. Numerous mitoses are seen. ([*B, C*] *Courtesy of* Roberto Novoa, MD.)

that molecular targets inhibiting these mutational pathway may hold promise for the development of personalized targeted adjuvant treatment in patients with unresectable or metastasized PDS tumors.[15,16,18,19] However, despite advances in understanding the oncogenetics of these tumors, the diverse mutational profiles and copy-number alterations in these tumor subtypes pose a continued challenge to fully understand genetic mechanisms involved in their development.

HISTOPATHOLOGY

Although AFX and PDS tumors are thought to share a fibrohistiocytic mesenchymal lineage, these tumors are often very diverse and can display significant heterogeneity. Classic features include dense cellularity with haphazardly arranged, large, pleomorphic, and atypical-appearing spindle-shaped cells arising just beneath the epidermis and extending into the reticular dermis and sometimes superficial subcutaneous fat[3,6,20–22] (see **Fig. 2**A). Neoplastic cells often have hyperchromatic, irregular nuclei, and bizarre multinucleated giant cells are often present, as are atypical mitotic figures.[22] However, although these classic histopathologic features are well recognized, multiple histologic variants have been noted, including pseudoangiomatous,[3,6,23] pigmented,[3,24] clear cell,[3,25] granular,[3,26] myxoid,[3] and keloidal, among others.[3,27]

As mentioned above, AFX is considered by many to represent a superficial variant of PDS.[1–4,6,11,28] Histologic features of PDS are virtually identical to those of AFX, albeit with a few critical differentiating characteristics including deeper subcutaneous tissue invasion, tumor necrosis, perineural invasion, and/or lymphovascular invasion (see **Fig. 2**B, C).[1–4,6,11,28] Tumors are often large, ill-defined, asymmetric, and diffusely infiltrative, and may extend into deep subcutaneous adipose tissue, skeletal muscle, fascia, or galea.[1–4,6,11,22,28] Similar to AFX, PDS are composed of sheets of pleomorphic, bizarre-appearing epithelioid and spindle cells, with abundant cytoplasm and hyperchromatic nuclei with multiple nucleoli (see **Fig. 2**B, C).[1–4,6,11,22,28] Multinucleated giant cells are often seen, and numerous atypical mitoses are often present.[1–4,6,11,22,28] Ulceration is common and tumor necrosis is present in approximately 50% of cases.[1–4,6,11,28]

IMMUNOHISTOCHEMISTRY

It is critical to note that these histopathologic features are not distinctly unique to AFX or PDS tumors; nearly identical histopathologic findings can be seen other tumors such as spindle-celled squamous cell carcinomas (SCCs) and melanomas, including desmoplastic variants. Distinguishing these tumors from the other spindle-celled neoplasms is crucial for diagnosis and management. In most cases, a judicious initial IHC panel including SOX-10 and/or S100, cytokeratins, and desmin/caldesmon, will help to distinguish between the most commonly implicated tumors in the differential diagnosis, namely SCC, melanoma, and leiomyosarcoma. The addition of CD10 and/or procollagen-1 may be helpful as relatively reliable antigenic markers in AFX.[1–4,6,29] This initial panel may be expanded in more challenging cases when other tumors—such as angiosarcoma, dermatofibrosarcoma protuberans, among others—enter the differential diagnosis.[1–4,29–31] However, the challenge remains in the ability of IHC to reliably differentiate AFX from PDS tumors, as many attempted and presumed markers have demonstrated a high degree of variability in sensitivity and specificity in differentiating between tumor subtypes.[1,6,28,29,32–35] There is no widely accepted IHC marker that is able to reliably differentiate between these tumors, further reinforcing the modern conceptualization of AFX and PDS as intimately associated.[1,6,28,29,32–35]

RISK STRATIFICATION

Atypical fibroxanthoma is a relatively low-grade cutaneous neoplasm with rare metastatic potential when strict diagnostic criteria are applied.[1–4,6,8–10,36–38] Reports of AFX metastases have been occasionally described in the literature, with cited rates ranging from less than 1% to 5%.[1–4,6,8–10,36–38] On further analysis of those reports, however, these cases demonstrated histopathologic features similar to AFX but often with deeper and more extensive subcutaneous invasion, necrosis, and/or lymphovascular or perineural invasion,[1–4,6–8,10,36–38] features that are now better regarded as meeting criteria for a diagnosis of PDS. As a recently described term, there is a relative paucity of literature regarding the rates of local recurrence and distant metastases for PDS. Historical rates of local recurrence and distant metastasis for its precursors termed MFH and UPS are widely variable. This is likely due to inclusion of neoplasms that would not uniformly meet current diagnostic criteria for PDS. From a comprehensive review of the literature, 2 recently reported case series investigated the clinical course of PDS tumors, demonstrating markedly higher rates of local recurrence and metastasis compared with AFX, with ranges from 20% to 28% and 10% to 20%, respectively.[2,39] As suspected from their histopathologic appearance, this suggests that, within the AFX/PDS tumor spectrum, tumors that display histopathologic criteria consistent with PDS are likely to be intrinsically higher risk, perhaps analogous to high-risk

cutaneous SCC, whereas features such as perineural invasion, poor histologic differentiation, and deeper depth of invasion are well-known harbingers of increased morbidity.[40,41] However, adequate surgical margin control was inconsistently achieved in these series.

ADDITIONAL WORKUP

With regard to further workup, evidence-based recommendations regarding imaging or sentinel lymph node biopsy are lacking, given a paucity of available data. In general, routine preoperative imaging is usually not indicated or performed in superficial AFX tumors with minimal high-risk histologic features. However, given our developing understanding of the similarities and critical difference in the clinical behavior of these tumors, the role of perioperative radiographic imaging may be helpful in certain cases, particularly in those where the depth of local infiltration may involve bone or critical anatomic structures. The usefulness of sentinel lymph node biopsy (SLNB) in the management of AFX or PDS is also unknown. However, an approximate 10% risk of regional metastasis is often used as a rough cutoff for performing SLNB in melanoma and SCC.[42] Assuming technical equivalence, applying this standard to AFX or PDS tumors would indicate that SLNB would not be helpful in cases of AFX but may be of benefit for PDS in select cases. Further prospective studies are clearly indicated but hampered by the rarity of these tumors.

MANAGEMENT
Tumor Extirpation

Historically, the standard of care in the treatment of AFX has been wide local excision (WLE).[1–4,6–8,36–38,43,44] However, defined margins for WLE remain unclear and local recurrence rates have been variable, ranging from 3% to 20% in the published literature.[1,6,7,36–38,44–46] With the advent of modern micrographic techniques using fresh frozen tissue for histopathologic analysis of tumor margin status, Mohs micrographic surgery (MMS) has been increasingly used for these tumors because of its well-known advantages in comprehensive margin analysis (**Fig. 1**). Several comparative analyses have investigated the outcomes of MMS compared with WLE in the treatment of AFX, and have demonstrated a lower rate of local recurrence with greater tissue preservation using MMS.[36–38,43–46] With regard to the optimal management of PDS tumors, however, evidence-based recommendations are lacking due to the paucity of available data surrounding these tumors and the relative novelty in terminology. In the aforementioned studies that investigated the clinical behaviors of PDS tumors, demonstrating rates of local recurrence and metastasis, ranging from 20% to 28% and 10% to 20%, respectively, these series of AFX/PDS tumors focused on histology rather than clinical management. Mohs micrographic surgery was not used for the treatment of any of these tumors, and most PDS tumors that recurred and metastasized had been incompletely excised. Comprehensive margin control, such as that provided by MMS, is thus considered paramount, akin to management of high-risk SCCs. However, consensus guidelines and prospective studies remain lacking given the paucity of data, relative rarity of tumor type, and the new emergence of PDS as a histopathological entity.[1–4,6,8,12,36–39,47]

Adjuvant Therapy

In the setting of unresectable, recurrent, or metastatic disease, adjuvant treatment with radiation and/or chemotherapy may be warranted, although evidence for efficacy is lacking. Historically, radiation therapy has been used both for AFX and PDS, and is likely most effectively used as an adjuvant treatment in the setting of unresectable, locally recurrent, or regionally metastatic disease.[1,8,9,36,48,49] However, there are no clear recommendations or guidelines on the role of radiation therapy in AFX or PDS; optimal dosing, fractionation, type, and frequency are not well described and determined on a case-by-case basis.

Traditional chemotherapy has been largely ineffectual in treating metastatic disease of the AFX/PDS/UPS lineage; however, recently identified genetic mutations involved in tumorigenesis may be helpful in guiding potential molecular therapies. In particular, as mentioned earlier, activating RAS mutations seems to be a distinguishing feature of more aggressive tumors,[15,16,18,19] and thus targeted molecular inhibitors of the RAS pathway may hold promise in the treatment of unresectable or metastatic disease. Future studies are needed to investigate the clinical efficacy of these and other potential drugs in treating unresectable and/or disseminated disease.

Surveillance and Follow-Up

Following the diagnosis of AFX or PDS, it is important to perform a full-body skin examination to evaluate for other skin cancers, because these are exceedingly common in this patient population. A complete review of systems and a regional nodal physical examination should also be performed to help detect clinical signs of metastatic disease. After definitive management, routine surveillance with follow-up every 6 months is recommended to assess for local recurrence, metastases, and the potential development of other skin cancers. In the rare setting of metastatic disease, a multidisciplinary approach is optimal with treatment individualized to the patient.

SUMMARY

Atypical fibroxanthoma and PDS tumors share many clinical, histopathologic, and oncogenic features, and are likely a part of a fibrohistiocytic mesenchymal tumor spectrum. In cutaneous oncology, differentiating between AFX and PDS is pivotal, as tumors with histologic features consistent with PDS seem to be higher risk for local recurrence and distant metastatic disease.

With regard to management, surgery remains the gold standard. In AFX, surgical excision with the Mohs micrographic technique offers superior tumor control rates with lower rates of local recurrence and greater tissue preservation compared with local excision. Mohs micrographic surgery should be considered first-line in the treatment of AFX. In the setting of PDS, optimal management is less clear, given the paucity of available data. However, because of the greater recurrence rate and higher metastatic potential, extirpation with complete tumor margin control is critical. In addition, these patients should be carefully monitored on a more frequent basis due to the higher risk of recurrence and metastasis. Although there are no standard clinical guidelines for these patients, in our practice we extrapolate from guidelines formulated for patients with high-risk SCC and see these patients every 3 to 6 months, especially for the first 2 years after diagnosis and treatment.

The roles of imaging and SLNB in management and clinical outcomes of AFX and PDS remain unclear. In reality, these tools are unlikely to be helpful in most cases of AFX, in which depth of infiltration is confined to at most the superficial subcutis, and the risk of distant spread is minimal. In the setting of PDS, however, emerging literature indicates that these tumors are deeper and inherently higher risk, and thus radiographic imaging and SLNB may be helpful in a select case-by-case basis.

In settings of advanced unresectable disease, radiation therapy or chemotherapy may provide additional benefit. Radiation therapy may be more ideal in settings of residual unresectable, locally recurrent, or regionally metastatic disease. Targeted molecular therapies may, in the relatively near future, offer benefits beyond those provided by traditional chemotherapies for disseminated disease. However, further studies are needed to establish best management practices. In the unfortunate setting of metastatic disease, a multidisciplinary approach is optimal.

Following the diagnosis of AFX or PDS, a complete review of systems and a regional nodal physical examination should be performed. After definitive management, patients should be carefully monitored on a more frequent basis due to the risk of recurrence and metastasis; although there are no standard clinical guidelines for these patients, we surveil patients every 3 to 6 months, especially for the first 2 years after diagnosis and treatment.

REFERENCES

1. Iorizzo LJ, Brown MD. Atypical fibroxanthoma: a review of the literature. Dermatol Surg 2011;37: 146–57.
2. Miller K, Goodlad JR, Brenn T. Pleomorphic dermal sarcoma. Adverse histologic features predict aggressive behavior and allow distinction from atypical fibroxanthoma. Am J Surg Pathol 2012;36: 1317–26.
3. Brenn T. Pleomorphic dermal neoplasms: a review. Adv Anat Pathol 2014;21:108–30.
4. McCalmont TH. AFX: what we now know. J Cutan Pathol 2011;38:853.
5. Lai K, Harwood CA, Purdie KJ, et al. Genomic analysis of atypical fibroxanthoma. PLoS One 2017; 12(11):e0188272.
6. Soleymani T, Hollmig ST. Conception and management of a poorly understood spectrum of dermatologic neoplasms: atypical fibroxanthoma, pleomorphic dermal sarcoma, and undifferentiated pleomorphic sarcoma [review]. Curr Treat Options Oncol 2017;18(8):50.
7. Fretzin DF, Helwig EB. Atypical fibroxanthoma of the skin. A clinicopathologic study of 140 cases. Cancer 1973;31:1541–52.
8. Helwig EB, May D. Atypical fibroxanthoma of the skin with metastasis. Cancer 1986;57:368–76.
9. Cooper JZ, Newman SR, Scott GA, et al. Metastasizing atypical fibroxanthoma (cutaneous malignant histiocytoma): report of five cases. Dermatol Surg 2005;31:221, 5; [discussion: 225].
10. Weiss SW, Goldblum JR. Malignant fibrous histiocytoma (pleomorphic undifferentiated sarcoma). In: Enzinger & Weiss's soft tissue tumors. 5th edition. Philadelphia: Mosby: Elsevier; 2008. p. 403–27.
11. Fletcher CD. Pleomorphic malignant fibrous histiocytoma: fact or fiction? A critical reappraisal based on 159 tumors diagnosed as pleomorphic sarcoma. Am J Surg Pathol 1992;16:213–28.
12. McCalmont TH. Correction and clarification regarding AFX and pleomorphic dermal sarcoma. J Cutan Pathol 2012;39:8.
13. Vallés-Torres J, Izquierdo-Villarroya MB, Vallejo-Gil JM, et al. Cardiac undifferentiated pleomorphic sarcoma mimicking left atrial myxoma. J Cardiothorac Vasc Anesth 2018. https://doi.org/10.1053/j.jvca.2018.02.010.
14. Li X, Zhang Z, Latif M, et al. Synovium as a widespread pathway to the adjacent joint in undifferentiated high-grade pleomorphic sarcoma of the tibia: a case report. Medicine (Baltimore) 2018;97(8):e9870.
15. Helbig D, Quaas A, Mauch C, et al. Copy number variations in atypical fibroxanthomas and pleomorphic dermal sarcomas. Oncotarget 2017;8(65): 109457–67.
16. Griewank KG, Schilling B, Murali R, et al. TERT promoter mutations are frequent in atypical fibroxanthomas and pleomorphic dermal sarcomas. Mod Pathol 2014;27(4):502–8.
17. Winchester D, Lehman J, Tello T, et al. Undifferentiated pleomorphic sarcoma: factors predictive of adverse outcomes. J Am Acad Dermatol 2018. https://doi.org/10.1016/j.jaad.2018.05.022.
18. Griewank KG, Wiesner T, Murali R, et al. Atypical fibroxanthoma and pleomorphic dermal sarcoma harbor frequent NOTCH1/2 and FAT1 mutations and similar DNA copy number alteration profiles. Mod Pathol 2018;31(3):418–28.
19. Helbig D, Ihle MA, Putz K, et al. Oncogene and therapeutic target analyses in atypical fibroxanthomas and pleomorphic dermal scarcomas. Oncotarget 2016;7(16):21763–74.
20. Weedon D, Kerr JF. Atypical fibroxanthoma of skin: an electron microscope study. Pathology 1975;7: 173–7.
21. Barr RJ, Wuerker RB, Graham JH. Ultrastructure of atypical fibroxanthoma. Cancer 1977;40:736–43.
22. Aasi SZ, Leffell DJ, Lazova RZ. Atlas of practical Mohs histopathology. New York: Springer; 2013.
23. Thum C1, Husain EA, Mulholland K, et al. Atypical fibroxanthoma with pseudoangiomatous features: a histological and immunohistochemical mimic of cutaneous angiosarcoma. Ann Diagn Pathol 2013; 17(6):502–7.
24. Diaz-Cascajo C, Weyers W, Borghi S. Pigmented atypical fibroxanthoma: a tumor that may be easily mistaken for malignant melanoma. Am J Dermatopathol 2003;25:1–5.
25. Patterson JW, Konerding H, Kramer WM. "Clear cell" atypical fibroxanthoma. J Dermatol Surg Oncol 1987;13:1109–14.
26. Wright NA, Thomas CG, Calame A, et al. Granular cell atypical fibroxanthoma: case report and review of the literature. J Cutan Pathol 2010;37:380–5.
27. Kim J, McNiff JM. Keloidal atypical fibroxanthoma: a case series. J Cutan Pathol 2009;36:535–9.
28. Hollmig ST, Rieger KE, Henderson MT, et al. Reconsidering the diagnostic and prognostic utility of LN-2 for undifferentiated pleomorphic sarcoma and

atypical fibroxanthoma. Am J Dermatopathol 2013; 35(2):176–9.

29. De Feraudy S, Mar N, McCalmont TH. Evaluation of CD10 and procollagen 1 expression in atypical fibroxanthoma and dermatofibroma. Am J Surg Pathol 2008;32:1111–22.

30. Mauzo SH, Milton DR, Prieto VG, et al. Summary of expression of SPARC protein in cutaneous vascular neoplasms and mimickers. Ann Diagn Pathol 2018; 34:151–4.

31. Mohanty SK, Sharma S, Pradhan D, et al. Microphthalmia-associated transcription factor (MiTF): promiscuous staining patterns in fibrohistiocytic lesions is a potential pitfall. Pathol Res Pract 2018; 214(6):821–5. https://doi.org/10.1016/j.prp.2018.05.001.

32. Monteagudo C, Calduch L, Navarro S, et al. CD99 immunoreactivity in atypical fibroxanthoma: a common feature of diagnostic value. Am J Clin Pathol 2002;117:126–31.

33. Hartel PH, Jackson J, Ducatman BS, et al. CD99 immunoreactivity in atypical fibroxanthoma and pleomorphic malignant fibrous histiocytoma: a useful diagnostic marker. J Cutan Pathol 2006; 33(Suppl 2):24–8.

34. Lazova R, Moynes R, May D, et al. LN-2 (CD74). A marker to distinguish atypical fibroxanthoma from malignant fibrous histiocytoma. Cancer 1997;79: 2115–24.

35. Hanlon A1, Stasko T, Christiansen D, et al. LN2, CD10, and Ezrin do not distinguish between atypical fibroxanthoma and undifferentiated pleomorphic sarcoma or predict clinical outcome. Dermatol Surg 2017;43(3):431–6.

36. Ang GC, Roenigk RK, Otley CC, et al. More than 2 decades of treating atypical fibroxanthoma at Mayo Clinic: what have we learned from 91 patients? Dermatol Surg 2009;35:765–72.

37. Seavolt M, McCall M. Atypical fibroxanthoma: review of the literature and summary of 13 patients treated with Mohs micrographic surgery. Dermatol Surg 2006;32:435–41.

38. Davis JL, Randle HW, Zalla MJ, et al. A comparison of Mohs micrographic surgery and wide excision for the treatment of atypical fibroxanthoma. Dermatol Surg 1997;23:105–10.

39. Tardío JC, Pinedo F, Aramburu JA, et al. Pleomorphic dermal sarcoma: a more aggressive neoplasm than previously estimated. J Cutan Pathol 2016; 43(2):101–12.

40. Karia PS, Jambusaria-Pahlajani A, Harrington DP, et al. Evaluation of American Joint Committee on Cancer, International Union Against Cancer, and Brigham and Women's Hospital tumor staging for cutaneous squamous cell carcinoma. J Clin Oncol 2014;32(4):327–34.

41. Duran J, Morgan FC, Karia PS, et al. An evaluation of high-stage cutaneous squamous cell carcinoma outcomes by gender. Br J Dermatol 2016. https://doi.org/10.1111/bjd.15208.

42. Schmitt AR, Brewer JD, Bordeaux JS, et al. Staging for cutaneous squamous cell carcinoma as a predictor of sentinel lymph node biopsy results: meta-analysis of American Joint Committee on Cancer criteria and a proposed alternative system. JAMA Dermatol 2014;150:19–24.

43. Stadler FJ, Scott GA, Brown MD. Malignant fibrous tumors. Semin Cutan Med Surg 1998;17:141–52.

44. Brown MD, Swanson NA. Treatment of malignant fibrous histiocytoma and atypical fibrous xanthomas with micrographic surgery. J Dermatol Surg Oncol 1989;15:1287–92.

45. Gonzalez-Garcia R, Nam-Cha SH, Munoz-Guerra MF, et al. Atypical fibroxanthoma of the head and neck: report of 5 cases. J Oral Maxillofac Surg 2007;65:526–31.

46. Huether MJ, Zitelli JA, Brodland DG. Mohs micrographic surgery for the treatment of spindle cell tumors of the skin. J Am Acad Dermatol 2001;44: 656–9.

47. Lum DJ, King AR. Peritoneal metastases from an atypical fibroxanthoma. Am J Surg Pathol 2006;30: 1041.

48. McCoppin HH1, Christiansen D, Stasko T, et al. Clinical spectrum of atypical fibroxanthoma and undifferentiated pleomorphic sarcoma in solid organ transplant recipients: a collective experience. Dermatol Surg 2012;38(2):230–9.

49. Hager S, Makowiec F, Henne K, et al. Significant benefits in survival by the use of surgery combined with radiotherapy for retroperitoneal soft tissue sarcoma. Radiat Oncol 2017;12(1):29.

Extramammary Paget Disease

Bradley G. Merritt, MD[a], Catherine A. Degesys, MD[a],*, David G. Brodland, MD[b,c,d,e]

KEYWORDS

- Extramammary paget disease • Mohs micrographic surgery • CK7 staining

KEY POINTS

- Extramammary Paget disease (EMPD) is an intraepidermal adenocarcinoma most often limited to the epidermis, with typical cases affecting genital skin.
- In patients with invasive disease, prognosis is based on the degree of invasion, with tumors less than 1 mm deep having low mortality.
- Careful evaluation for an underlying malignancy should be carried out to exclude life-threatening disease.
- Mohs surgery has proven effective in the treatment of EMPD, and the implementation of CK7 immunostaining assists in reducing the recurrence rate.
- Alternative treatments, including topical treatment with imiquimod and 5-fluorouracil, and photodynamic therapy, may be effective in select cases of EMPD.

INTRODUCTION

Extramammary Paget disease (EMPD) is a rare, intraepithelial adenocarcinoma that affects anatomic regions with abundant apocrine sweat glands. The disease exists most commonly in a primary form, originating in the epidermis or cutaneous adnexa. Less often, EMPD occurs in association with an underlying malignancy (secondary EMPD), usually of the lower gastrointestinal or urinary tract. When limited to the epidermis, primary EMPD is not life-threatening, but invasive disease may portend a poor prognosis. Patients with primary EMPD have a better prognosis than those with secondary EMPD because of the association of the latter with internal malignancy, so it is important to perform a full evaluation to exclude coexistent internal malignancy. Surgical excision remains the mainstay of treatment of EMPD, and Mohs micrographic surgery (MMS) is considered the treatment of choice, allowing for precise margin control with reduced recurrence rates. Alternative treatments include topical 5-fluorouracil and imiquimod, photodynamic therapy, laser vaporization, chemotherapy, and radiation therapy but data are limited.

EPIDEMIOLOGY

EMPD is rare, with an incidence estimated to be 0.11 per 100,000 person years.[1] Of all cases of Paget disease (mammary and extramammary), EMPD accounts for 7% to 14%.[1] One of the largest registries including patients with mammary and extramammary Paget disease documents EMPD patients having invasive disease 21% of the time, compared with 44% of patients with invasive mammary Paget disease.[1] The age of onset of

Disclosure Statement: The authors have nothing to disclose.
[a] Department of Dermatology, University of North Carolina-Chapel Hill, 410 Market Street, Suite 400, Chapel Hill, NC 27516, USA; [b] Zitelli and Brodland PC, 5200 Centre Avenue, Suite 303, Pittsburgh, PA 15232, USA; [c] Department of Dermatology, The University of Pittsburgh Medical Center, Pittsburgh, PA, USA; [d] Department of Otolaryngology, The University of Pittsburgh Medical Center, Pittsburgh, PA, USA; [e] Department of Plastic Surgery, The University of Pittsburgh Medical Center, Pittsburgh, PA, USA
* Corresponding author.
E-mail addresses: ABBIE.DEGESYS@GMAIL.COM; CATHERINE.DEGESYS@UNCH.UNC.EDU

Dermatol Clin 37 (2019) 261–267
https://doi.org/10.1016/j.det.2019.02.002
0733-8635/19/© 2019 Elsevier Inc. All rights reserved.

derm.theclinics.com

EMPD is typically 64 to 75 years. White women and Asian men are affected at disproportionately high rates.[2] The vulva is the most commonly involved site of EMPD, accounting for approximately 65% of EMPD.[3]

ASSOCIATED MALIGNANCIES

Of patients with EMPD, 5% to 42% are reported to have an additional malignancy documented either before, simultaneously, or after development of EMPD. These cases are classified as secondary EMPD. These range from extragenital skin cancer to distant internal malignancies. The broad range of published percentages of second malignancy, wide-spectrum of associated malignancy, and elevated baseline risk for cancer in the aged population has led to controversy regarding the true association between internal malignancies and EMPD. One study reported the rate of internal malignancy is higher in patients with EMPD with a standardized incidence ratio of 1.7.[1] Of those patients with EMPD and an internal malignancy, slightly more than half present with the internal malignancy before their diagnosis of EMPD with a median time from diagnosis of primary malignancy until the diagnosis of EMPD ranging from 2.8 to 10.9 years. For patients diagnosed with EMPD before the diagnosis of an internal malignancy, the median time to diagnosis of the internal malignancy is 2.9 to 3.8 years.[1] However, a recent study of 199 patients suggests that there is no increased risk of breast, intestine, or urologic tract malignancy among patients with vulvar EMPD.[4]

In cases of EMPD with coexistent internal cancer, the location of EMPD is often correlated with the site of the underlying malignancy. Perianal EMPD is associated with lower gastrointestinal malignancy and penoscrotal EMPD is associated with urinary tract malignancy. Distant internal malignancies reported in association with EMPD include breast carcinoma, ovarian carcinoma, bile duct carcinoma, hepatocellular carcinoma, renal cell carcinoma, lung carcinoma, stomach carcinoma, and pancreatic carcinoma.[5,6] Additionally, secondary EMPD has been described in the setting of contiguous pagetoid spread from an underlying adenocarcinoma. Rates of contiguous spread from adjacent malignancy of up to 23.9% have been reported in the literature.[3,7-9] In particular, contiguous spread is more likely to occur from the vulva, urinary tract, and anorectal regions.

CLINICAL PRESENTATION

The diagnosis of EMPD is usually made after other diagnoses have been considered and treatment ineffective. The differential diagnosis includes Bowen disease, tinea cruris, contact dermatitis, lichen simplex chronicus, lichen planus, cutaneous T-cell lymphoma, psoriasis, and seborrheic dermatitis.[10] Onset is often insidious, and a high degree of clinical suspicion should be present in vulvar, perianal, genital, or axillary dermatoses that do not respond to typical therapy.

EMPD presents with a variety of clinical manifestations. Erythematous plaques and pruritus are most common. **Fig. 1** shows an example of the typical clinical presentation. Patients may later develop erosions and ulcerations, with a burning sensation and pain associated with more advanced lesions, especially in anogenital areas. The disease can also present with scale, nodules, verrucous lesions, and hypopigmentation to depigmentation. Diagnosis of vulvar EMPD is delayed by an average of 20 months, with most patients treated for fungal infection or vulvovaginitis first. Delayed diagnosis leads to a statistically significant increase in lesion size but not tumor depth. In a series of 56 patients, invasive disease was reported in 18%.[11] Perianal EMPD is less common than other subtypes, representing about 20% of cases of EMPD.[12] Its presence, however, is correlated more often with underlying malignancy, especially cancer of the anus or colorectum.[10] Associated internal malignancies include colon adenocarcinoma, prostate cancer, esophageal cancer, and lung cancer. Penoscrotal EMPD, like perianal EMPD, is more commonly associated with an underlying neoplasm in locally adjacent organs and structures, including cancer of the prostate, urethra, bladder, and testicles.

EMPD involving the genital region concomitant with the bilateral axillae has been reported, primarily in Japanese men.[13] Any patient with genital EMPD should undergo a thorough examination to exclude additional cutaneous involvement.

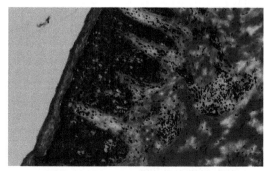

Fig. 1. Erythematous, scaling patch within the intergluteal cleft with clinical presentation consistent with extramammary Paget disease.

HISTOLOGY

A skin biopsy should be performed for any suspicious lesions that fail to respond to the typical treatments for other possible diagnoses. EMPD must be confirmed by histology. Typical findings include intraepidermal aggregates of pale-staining cells that are larger than keratinocytes and contain pleomorphic nuclei with pronounced atypia, prominent nucleoli, and mitotic figures.[14,15]

UNIFOCAL OR MULTIFOCAL DISEASE?

Uncertainty exists as to whether EMPD grows in a contiguous pattern or with field cancerization and multiple foci.[16] Many reports exist describing a presumed multifocal phenomenon, most of these rely on standard hematoxylin and eosin for margin evaluation.[16] With immunostaining using cytokeratin 7 (CK7), EMPD shows significant involvement not seen on routine hematoxylin and eosin staining. Margin control of EMPD with Mohs surgery using CK7 can reveal a digitate, often haphazard growth pattern.[16] With standard excision or Mohs surgery without the use of CK7 immunostaining, these haphazard extensions may be missed, giving the impression of multicentric disease.[16] This can lead to misinterpreting recurrence as a second primary tumor. Multiple foci of spontaneous or treatment-induced tumor regression could also lead to a false-negative margin.[17]

Given the potential for concurrent internal malignancy in EMPD, multiple separate skin lesions may occur, perhaps because of a common genetic predisposition for malignant degeneration. Nonetheless, better margin evaluation and reduced recurrence rates demonstrated with Mohs surgery and CK7 staining support this treatment modality and the idea of contiguous growth of EMPD.

PROGNOSIS

Patients with primary EMPD have a significantly better prognosis in regards to mortality than those with secondary EMPD because of the absence of coexistent malignancy. Primary EMPD confined to the epidermis has an excellent prognosis. Although evidence is limited, primary EMPD restricted to the epidermis is reported to have no risk of metastasis.[2] Prognosis of invasive EMPD is closely related to depth of invasion from the dermoepidermal junction, with invasion less than 1 mm carrying minimal risk of nodal involvement. Microscopic invasive disease (<1 mm) is also believed to have no adverse impact on survival. EMPD greater than 1 mm depth has an increased risk of nodal involvement and metastasis. Reported percentages of survival vary in the literature, but those with local or distant metastases have reduced survival rates. One study reported 5-year disease-specific survival rates of invasive EMPD by type: localized EMPD 94.9%, regional lymph node involvement with EMPD 84.9%, and distant metastases 52.5%.[18]

Patients with secondary EMPD have mortality rates exceeding 50%, because of internal malignancy. However, as treatments for the respective internal malignancies improve, this mortality rate will likely be reduced. Of patients with secondary EMPD, those with internal malignancy diagnosed before developing EMPD have a relative excess risk of death of 3.2 compared with patients with EMPD without an underlying tumor. Patients who are diagnosed with a secondary malignancy after the diagnosis of EMPD have a relative excess risk of 2.5.[1] This may be explained by the fact that internal malignancy is diagnosed sooner because of screening in the setting of EMPD.

EVALUATION FOR INTERNAL MALIGNANCY

After confirmation of the diagnosis of EMPD by histology, a work-up to exclude underlying associated malignancies is prudent. A comprehensive review of systems and complete physical examination should be carried out, including careful palpation of lymph nodes. Bilateral "underpants pattern" erythema has been associated with pronounced lymphovascular invasion and should alert the clinician to the likelihood of nodal disease.[19] In cases where extent of the tumor is questionable, multiple scouting biopsies may be helpful to establish a more accurate estimate of the margins.

Clear screening guidelines for patients diagnosed with EMPD are lacking, but a recent study out from the Mayo Clinic evaluating 161 patients proposed a screening algorithm. First is a thorough review of systems and physical examination to evaluate for internal malignancy and lymphadenopathy, including breast examination. Second, all patients should undergo age-related cancer screening, urine cytology examination, and colonoscopy. For men, a prostate-specific antigen and digital rectal examination should be performed and for women, a Papanicolaou test and mammography should be performed.[8]

EXTRAMAMMARY PAGET DISEASE TREATMENT

Surgical excision of EMPD remains the mainstay of treatment. Mohs surgery is often used because of the ability to evaluate 100% of the margin while minimizing tissue loss and morbidity. EMPD of the vulva has been treated surgically with methods ranging from vulvectomy (partial or total) to wide local excision with margins of 1 to 3 cm. Vulvectomy, although the most extensive and morbid procedure, has the lowest reported recurrence rate in some series (15%), compared with 43% recurrence for wide local excision. Perianal and scrotal EMPD have a higher rate of recurrence after wide local excision, some series reporting a rate up to 50%, although some have achieved a lower recurrence rate of 9.9% using a combination of 3-cm margins and intraoperative standard frozen sections.[20–22] Some studies have shown that margin status is predictive of recurrence, with positive margins leading to higher rates of recurrence. Many other series, however, document recurrence of EMPD independent of margin status, with patients who have reportedly clear margins as likely to develop recurrent disease. This reiterates the idea that many of the previously reported negative margins might have been false-negatives on hematoxylin and eosin, supported by the striking margin involvement often detected when adding CK7 immunostaining to Mohs surgery.

Mohs Surgery for Extramammary Paget Disease Without Immunostaining

Multiple case series have been published that confirm the efficacy of Mohs surgery for EMPD. Published series using Mohs surgery with hematoxylin and eosin staining demonstrate a recurrence rate ranging from 0% to 28%, with varying duration of follow-up.[2,17,23–25] In a meta-analysis published in 2013, it was determined that the overall recurrence rate for EMPD after MMS (without CK7 immunostaining) was 12.2% corresponding to an estimated 5-year disease-free rate of 83.6% as determined via Kaplan-Meier analysis. There was a statistically significantly lower rate of recurrence than wide local excision.[24] A recent comparison of men and women with genital EMPD treated with Mohs surgery without immunostaining or a variety of alternatives including wide local excision with margins up to 3 cm, vulvectomy, and hemivulvectomy found a recurrence rate of 18% in the Mohs surgery group versus 36% in the collective group treated with wide local excision, vulvectomy, or hemivulvectomy.[2]

Mohs Surgery with CK7 Immunostaining

CK7 has proven to be a sensitive marker for detecting the presence of neoplastic cells in EMPD, with near 100% positivity in primary and secondary EMPD. Over the past decade, CK7 has been increasingly implemented in Mohs surgery, improving the detection of subtle disease

that would otherwise go unseen. **Figs. 2** and **3** demonstrate an example where EMPD is unapparent on hematoxylin and eosin–stained frozen section, but apparent on CK7-stained frozen section. In cases treated with Mohs surgery using CK7 in addition to hematoxylin and eosin, hematoxylin and eosin–negative but CK7-positive foci are visualized in about 65% of cases (authors' experience). This suggests that the false-negative rate may be 65% when not using Mohs surgery with CK7, a possible explanation for the higher recurrence rate of EMPD compared with basal cell and squamous cell carcinomas treated with Mohs surgery. In the largest retrospective, multicenter cohort study of patients with EMPD treated with MMS plus CK7, the local recurrence rate was found to be 2.3% and 5.3% for primary and recurrent tumors, respectively. The mean follow-up time was 44.1 months and the study demonstrates the lowest local recurrence rate with adequate follow-up to date. Similarly, the 5-year tumor-free rates of 97.1% and 80.0% for primary and recurrent tumors are the highest reported to date. There were two total recurrences in the study. In both of these cases, the entire specimen was not processed by the Mohs technique. If only the tumors treated entirely by Mohs technique with CK7 immunostain are considered, the recurrence rate would be 0%.[25] The authors recommend processing the central portion (debulking specimen) via vertical section and CK7 immunostain to evaluate depth of invasion.

Peripheral In-Continuity Tissue Examination Using Frozen Section Technique

Peripheral in-continuity tissue examination with frozen sections has been used for large tissue areas, greater than 8 cm, with superficial/intraepidermal involvement and no histologic or clinical evidence of invasive disease.[26–28] In this

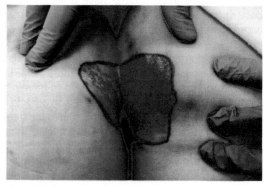

Fig. 2. Intraepidermal aggregates of pale-staining cells within the epidermis (hematoxylin and eosin, original magnification ×100).

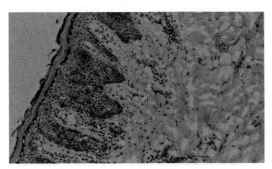

Fig. 3. Pagetoid cells easily highlighted on CK-7 immunostain (original magnification ×100).

modification, the peripheral margin of the tumor is initially excised using the en face margin, as with the Mohs technique, to remove 2- to 3-mm-wide strips of epidermis, dermis, and subcutaneous tissue. These peripheral pieces are processed and evaluated using CK7 immunostaining to augment hematoxylin and eosin staining. After clearing the margin peripherally, the remaining central island of tumor, containing skin, adnexa, and superficial subcutaneous tissue, is excised at the level of the midsubcutaneous tissue. This ensures removal of the epidermal tumor, along with any tumor that may extend down the adnexa. Exhaustive histologic evaluation with immunostains may or may not be undertaken of the deep margin.

This modification has been performed as an alternative to save time and expense of microscopic examination of extremely large tissue areas. This method is not suitable for EMPD with histologic or clinical evidence of invasive disease.[26–28]

ALTERNATIVE TREATMENT OPTIONS

Imiquimod has been used off-label for the treatment of intraepithelial EMPD, with case reports of successful treatment of primary and recurrent tumor clinically and histologically.[29] Practitioners should be admonished that when using a topical treatment that may partially treat a clinically indistinct tumor, leading to discontinuous growth. Using this approach may unintentionally render all histologically based margin examination surgical techniques to be less effective because of fragmentation of the tumor. Because of the short duration of follow-up of most reported cases treated with 5% imiquimod, no definitive conclusion can be reached regarding the long-term efficacy. Presently, its use may be best reserved for patients who refuse or are unable to tolerate surgical treatment. 5-Fluorouracil has also been explored as a potential surgery-sparing treatment in EMPD and has the same limitations in efficacy and evidence

as imiquimod. Although case reports suggest clinical clearance of tumor after 5-fluorouracil treatment, histologic persistence has been noted. The clinician should recognize that when considering treatment with a topical therapy its efficacy is unproven and it can mask persistent tumor including deeper, potentially invasive disease.[30]

Photodynamic therapy with topical aminolevulinic acid or intravenous porfimer sodium followed by treatment with a 632.8-nm argon-pumped dye laser has been used for noninvasive EMPD. Results of a retrospective series found 78% (seven of nine) of patients treated with intravenous porfimer photosensitization and argon laser to be disease free at follow-up (12–96 months).[31] The tumor diameter ranged from less than 1.5 cm to 8.5 cm.

Destruction of EMPD with carbon dioxide laser vaporization has been documented; however, studies have been disappointing. In a study of 52 patients with EMPD treated with wide local excision, laser alone, or a combination of the two showed significantly increased recurrence rates in the laser alone group.[32] One concern is that to obtain cosmetically acceptable results, the deeper portions of the adnexal structures must be left intact, which increases likelihood of residual disease.

Radiation therapy has been used as a treatment of primary EMPD, following surgical excision of EMPD with the aim of reducing local recurrence and as a treatment of recurrent disease. Intraepidermal and invasive EMPD have been treated with radiation therapy, primarily disease located in the anogenital region. Patients in most published series have generally been considered poor surgical candidates, and therefore, recurrence rates likely reflect a higher-risk subset of patients with a worse prognosis. Patients with secondary EMPD have an extremely poor prognosis, regardless of treatment with radiation therapy. In a 2002 review of the existing literature on radiation therapy for perianal Paget disease, 43 cases were analyzed.[33] Of the patients with primary EMPD, recurrence after radiation therapy was 35%, compared with a recurrence of 77% in patients with secondary EMPD. In this review, 5-year survival was 20% for invasive perianal EMPD and 94% for noninvasive EMPD. Radiation therapy, like topical treatments, is most applicable in patients who are unsuitable candidates for surgical intervention.

CHEMOTHERAPY FOR EXTRAMAMMARY PAGET DISEASE: LOCAL AND SYSTEMIC

Systemic chemotherapy has shown little efficacy in the treatment of metastatic disease. Several regimens have been used to treat metastatic EMPD, including low-dose 5-fluorouracil/cisplatin, FECOM (5-fluorouracil, epirubicin, carboplatin, vincristine, and mitomycin C), docetaxel mono-therapy, S-1 monotherapy, docetaxel and S-1 combination therapy, and PET (cisplatin, epirubi-cin, and paclitaxel).[34] Complete cure has not been obtained, but improved quality of life has been achieved with minimal treatment-related morbidity.

SUMMARY

EMPD is a cutaneous adenocarcinoma most often limited to the epidermis, with typical cases affecting genital skin in women and men. In pa-tients with invasive disease, prognosis is based on the degree of invasion, with tumors less than 1 mm deep having low mortality. Careful evalua-tion for an underlying malignancy, most often co-lon or genitourinary, should be carried out to exclude life-threatening disease. Mohs surgery has proven effective in the treatment of EMPD with the best reported cure rates. The implementa-tion of CK7 shows promise in further reducing the recurrence rate. Other histologically based margin evaluation techniques using immunostaining are likely to provide better cure rates than has stan-dard wide excision.

REFERENCES

1. Siesling S, Elferink MA, van Dijck JA, et al. Epidemi-ology and treatment of extramammary Paget dis-ease in the Netherlands. Eur J Surg Oncol 2007; 33:951–5.
2. Lee KY, Roh MR, Chung WG, et al. Comparison of Mohs micrographic surgery and wide excision for extramammary Paget's disease: Korean experience. Dermatol Surg 2009;35:34–40.
3. Chanda JJ. Extramammary Paget's disease: prog-nosis and relationship to internal malignancy. J Am Acad Dermatol 1985;13(6):1009–14.
4. Van der Linden M, Schuurman M, Bulten J, et al. Stop routine screening for associated malignancies in cutaneous noninvasive vulvar Paget disease? Br J Dermatol 2018;179(6):1315–21.
5. Hayashibara Y, Ikeda S. Extramammary Paget's dis-ease with internal malignancies. Gan To Kagaku Ryoho 1988;15:1569–75.
6. Nakano S, Narita R, Tabaru A, et al. Bile duct cancer associated with extramammary Paget's disease. Am J Gastroenterol 1995;90:507–8.
7. Parker L, Parker J, Bodurka-Bevers D. Paget's dis-ease of the vulva: pathology, pattern of involvement, and prognosiss. Gynecol Oncol 2000;77(1):183–9.
8. Schmitt AR, Long BJ, Weaver AL. Evidence-based screening recommendations for occult cancers in the setting of newly diagnosed extramammary Pa-get disease. Mayo Clin Proc 2018;93(7):877–83.
9. Isik O, Aytac E, Brainard M. Perianal Paget's dis-ease: three decades experience of a single institu-tion. Int J Colorectal Dis 2016;31(1):29–34.
10. Kyriazanos ID, Stamos NP, Miliadis L, et al. Extra-mammary Paget's disease of the perianal region: a review of the literature emphasizing the operative management technique. Surg Oncol 2011;20(2): e61–71.
11. Shaco-Levy R, Bean SM, Vollmer RT, et al. Paget disease of the vulva: a study of 56 cases. Eur J Ob-stet Gynecol Reprod Biol 2010;149(1):86–91.
12. Minicozzi A, Borzellino G, Momo R, et al. Perianal Paget's disease: presentation of six cases and liter-ature review. Int J Colorectal Dis 2010;25:1–7.
13. Kitajima S, Yamamoto K, Tsuji T, et al. Triple extra-mammary Paget's disease. Dermatol Surg 1997; 23:1035–8.
14. Perrotto J, Abbott JJ, Ceilley RI, et al. The role of immunohistochemistry in discriminating primary from secondary extramammary Paget disease. Am J Dermatopathol 2010;32:137–43.
15. Jones RE Jr, Austin C, Ackerman AB. Extramam-mary Paget's disease. A critical reexamination. Am J Dermatopathol 1979;1:101–32.
16. Hendi A, Perdikis G, Snow JL. Unifocality of extra-mammary Paget disease. J Am Acad Dermatol 2008;59:811–3.
17. Coldiron BM, Goldsmith BA, Robinson JK. Surgical treatment of extramammary Paget's disease. A report of six cases and a reexamination of Mohs mi-crographic surgery compared with conventional sur-gical excision. Cancer 1991;67:933–8.
18. Karam A, Dorigo O. Treatment outcomes in a large cohort of patients with invasive extramammary Pa-get's disease. Gynecol Oncol 2012;125:346–51.
19. Murata Y, Kumano K, Tani M. Underpants-pattern er-ythema: a previously unrecognized cutaneous mani-festation of extramammary Paget's disease of the genitalia with advanced metastatic spread. J Am Acad Dermatol 1999;40(6 Pt 1):949–56.
20. Zollo JD, Zeitouni NC. The Roswell Park Cancer Institute experience with extramammary Paget's dis-ease. Br J Dermatol 2000;142:59–65.
21. Zhu Y, Ye DW, Chen ZW, et al. Frozen section-guided wide local excision in the treatment of peno-scrotal extramammary Paget's disease. BJU Int 2007;100:1282–7.
22. Thomas CJ, Wood GC, Marks VJ. Mohs micro-graphic surgery in the treatment of rare aggressive cutaneous tumors: the Geisinger experience. Der-matol Surg 2007;33:333–9.
23. O'Connor WJ, Lim KK, Zalla MJ, et al. Comparison of Mohs micrographic surgery and wide excision for

extramammary Paget's disease. Dermatol Surg 2003;29:723–7.

24. Bae J, Choi Y, Kim H, et al. Mohs micrographic surgery for extramammary Paget disease: a pooled analysis of individual patient data. Dermatol Surg 2013;68(4):632–7.

25. Brodland DG, Etzkorn JR, Terushkin V, et al. Intraoperative immunostaining for cytokeratin-7 during Mohs micrographic surgery demonstrates low local recurrence rates in extramammary Paget's disease. Dermatol Surg 2018;44(3):354–64.

26. Hendi A, Brodland D, Zitelli J. Extramammary Paget's disease: surgical treatment with Mohs micrographic surgery. J Am Acad Dermatol 2004;51(5):767–73.

27. Woods J, Farrow G. Peripheral tissue examination for malignant lesions of the skin. Mayo Clin Proc 1991;66:207–9.

28. Hagerty R, Worsham G, Rutland ED, et al. Peripheral in-continuity tissue examination. Plast Reconstr Surg 1989;83(3):539–45.

29. Cohen PR, Schulze KE, Tschen JA, et al. Treatment of extramammary Paget disease with topical imiquimod cream: case report and literature review. South Med J 2006;99:396–402.

30. Brown RS, McCormack M, Lankester KJ, et al. Spontaneous apparent clinical resolution with histologic persistence of a case of extramammary Paget's disease: response to topical 5-fluorouracil. Cutis 2000;66:454–5.

31. Housel JP, Izikson L, Zeitouni NC. Noninvasive extramammary Paget's disease treated with photodynamic therapy: case series from the Roswell Park Cancer Institute. Dermatol Surg 2010;36:1718–24.

32. Louis-Sylvestre C, Haddad B, Paniel BJ. Paget's disease of the vulva: results of different conservative treatments. Eur J Obstet Gynecol Reprod Biol 2001;99(2):253–5.

33. Brown RS, Lankester KJ, McCormack M, et al. Radiotherapy for perianal Paget's disease. Clin Oncol (R Coll Radiol) 2002;14:272–84.

34. Fukuda K, Funakoshi T. Metastatic extramammary Paget's disease: pathogenesis and novel therapeutic approach. Front Oncol 2018;8:38.

Merkel Cell Carcinoma
Updates on Staging and Management

Christine Cornejo, MD[a], Christopher J. Miller, MD[b],*

KEYWORDS

- Merkel cell carcinoma • Merkel cell polyomavirus • Staging • Sentinel lymph node biopsy
- Wide local excision • Mohs micrographic surgery • Immune checkpoint inhibitors

KEY POINTS

- Accurate staging of Merkel cell carcinoma allows clinicians to counsel patients about prognosis, design treatment plans, and determine eligibility for clinical trials.
- Sentinel lymph node biopsy provides important prognostic information and can identify patients who may benefit from systemic medications to improve survival.
- Treatment depends on the pathologic characteristics of the primary tumor and the extent of disease.
- Merkel cell carcinoma is associated with a high risk of local, regional, and distant recurrence and long-term surveillance is important.

INTRODUCTION

Merkel cell carcinoma (MCC) is an aggressive neuroendocrine carcinoma with a high rate of metastasis and 5-year overall survival (OS) ranging from 50.6% for patients with local disease to 13.5% for patients with distant metastases.[1] Most MCCs present as rapidly growing red or violaceous firm nodules on the sun-exposed skin of fair-skinned Caucasians older than 60 years.[1] Approximately 5% of MCC are found in the lymph nodes (LNs) without a primary tumor on the skin.[1] The risk for MCC is higher in patients who are immunosuppressed from hematologic malignancy, human immunodeficiency virus/AIDS, or medications for solid organ transplants and autoimmune disease.[2] MCCs are caused by either monoclonal integration of Merkel cell polyomavirus (MCPyV) or somatic mutations from ultraviolet light.[3] The incidence of MCC increased more than 5-fold between 1986 and 2011 in the United States and continues to

increase in Australia and many European countries.[2,4,5] The American Joint Committee on Cancer (AJCC) updated staging criteria in 2017, and the National Comprehensive Cancer Network updated clinical practice guidelines on August 31, 2018. This article reviews the most recent evidence-based updates on staging and management.

ESTABLISHING THE DIAGNOSIS OF MERKEL CELL CARCINOMA

MCC is unsuspected by clinical examination in 99% of cases; therefore, biopsy is necessary to establish a pathologic diagnosis.[6] Hematoxylin and eosin stains of MCC typically show small, round, blue cells with sparse cytoplasm, abundant mitoses, and dense core granules in the cytoplasm.[2] The histologic differential diagnosis includes other small round blue cell tumors, particularly metastatic small cell carcinoma of the lung.

Disclosure Statement: The authors have nothing to disclose.
[a] Department of Dermatology, University of Pennsylvania, 2 Maloney Building, 3600 Spruce Street, Philadelphia, PA 19104, USA; [b] Department of Dermatology, Perelman Center for Advanced Medicine, University of Pennsylvania, 1st Floor South Pavilion, 3400 Civic Center Boulevard, Suite 1-330S, Philadelphia, PA 19104, USA
* Corresponding author.
E-mail address: christopher.miller@uphs.upenn.edu

Dermatol Clin 37 (2019) 269–277
https://doi.org/10.1016/j.det.2019.03.001
0733-8635/19/© 2019 Elsevier Inc. All rights reserved.

derm.theclinics.com

Immunohistochemistry is helpful to distinguish MCC from its histologic mimickers. Primary cutaneous MCC is cytokeratin 20 positive with a perinuclear dotlike pattern and thyroid transcription factor 1 negative. Positive staining with neuroendocrine markers, such as chromogranin, synaptophysin, CD56, neuron-specific enolase, and neurofilament, also support a diagnosis of MCC.

Merkel Cell Polyomavirus Antibody Testing

Baseline determination of Merkel virus oncoprotein antibody titer or quantitation of MCPyV oncoproteins can assist with risk stratification and subsequent detection of recurrent disease. Antibodies to MCPyV capsid proteins, which mark previous viral exposure, are detectable in 90% of patients with MCC and more than 60% of healthy adults.[7] Although high antibody titers to MCPyV capsid protein at presentation may portend a more favorable prognosis, these titers do not correlate with MCC tumor burden and cannot be used to assess response to treatment.[8] In contrast, antibodies to MCPyV oncoprotein, which are present in more than 50% of patients with MCC and only rarely detectable in healthy adults, correlate with MCC tumor burden. Additionally, MCC patients without MCPyV oncoproteins (seronegative) may have a higher risk of recurrence than seropositive patients.[9] Although this testing may be considered as part of the initial workup or as surveillance, it is not considered part of the routine staging evaluation. MCC oncoprotein serology testing is now clinically available (AMERK; https://www.merkelcell.org/serology).

STAGING

After establishing a diagnosis of MCC, an additional workup with a physical examination, imaging, and surgery is necessary to establish the AJCC stage. Accurate staging is important to counsel patients about prognosis, design treatment plans, and determine eligibility for clinical trials. Before 2010, nonuniform criteria from 5 separate staging systems made it difficult to compare results from different studies of MCC. In 2010, the AJCC introduced the first consensus staging system for MCC based on data from the National Cancer Database.[10,11]

The AJCC categorizes MCC patients with similar survival outcomes using the TNM Staging System, which is based on the extent of the primary tumor (T), the extent of spread to nearby LNs (N), and the presence of metastasis to sites other than the LNs near the primary tumor (M). The T, N, and M stages are combined to assign an overall stage of I and II for MCC localized to the skin, III for MCC with metastasis to LNs near the primary tumor or if no primary tumor is detected, and IV for metastasis to sites other than the regional LNs (**Table 1**). These stages are subdivided into smaller patient populations with similar prognoses. The TNM staging for MCC includes clinical staging categories, based on physical examination and imaging studies, and was updated in 2017 in the eighth edition to include pathologic staging categories based on the pathology of the LNs (pN) and distant metastases (M).[10] Pathologic staging of metastases to LNs or distant sites provides more accurate prognostic information compared with clinical examination, because pathology is necessary to detect microscopic tumor or confirm the diagnosis of suspected metastasis.[1]

STAGING THE PRIMARY TUMOR (T STAGE)

Sixty-five percent of MCCs present with local disease and no clinical or pathologic evidence of metastasis to regional LNs or distant sites.[1] The AJCC T stage (primary tumor) is based on a combination of the clinical diameter of the tumor and the anatomic depth of invasion, based on clinical examination and pathology. The size of the tumor, measured in centimeters before biopsy or excision, stratifies prognosis. The 5-year OS is 55.8% for T1 primary tumors (≤2 cm clinical diameter) versus 41.1% for T2 (>2 cm but ≤5 cm) and T3 (>5 cm) primary tumors.[1] Clinical or pathologic evidence of invasion to fascia, muscle, cartilage, or bone (T4 primary tumors) lowers the 5-year OS to 31.8%.[1]

Table 1
Prognostic clinical and pathologic stage groups

Stage	Primary Tumor	LN	Metastasis	5-y OS[a]
0	Tis	N0	M0	
I	T1	(p)N0	M0	62.8%
IIA	T2-3	(p)N0	M0	54.6%
IIB	T4	(p)N0	M0	34.8%
III	T0-4	N1-3	M0	
IIIA[b]	T1-4	pN1a(sn) or pN1a	M0	40.3%
	T0	pN1b	M0	
IIIB[b]	T1-4	N1b-3	M0	26.8%
IV	T0-4	Any N	M1	13.5%

Abbreviation: TNM, tumor, node, metastasis.
[a] The 5-year OS is based on pathologic stage.[1]
[b] Stages IIIA and IIIB only apply to pathologic staging criteria.

STAGING THE REGIONAL LYMPH NODES (N STAGE)

After establishing the T stage, a complete examination of the regional LNs should be performed. Clinical LN status will determine the method of node sampling for pathologic analysis, which should include immunohistochemistry (**Fig. 1**).[12] The AJCC divides regional LN staging into clinical (N) and pathologic (pN) stages depending on whether the LNs were evaluated by clinical examination or pathology and whether in-transit metastases are present with or without LN metastases (see **Table 1**).

Pathologic nodal evaluation improves prognostication, and sentinel LN (SLN) status can help to guide management and improve regional control.[11] The incidence of occult nodal metastases in patients without clinically apparent lymphadenopathy is high (approximately 25%–30%).[13–18] Patients with primary tumors 2 cm or smaller who have no pathologic evidence of regional LN disease have better 5-year OS (62.8%) than patients whose node-negative status was determined only by skin examination (45%).[1] Therefore, consensus guidelines recommend consideration of SLN biopsy (SLNB) in all patients with MCC without clinically detectable nodes, unless surgery is contraindicated or declined.

There are no clinical or pathologic factors that can identify a patient population at sufficiently low enough risk for occult nodal metastasis to safely omit SLNB.[15] However, factors that can predict SLN positivity include increasing clinical tumor size and pathologic features of increasing tumor thickness, increasing mitotic rate, and infiltrative tumor growth.[19,20] Although larger tumors have higher rates of lymphatic spread, small tumors also carry a notable risk of occult nodal disease (up to 14% in 0.5-cm tumors).[1,19,20]

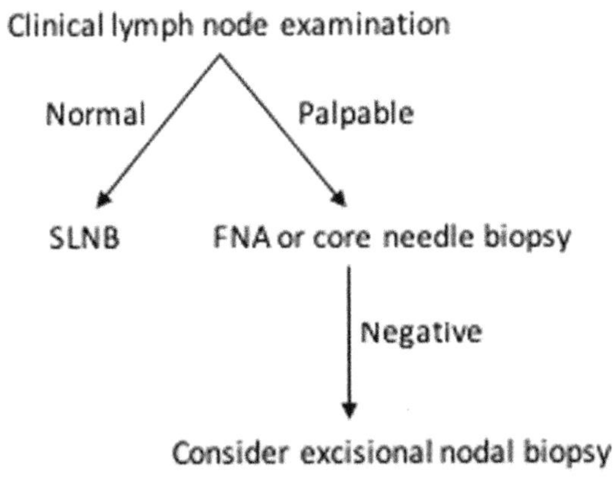

Despite the role of the SLNB in providing important prognostic information, there is controversy regarding the impact of SLN status on survival, particularly disease-specific survival (DSS). Several studies have shown SLN status to be a strong predictor of OS and disease-free survival.[11,14,15,18,21–23] However, no significant association between DSS and SLN status was seen in studies from Memorial Sloan-Kettering Cancer Center (n = 153) or the Mayo Clinic (n = 150).[15,24] A study of 4543 MCC patients from the Surveillance, Epidemiology, and End Results database found an association between improved DSS and use of SLNB and/or lymph node dissection on univariate but not on multivariate analysis.[21] As reported in other studies of SLNB in MCC, it is possible that the patients with a positive SLNB may have been selected for further adjuvant therapy, leading to improved DSS.[21,24] Although the precise effect on DSS remains unclear, SLNB may identify patients who could benefit from treatments to improve survival. A clinical trial investigating adjuvant avelumab, an anti–programmed death receptor ligand-1 (PD-L1) antibody, in patients with histologically confirmed LN disease is currently underway (ADAM; NCT03271372).

STAGING FOR DISTANT METASTASES (M STAGE)

The AJCC staging for MCC subdivides M stage based on the location of the distant metastases and whether the metastases were confirmed clinically (physical examination or imaging) versus pathologically. Metastases to the skin and distant LNs may be detectable by clinical examination, but imaging is usually necessary to find internal metastases.

All patients with pathologic evidence of LN involvement should have careful evaluation for occult distant metastatic disease with whole body PET with fluorodeoxyglucose tracer combined with computed tomography scans or neck, chest, abdomen, and pelvis computed tomography scanning with contrast. Imaging is also encouraged in patients with unresectable disease or whenever metastasis is suspected based on patients' signs and/or symptoms.[12,18] In patients who have surgically resectable disease and no clinical signs of nodal or metastatic spread, imaging is not routinely recommended for staging purposes.[12]

The ideal imaging modality may depend on the clinical scenario. Whole-body PET with fluorodeoxyglucose offers improved sensitivity compared with computed tomography scanning

Clinical lymph node examination

Fig. 1. LN staging evaluation. FNA, fine needle aspiration; SNLB, sentinel LN biopsy.

alone, with an added impact on management in 37% of patients.[25] MRI of the brain is considered by some clinicians for patients with suspected intracranial metastases.

Merkel Cell Carcinoma Management

The treatment of MCC depends on the pathologic characteristics of the primary tumor and the extent of disease, particularly the presence or absence of clinically involved LNs or distant metastases. Initial management typically involves treatment of the primary tumor and tumor bed and staging of the regional LNs with SLNB. If there is evidence of metastatic disease, a tumor board meeting to discuss options for palliation, surgery, radiation, chemotherapy, immunotherapy, and/or enrollment into a clinical trial based on the clinical scenario is recommended.

MANAGEMENT OF THE PRIMARY TUMOR AND TUMOR BED
Surgery

Wide local excision (WLE) is the most common method of surgery for primary MCC.[26,27] Mohs micrographic surgery (MMS) is another surgical option for MCC and is more commonly performed at academic centers and on smaller tumors (T1) in the head and neck region.[28,29] Compared with WLE, MMS offers the advantage of complete histologic control of the peripheral and deep margins while secondarily sparing normal tissue. The reported local recurrence rates after MMS have ranged from 5% to 22%, compared with 25% to 40% for WLE.[26,27,30–33] Survival outcomes for MMS are comparable with those for WLE.[28,29,34]

The goal of primary tumor resection is to obtain histologically negative margins when clinically feasible, with clearance of the tumor being more important than the actual surgical margin taken.[12] The current NCCN guidelines recommend wide excision with 1- to 2-cm margins to investing fascia of muscle or pericranium when clinically feasible or MMS as surgical options for primary tumor resection.[12] If MMS is performed, the central portion of the tumor should be sent for permanent sections.

Definitive excision, regardless of the surgical approach, should be coordinated with and occur after SLNB, if indicated, to avoid any alteration of the lymphatic drainage patterns. Any reconstruction involving extensive undermining or tissue movement should be delayed until negative histologic margins are verified. If adjuvant radiation therapy is planned, extensive tissue movement should be minimized and closure should be chosen to allow for expeditious initiation of radiation therapy.

Radiation Monotherapy

Radiation monotherapy for the treatment of primary tumors is an alternative to surgery in patients who are poor surgical candidates or at risk for significant surgical morbidity.[35] There are limited outcome data on radiation monotherapy for MCC. Although the in-field control ranges from 75% to 100%, distant recurrence is increased, and the rates of cancer-specific and OS are decreased compared with complete surgical resection.[36] However, these rates are likely influenced by other non–treatment-related factors, because patients selected for radiation monotherapy often have inoperable tumors or have comorbidities that preclude surgical resection and may lower OS.

Adjuvant Radiation for Localized Merkel Cell Carcinoma

Adjuvant radiation to the primary tumor bed after resection is associated with improved locoregional control and a trend toward improved disease-free survival in multiple retrospective studies.[17,23,37–40] In particular, adjuvant radiation can be highly effective for local control after subtotal resection or microscopically positive margins.[41] However, the use of adjuvant radiation to the primary tumor bed in patients who have established clear surgical margins is controversial. Adjuvant radiation was not associated with improved local control after margin-negative WLE in 1 study,[13] and another study failed to show a significant difference in OS, relapse-free survival, or disease-free survival after adjuvant postoperative radiation therapy in patients with stage IA MCC who achieved clear histologic margins after MMS.[32]

Adjuvant radiation may not be essential for patients who have low-risk tumors and are histologically free of disease at the primary tumor site. The NCCN guidelines state that clinical observation without adjuvant radiotherapy may be considered for a subset of immunocompetent patients with low-risk tumors that are small (ie, <1 cm), widely excised, and free of lymphovascular invasion.[12] If patients undergo adjuvant radiation therapy, recommended doses increase according to the tumor burden.

MANAGEMENT OF REGIONAL LYMPH NODES

SLN status is important for accurate staging; however, the optimal treatment after SLNB, regardless of nodal status, has not been defined. Current data suggest that patients with negative SLNB can be safely observed without adjuvant radiation to the regional LN basin.[14,16,17] However, adjuvant radiation can be considered in patients at risk for false-negative SLNB (ie, previous WLE, failure to perform appropriate immunohistochemistry on SLNs, or tumors involving the head and neck).[12] Adjuvant radiation to regional nodes can also be considered for patients who have early stage disease, are clinically node negative, and either decline or are not candidates for SLNB.[17,37]

For patients with clinically or pathologically positive nodal disease, a multidisciplinary tumor meeting for a discussion of nodal dissection and/or radiation and a consideration for adjuvant systemic therapy is recommended. Data comparing outcomes for complete LN dissection (CLND), radiation, and combination therapy in the management of nodal disease are limited. In patients with clinically evident nodal disease, adjuvant radiation has been reported to improve regional recurrence rates; however, it is unclear if these findings also apply to subclinical disease detected by SLNB.[42] Generally, rates of regional recurrence after radiation and CLND are similar, with no additional benefit from adjuvant radiation after CLND.[15] Complete nodal dissection offers the advantage of pathologic examination of the entire nodal basin, which may provide further prognostic information that could help to guide management and is more strongly favored in patients with clinically apparent disease compared with those with occult LN involvement. In patients who cannot undergo surgery for nodal disease, radiation offers excellent regional control.[43] Consensus guidelines recommend adjuvant radiation to the draining nodal basin after CLND in patients with multiple involved nodes or histologic evidence of extracapsular tumor extension.[12]

Patients with SLN-positive disease who undergo either CLND or adjuvant radiation to the nodal basin have OS and DSS similar to patients with SLN-negative disease, highlighting the importance of treating nodal disease.[15] Until specific guidelines for patients with nodal disease are better established, the risks and benefits of each treatment option should be discussed with patient, and final treatment decisions may vary based on site-specific morbidity, tumor characteristics, and patient comorbidities. At present, systemic therapies are not considered first line in the management of nodal disease. However, with emerging data demonstrating the efficacy of immunotherapies for MCC, standards for managing regional LNs may change.

METASTATIC DISEASE

For patients with metastatic disease, consensus guidelines recommend a multidisciplinary tumor board meeting to discuss enrollment in a clinical trial, palliation, surgery, radiation, and/or systemic therapy (chemotherapy or immunotherapy) based on the clinical scenario. Emerging data suggest that immunotherapies have the potential to improve outcomes in patients with metastatic MCC and may provide new treatment options for this patient population. In particular, PD-1/PD-L1–based immunotherapy is likely to be considered the new standard of care for first-line treatment of patients with metastatic MCC. Response rates to immunotherapy are higher in treatment-naïve patients and lower in those treated with prior chemotherapy, likely owing to the well-characterized immunosuppressive effects of chemotherapy, and this factor should be considered when making treatment decisions. Presently, enrollment in a clinical trial should still be the preferred choice, whenever available and appropriate.[12]

SYSTEMIC THERAPIES
Chemotherapy

Until recently, the options for systemic therapies for MCC have been limited to cytotoxic chemotherapies, used alone or in combination. These agents have been used primarily as palliation in patients with advanced MCC because their use has not been associated with survival benefit.[38,44] Although initial response rates range from 53% to 76%, progression-free survival is short (median, 3–8 months), and disease progresses in 90% of patients at 10 months.[45] There is also significant morbidity and mortality associated with chemotherapy-related toxicities. Given the unclear benefit, considerable toxicities in elderly patients, and the potential to decrease efficacy of subsequent checkpoint immunotherapy, adjuvant chemotherapy is not routinely recommended.[46] The NCCN guidelines specify that adjuvant chemotherapy may be indicated in patients with disseminated disease based on clinical judgment for patients with contraindications to checkpoint immunotherapy.[12]

Immune Checkpoint Inhibitors

Increased expression of PD-L1 on the surface of MCC tumor cells, particularly those that are MCPyV positive, and PD-1 in the tumor microenvironment have been demonstrated.[47] Given the increased PD-1/PD-L1 axis expression seen in MCC, there has been considerable interest in investigating the use of PD-1 and PD-L1 immune checkpoint inhibitors in the management of MCC.

Initial studies, which focused on immune checkpoint inhibitors in patients with metastatic MCC, have led to the addition of avelumab, nivolumab, and pembrolizumab to the list of treatment options for disseminated MCC in the 2018 NCCN guidelines.[48–50] Clinical trials are also looking at the safety and efficacy of immune checkpoint inhibitors as systemic adjuvant therapy in high-risk patients with MCC and as a combined therapy with other agents, including other immunotherapeutics and/or radiation.

Overall, inhibitors of the PD-1/PD-L1 axis lead to durable responses that are associated with improved quality of life.[51] Treatment-related adverse effects seem to be similar to those experienced by patients receiving PD-1/PD-L1 inhibitors for other tumor types and compare favorably with those of cytotoxic chemotherapy. For eligible patients, no clear data favor use of one PD-1 or PD-L1 inhibitor over another. Objective responses are seen regardless of PD-L1 or MCPyV tumor status, although a trend for higher ORR was seen in patients with PD-L1–positive tumors treated with avelumab.[48] Presently, testing for MCPyV status (by immunohistochemistry or serology) or PD-L1 expression (by immunohistochemistry) has limited usefulness in patient selection for PD-1/PD-L1 blockade and is not routinely supported.

Other Immunotherapies and Targeted Molecular Therapies

Several additional immunotherapies and targeted molecular therapies with varying levels of success have been described in case reports and are being investigated in clinical trials, including adoptive T-cell transfer, nanoparticle albumin-bound antigen natural killer T-cell MCC vaccine, intralesional interferon, IL-12 DNA electroporation, tyrosine kinase inhibitors, and Toll-like receptor-4 agonists as listed in **Box 1**.[52–66] Results from nonimmune therapy trials are especially relevant to patients who are not eligible for immunotherapy (see **Box 1**).

SURVEILLANCE

MCC is associated with a high risk of local, regional, and distant recurrence. Follow-up visits with complete skin and LN examination is recommended every 3 to 6 months for 2 to 3 years and every 6 to 12 months thereafter if the patient is free of disease.[12] Immunosuppressed patients are at a higher risk for recurrence and, as such, more frequent follow-up may be indicated. Immunosuppressive treatments should be minimized as clinically feasible.

Decisions regarding surveillance imaging should be based on patient-specific risk factors or symptoms because guidelines for imaging

---

Box 1
Other investigational therapies for MCC

Cellular immunotherapy

Adoptive T-cell therapy[52,54]

Nab antigen natural killer T-cell (NANT) vaccine[a]

Intralesional immunotherapy

Tumor necrosis factor (TNF)[55,56]

Class I interferon[53,57–59]

Talimogene laherparepvec (T-vec)[60]

Toll-like receptor (TLR)-4 agonist[61]

IL-12 electroporation[62]

Targeted molecular therapy

Phosphoinositide 3-kinase (PI3K) inhibitor (idelasisib)[63]

Multitargeted tyrosine kinase inhibitor (pazopanib[64] and cabozantinib[65])

Somatostatin analog (lanreotide)[66]

Abbreviation: Nab, nanoparticle albumin-bound.

[a] QUILT-3.045: NANT Merkel Cell Carcinoma (MCC) Vaccine: Combination Immunotherapy in Subjects With MCC Who Have Progressed on or After PD-L1 Therapy (not yet recruiting; NCT03167164).

---

frequency do not exist. Routine surveillance imaging should be considered for high-risk patients, including those with nodal disease, high-risk tumor characteristics, or immunosuppression. In the absence of other concerning signs of symptoms, routine surveillance imaging is not typically advised for immunocompetent patients with small primary tumors (<2 cm) and negative SLNB.[67] The NCCN guidelines indicate that quantitation of MCPyV oncoprotein can help to inform decisions regarding radiologic surveillance in patients with MCC. Seronegative patients may have a higher risk of recurrence and in seropositive patients, an increasing titer may be an early indicator of recurrence (positive predictive value, 66%), whereas a decreasing titer is reassuring (negative predictive value, 97%).[9,68] For seropositive patients, imaging could be reserved for those who report a change in clinical symptoms or have an increasing MCPyV oncoprotein antibody titer. Prompt recognition and treatment of metastatic disease may allow patients to start immunotherapy at a time of lower disease burden, which may be associated with better outcomes.

SUMMARY

As research improves our understanding of the biology and treatment of MCC, guidelines to manage these aggressive tumors will continue to evolve.[3] The eighth edition of the AJCC Staging System provides important prognostic information for patients, but the rising incidence of MCC increases the urgency for more research to improve outcomes.

REFERENCES

1. Harms KL, Healy MA, Nghiem P, et al. Analysis of prognostic factors from 9387 Merkel cell carcinoma cases forms the basis for the new 8th edition AJCC staging system. Ann Surg Oncol 2016;23(11): 3564–71.
2. Tetzlaff MT, Nagarajan P. Update on Merkel cell carcinoma. Head Neck Pathol 2018;12(1):31–43.
3. Harms PW, Harms KL, Moore PS, et al. The biology and treatment of Merkel cell carcinoma: current understanding and research priorities. Nat Rev Clin Oncol 2018;15(12):763–76.
4. Kieny A, Cribier B, Meyer N, et al. Epidemiology of Merkel cell carcinoma. A population-based study from 1985 to 2013, in northeastern of France. Int J Cancer 2018;144(4):741–5.
5. Youlden DR, Soyer HP, Youl PH, et al. Incidence and survival for Merkel cell carcinoma in Queensland, Australia, 1993-2010. JAMA Dermatol 2014;150(8): 864–72.
6. Heath M, Jaimes N, Lemos B, et al. Clinical characteristics of Merkel cell carcinoma at diagnosis in 195 patients: the AEIOU features. J Am Acad Dermatol 2008;58(3):375–81.
7. Touze A, Le Bidre E, Laude H, et al. High levels of antibodies against Merkel cell polyomavirus identify a subset of patients with Merkel cell carcinoma with better clinical outcome. J Clin Oncol 2011;29(12): 1612–9.
8. Samimi M, Molet L, Fleury M, et al. Prognostic value of antibodies to Merkel cell polyomavirus T antigens and VP1 protein in patients with Merkel cell carcinoma. Br J Dermatol 2016;174(4):813–22.
9. Paulson KG, Lewis CW, Redman MW, et al. Viral oncoprotein antibodies as a marker for recurrence of Merkel cell carcinoma: a prospective validation study. Cancer 2017;123(8):1464–74.
10. Bichakjian CK, Nghiem P, Johnson T, et al. Merkel cell carcinoma. In: Amin MB, ES, Greene FL, et al, editors. AJCC cancer staging manual. 8th edition. New York: Springer International Publishing; 2017. p. 549–62.
11. Lemos BD, Storer BE, Iyer JG, et al. Pathologic nodal evaluation improves prognostic accuracy in Merkel cell carcinoma: analysis of 5823 cases as the basis of the first consensus staging system. J Am Acad Dermatol 2010;63(5):751–61.
12. Bichakjian CK, Olencki T, Aasi SZ, et al. Merkel cell carcinoma, version 1.2018 clinical practice guidelines in oncology. J Natl Compr Canc Netw 2018; 16(6):742–74.
13. Allen PJ, Bowne WB, Jaques DP, et al. Merkel cell carcinoma: prognosis and treatment of patients from a single institution. J Clin Oncol 2005;23(10): 2300–9.
14. Gunaratne DA, Howle JR, Veness MJ. Sentinel lymph node biopsy in Merkel cell carcinoma: a 15-year institutional experience and statistical analysis of 721 reported cases. Br J Dermatol 2016;174(2): 273–81.
15. Sims JR, Grotz TE, Pockaj BA, et al. Sentinel lymph node biopsy in Merkel cell carcinoma: the Mayo Clinic experience of 150 patients. Surg Oncol 2018;27(1):11–7.
16. Karunaratne YG, Gunaratne DA, Veness MJ. Systematic review of sentinel lymph node biopsy in Merkel cell carcinoma of the head and neck. Head Neck 2018;40(12):2704–13.
17. Strom T, Naghavi AO, Messina JL, et al. Improved local and regional control with radiotherapy for Merkel cell carcinoma of the head and neck. Head Neck 2017;39(1):48–55.
18. Gupta SG, Wang LC, Penas PF, et al. Sentinel lymph node biopsy for evaluation and treatment of patients with Merkel cell carcinoma: the Dana-Farber experience and meta-analysis of the literature. Arch Dermatol 2006;142(6):685–90.
19. Smith FO, Yue B, Marzban SS, et al. Both tumor depth and diameter are predictive of sentinel lymph node status and survival in Merkel cell carcinoma. Cancer 2015;121(18):3252–60.
20. Iyer JG, Storer BE, Paulson KG, et al. Relationships among primary tumor size, number of involved nodes, and survival for 8044 cases of Merkel cell carcinoma. J Am Acad Dermatol 2014;70(4):637–43.
21. Sridharan V, Muralidhar V, Margalit DN, et al. Merkel cell carcinoma: a population analysis on survival. J Natl Compr Canc Netw 2016;14(10):1247–57. Was 23.
22. Sadeghi R, Adinehpoor Z, Maleki M, et al. Prognostic significance of sentinel lymph node mapping in Merkel cell carcinoma: systematic review and meta-analysis of prognostic studies. Biomed Res Int 2014;2014:489536.
23. Servy A, Maubec E, Sugier PE, et al. Merkel cell carcinoma: value of sentinel lymph-node status and adjuvant radiation therapy. Ann Oncol 2016;27(5): 914–9. WAS 39.
24. Fields RC, Busam KJ, Chou JF, et al. Recurrence and survival in patients undergoing sentinel lymph node biopsy for Merkel cell carcinoma: analysis of

153 patients from a single institution. Ann Surg Oncol 2011;18(9):2529–37. Was 21.

25. Siva S, Byrne K, Seel M, et al. F-18-FDG PET provides high-impact and powerful prognostic stratification in the staging of Merkel cell carcinoma: a 15-year institutional experience. J Nucl Med 2013; 54(8):1223–9.

26. O'Connor WJ, Roenigk RK, Brodland DG. Merkel cell carcinoma. comparison of Mohs micrographic surgery and wide excision in eighty-six patients. Dermatol Surg 1997;23(10):929–33.

27. Gollard R, Weber R, Kosty MP, et al. Merkel cell carcinoma - review of 22 cases with surgical, pathologic, and therapeutic considerations. Cancer 2000;88(8):1842–51.

28. Singh B, Qureshi MM, Truong MT, et al. Demographics and outcomes of stage I and II Merkel cell carcinoma treated with Mohs micrographic surgery compared with wide local excision in the National Cancer Database. J Am Acad Dermatol 2018;79(1):126–34.e3.

29. Shaikh WR, Sobanko JF, Etzkorn JR, et al. Utilization patterns and survival outcomes after wide local excision or Mohs micrographic surgery for Merkel cell carcinoma in the United States, 2004-2009. J Am Acad Dermatol 2018;78(1):175–7.e3.

30. Kline L, Coldiron B. Mohs micrographic surgery for the treatment of Merkel cell carcinoma. Dermatol Surg 2016;42(8):945–51.

31. Snow SN, Larson PO, Hardy S, et al. Merkel cell carcinoma of the skin and mucosa: report of 12 cutaneous cases with 2 cases arising from the nasal mucosa. Dermatol Surg 2001;27(2):165–70.

32. Boyer JD, Zitelli JA, Brodland DG, et al. Local control of primary Merkel cell carcinoma: review of 45 cases treated with Mohs micrographic surgery with and without adjuvant radiation. J Am Acad Dermatol 2002;47(6):885–92.

33. Lamb EP, Shaw FR, Fleming MD. Investigation of the diagnostic precision and utility of sentinel lymph node biopsy in the treatment of patients with Merkel cell carcinoma. Am Surg 2018;84(5):173–5.

34. Su C, Bai HX, Christensen S. Relative survival analysis in patients with stage I-II Merkel cell carcinoma treated with Mohs micrographic surgery or wide local excision. J Am Acad Dermatol 2018. [Epub ahead of print].

35. Harrington C, Kwan W. Outcomes of Merkel cell carcinoma treated with radiotherapy without radical surgical excision. Ann Surg Oncol 2014;21(11):3401–5.

36. Veness M, Howle J. Radiotherapy alone in patients with Merkel cell carcinoma: the Westmead Hospital experience of 41 patients. Australas J Dermatol 2015;56(1):19–24.

37. Jouary T, Leyral C, Dreno B, et al. Adjuvant prophylactic regional radiotherapy versus observation in stage I Merkel cell carcinoma: a multicentric prospective randomized study. Ann Oncol 2012; 23(4):1074–80.

38. Bhatia S, Storer BE, Iyer JG, et al. Adjuvant radiation therapy and chemotherapy in Merkel cell carcinoma: survival analyses of 6908 cases from the National Cancer Data Base. J Natl Cancer Inst 2016; 108(9) [pii:djw042].

39. Takagishi SR, Marx TE, Lewis C, et al. Postoperative radiation therapy is associated with a reduced risk of local recurrence among low risk Merkel cell carcinomas of the head and neck. Adv Radiat Oncol 2016;1(4):244–51.

40. Chen MM, Roman SA, Sosa JA, et al. The role of adjuvant therapy in the management of head and neck Merkel cell carcinoma an analysis of 4815 patients. JAMA Otolaryngol Head Neck Surg 2015; 141(2):137–41.

41. Harrington C, Kwan W. Radiotherapy and conservative surgery in the locoregional management of Merkel cell carcinoma: the British Columbia Cancer Agency Experience. Ann Surg Oncol 2016;23(2): 573–8.

42. Lee J, Poon I, Balogh J, et al. A review of radiotherapy for Merkel cell carcinoma of the head and neck. J Skin Cancer 2012;2012:563829.

43. Fang LC, Lemos B, Douglas J, et al. Radiation monotherapy as regional treatment for lymph node-positive Merkel cell carcinoma. Cancer 2010; 116(7):1783–90.

44. Fochtmann-Frana A, Haymerle G, Loewe R, et al. Incurable, progressive Merkel cell carcinoma: a single-institution study of 54 cases. Clin Otolaryngol 2018;43(2):678–82.

45. Iyer JG, Blom A, Doumani R, et al. Response rates and durability of chemotherapy among 62 patients with metastatic Merkel cell carcinoma. Cancer Med 2016;5(9):2294–301.

46. Paulson KG, Bhatia S. Advances in immunotherapy for metastatic Merkel cell carcinoma: a clinician's guide. J Natl Compr Canc Netw 2018;16(6):782–90.

47. Mitteldorf C, Berisha A, Tronnier M, et al. PD-1 and PD-L1 in neoplastic cells and the tumor microenvironment of Merkel cell carcinoma. J Cutan Pathol 2017;44(9):740–6.

48. Kaufman HL, Russell JS, Hamid O, et al. Updated efficacy of avelumab in patients with previously treated metastatic Merkel cell carcinoma after >/ =1 year of follow-up: JAVELIN Merkel 200, a phase 2 clinical trial. J Immunother Cancer 2018;6(1):7.

49. D'Angelo SP, Russell J, Lebbe C, et al. Efficacy and safety of first-line avelumab treatment in patients with stage IV metastatic Merkel cell carcinoma: a preplanned interim analysis of a clinical trial. JAMA Oncol 2018;4(9):e180077.

50. Topalian SL, Bhatia S, Hollebecque A, et al. Abstract CT074: non-comparative, open-label, multiple cohort, phase 1/2 study to evaluate nivolumab

(NIVO) in patients with virus-associated tumors (CheckMate 358): efficacy and safety in Merkel cell carcinoma (MCC). Cancer Res 2017;77(13 Suppl):CT074.

51. Kaufman HL, Hunger M, Hennessy M, et al. Non-progression with avelumab treatment associated with gains in quality of life in metastatic Merkel cell carcinoma. Future Oncol 2018;14(3):255–66.

52. Chapuis AG, Afanasiev OK, Iyer JG, et al. Regression of metastatic Merkel cell carcinoma following transfer of polyomavirus-specific T cells and therapies capable of re-inducing HLA class-I. Cancer Immunol Res 2014;2(1):27–36.

53. Wahl RU, Braunschweig T, Ghassemi A, et al. Immunotherapy with imiquimod and interferon alfa for metastasized Merkel cell carcinoma. Curr Oncol 2016;23(2):e150–3.

54. Paulson KG, Perdicchio M, Kulikauskas R. Augmentation of adoptive T-cell therapy for Merkel cell carcinoma with avelumab. J Clin Oncol 2017;35(Suppl 15) [abstract: 3044].

55. Ito Y, Kawamura K, Miura T, et al. Merkel cell carcinoma. A successful treatment with tumor necrosis factor. Arch Dermatol 1989;125(8):1093–5.

56. Hata Y, Matsuka K, Ito O, et al. Two cases of Merkel cell carcinoma cured by intratumor injection of natural human tumor necrosis factor. Plast Reconstr Surg 1997;99(2):547–53.

57. Durand JM, Weiller C, Richard MA, et al. Treatment of Merkel cell tumor with interferon-alpha-2b. Br J Dermatol 1991;124(5):509.

58. Biver-Dalle C, Nguyen T, Touze A, et al. Use of interferon-alpha in two patients with Merkel cell carcinoma positive for Merkel cell polyomavirus. Acta Oncol 2011;50(3):479–80.

59. Paulson KG, Tegeder A, Willmes C, et al. Downregulation of MHC-I expression is prevalent but reversible in Merkel cell carcinoma. Cancer Immunol Res 2014;2(11):1071–9.

60. Blackmon JT, Dhawan R, Viator TM, et al. Talimogene laherparepvec for regionally advanced Merkel cell carcinoma: a report of 2 cases. JAAD Case Rep 2017;3(3):185–9.

61. Bhatia S, Miller NJ, Lu H, et al. Intratumoral G100, a TLR4 agonist, induces anti-tumor immune responses and tumor regression in patients with Merkel cell carcinoma. Clin Cancer Res 2018;25(4): 1185–95.

62. Bhatia S, Iyer J, Ibrani D, et al. Intratumoral delivery of Interleukin-12 DNA via in vivo electroporation leads to regression of injected and non-injected tumors in Merkel cell carcinoma: final results of a phase 2 study. Eur J Cancer 2015;51:S104.

63. Shiver MB, Mahmoud F, Gao L. Response to idelalisib in a patient with stage IV Merkel cell carcinoma. N Engl J Med 2015;373(16):1580–2.

64. Nathan PD, Gaunt P, Wheatley K, et al. UKMCC-01: a phase II study of pazopanib (PAZ) in metastatic Merkel cell carcinoma. J Clin Oncol 2016;34(15): 9542.

65. Tarabadkar ES, Thomas H, Blom A, et al. Clinical benefit from tyrosine kinase inhibitors in metastatic Merkel cell carcinoma: a case series of 5 patients. Am J Case Rep 2018;19:505–11.

66. Fakiha M, Letertre P, Vuillez JP, et al. Remission of Merkel cell tumor after somatostatin analog treatment. J Cancer Res Ther 2010;6(3):382–4.

67. Frohm ML, Griffith KA, Harms KL, et al. Recurrence and survival in patients with Merkel cell carcinoma undergoing surgery without adjuvant radiation therapy to the primary site. JAMA Dermatol 2016; 152(9):1001–7.

68. Paulson KG, Carter JJ, Johnson LG, et al. Antibodies to Merkel cell polyomavirus T antigen oncoproteins reflect tumor burden in Merkel cell carcinoma patients. Cancer Res 2010;70(21): 8388–97.

Management of Skin Cancer in the Elderly

Michael Renzi Jr, MD[a], Josh Schimmel, BS[b], Ashley Decker, MD[c], Naomi Lawrence, MD[d],*

KEYWORDS

- Elderly • Skin cancer • Basal cell carcinoma • Squamous cell carcinoma • Functional assessment
- Quality of life • Karnofsky

KEY POINTS

- The increase in the incidence of skin cancer in the elderly population has had a significant impact on the delivery of health care to these patients.
- Clinicians should use a comprehensive approach that accounts for functional status, impact on quality of life, cost, and adverse outcomes when managing both high- and low-morbidity skin cancers in the elderly.
- Treatment of cutaneous malignancy is a shared decision, and clinicians must consider patient goals when selecting therapy.

INTRODUCTION

The commonly held definition of an elderly patient is one with the chronologic age of 65 years or older. In 2014, the US Census Bureau reported 43.1 million citizens aged 65 years and older and predicts this population will grow to 83.7 million by the year 2050.[1] As the average lifespan continues to increase, the country faces several paradigm shifts to address this burgeoning population. Such a demographic shift has a significant impact on the delivery of health care.

Skin cancer is the most common malignancy in the United States, with an incidence that continues to increase.[2,3] Approximately 1 in 5 Americans will be diagnosed with skin cancer in their lifetime. Most cutaneous malignancies are found among America's elderly population.[4,5] The management of skin cancer in the elderly population has become a source of debate in the current medical environment. Recent literature suggests that elderly patients may not live long enough to see benefits from treating their cutaneous malignancies, particularly nonmelanoma skin cancers (NMSC).[6,7] Although these concerns should be addressed, especially in a health care system that strives to better allocate resources, there are other factors in addition to age, that must be considered when treating skin cancers in the elderly.

MANAGEMENT OF LOW MORBIDITY SKIN CANCERS
Tumor Pathology

The type of cutaneous malignancy and histologic subtype will invariably be one of the first considerations when selecting a treatment modality (**Table 1**). Tumors characterized by high recurrence rates or frequent invasion of local structures will typically warrant a more aggressive treatment approach. For basal cell carcinomas, micronodular, basosquamous, infiltrative, and morpheaform subtypes, which are considered to have more aggressive growth patterns, a treatment with a higher cure rate, such as Mohs micrographic

Disclosure: The authors have no financial conflicts of interest to disclose.
[a] Division of Dermatology, Cooper University Hospital, 3 Cooper Plaza, Suite 504, Camden, NJ 08103, USA;
[b] Cooper Medical School of Rowan University, 3 Cooper Plaza, Suite 504, Camden, NJ 08103, USA; [c] Cooper University Hospital, 10000 Sagemore Drive #10103, Marlton, NJ 08053, USA; [d] Division of Dermatology, Cooper University Hospital, 10000 Sagemore Drive #10103, Marlton, NJ 08053, USA
* Corresponding author.
E-mail address: lawrence-naomi@cooperhealth.edu

Dermatol Clin 37 (2019) 279–286
https://doi.org/10.1016/j.det.2019.02.003
0733-8635/19/© 2019 Elsevier Inc. All rights reserved.

Table 1
Available treatment options for nonmelanoma skin cancers listed with individual benefits and drawbacks

Treatment	Benefits	Drawbacks
MMS	Highest cure rate for all pathologic subtypes, cosmetically appealing reconstruction	Long procedure time, costly
Simple excision (with paraffin margins)	Can treat all pathologic subtypes, shorter procedure time than Mohs, cosmetically appealing scar	Unable to check margins in real time
ED&C	Shortest procedure time, cheapest treatment modality	Can only be used for superficial subtypes, cosmetically unappealing scar, higher recurrence rate than excision
Topical medications (Imiquimod or 5%-Fluorouracil)	No procedure required, minimal scarring	Costly, can only be used for superficial subtypes, high recurrence rates
RT	Good for large tumors not amenable for surgery and patients who cannot tolerate surgery	Costly, not available at every institution, high recurrence rates
Hedgehog pathway inhibitors	Only oral therapy available for locally advanced/unrespectable tumors	Too costly for use in everyday practice, significant side effects, high rates of primary and secondary resistance to the drug

surgery (MMS), will be the preferred option.[8–10] The same is true for certain squamous cell carcinoma subtypes, including sclerosing, infiltrative, poorly differentiated, and spindle cell.[8] For low-risk, localized subtypes, less invasive treatments, including electrodessication and curettage (ED&C), or topical medications, such as imiquimod or 5%-fluorouracil, may be used.[9]

Tumor Location

Tumor location must also be considered in conjunction with tumor pathology, because anatomic location increases the risk for recurrence and local invasion.[9,10] Area H, as designated by the Appropriate Use Criteria (AUC), includes the mask area of the face, which contains locations known for such increased risk of local invasion and higher rates of reoccurence.[8–10] The AUC, set forth by the American Academy of Dermatology in collaboration with other dermatologic societies, is a useful tool to determine which lesions warrant treatment with MMS based on clinical and pathologic characteristics. Although such clinical criteria are useful in narrowing treatment options, clinicians must remember the AUC is just another tool to aid the process of selecting appropriate therapy. Not every lesion that meets AUC should be treated with MMS.

Characterizing Patient Health

Central to the debate regarding the optimal approach to managing cutaneous malignancy in the elderly is the dilemma of the optimal method to characterize patient health and life expectancy. The goal is to have a comprehensive understanding of a patient's overall health in order to avoid subjecting them to unnecessary and invasive procedures that will ultimately yield little benefit to survival or quality of life (QOL). Some researchers have suggested that age be used as a relative contraindication for treatment of cutaneous malignancies, especially NMSCs. These criteria are justified by the observation that in patients as old as 90 years of age, more than half of patients died within a year of excision due to unrelated causes.[7] In contrast, others have demonstrated that MMS is well tolerated in patients 90 years of age or older, with no procedure-related mortality and a median survival of 36.9 months after the procedure.[5] Such disparity in research using age as the primary delineating factor leads one to think that additional aspects of patient health should be considered when determining treatment.

One of the common practices in the characterization of patient health is the use of tools that weigh comorbid conditions in conjunction with age to assess for limited life expectancy (LLE). One frequently used tool is the Charlson comorbidity index (CCI).[4,6] Although the CCI provides insight into the overall severity of a patient's comorbid conditions, there are no established guidelines demonstrating what scores truly predict LLE. Studies have used CCI scores of 3+ to define LLE based on previous research showing 44% 2-year mortality, whereas others have demonstrated less than 40% probability of mortality at 2 years with a CCI score of 7+.[4,6,11] Perhaps one of the reasons for this index's lack of reliability is the inability to factor severity of disease when determining a score. As a result of the paucity of consistent evidence establishing which score is truly prognostic of LLE, comorbid conditions should not be the only consideration when selecting treatment of NMSC in the elderly.

The assessment of patient functionality is a common practice among oncologists and geriatricians when determining how aggressive to be in the treatment of the elderly.[12,13] Within dermatology, the assessment of patient functionality is valuable when selecting treatment of NMSC. The Karnofsky Performance Status (KPS) scale (**Table 2**) is a reliable and valid method that weighs the symptom burden of systemic disease with a patient's ability to carry out activities of daily living. As a result, functional assessment provides a more comprehensive view of patient health than comorbid conditions alone. Research assessing the utilization of KPS scores in the general dermatology and MMS environment has shown that patient functionality is informally assessed when determining treatment of NMSC.[14,15] Functional assessment has been shown to be a useful measure of overall patient health and is predictive of survival in the elderly.[16,17] Therefore, a functional assessment should be used in the treatment of every patient, even if informally (**Fig. 1**).

Impact on Quality of Life

Tumor location and impact on QOL are important considerations when selecting a treatment modality.[14,18] Tumor location as a pathologic consideration is discussed in a previous section; however, addressing tumor location in relation to its effect on appearance is critical to patient satisfaction. NMSCs that impact a patient's appearance can cause significant emotional distress, especially when they bleed. Large lesions can become disfiguring and embarrassing, causing patients to avoid social situations, further impacting QOL. Such concerns should be considered and addressed in the initial consultation, allowing the physicians to select a treatment modality that will most effectively manage this aspect of the negative emotional impact.

There are inherent cosmetic considerations when selecting a treatment, because certain modalities can leave scars as disfiguring as the skin cancers themselves. ED&C leaves large, depressed scars, which is why this treatment modality is best reserved for lesions on the trunk and extremities.[18] As a result, MMS is typically the treatment of choice when treating tumors on the head and neck, even in the Medicare population.[5,14]

Cost of Care

According to the US Surgeon General, the annual cost associated with the treatment of cutaneous malignancies is approximately $8.1 billion, of which $4.8 billion is attributed to NMSCs.[19] The cost associated with the treatment of an NMSC varies depending on the method of treatment, treatment facility, and associated pathology costs. For NMSCs, surgical treatments are on the more expensive end of the cost spectrum, with MMS costing slightly more than excision, with paraffin sections, though, less than excision with frozen sections.[10,20] Surgical treatment in the outpatient setting has been shown to be substantially less expensive than operating room cases.[21] ED&C is the least expensive treatment modality, with varying costs depending on the size of the lesion, but is

Table 2
The Karnofsky performance status scale
100	Normal; no complaints; no evidence of disease
90	Able to carry out normal activity; minor signs or symptoms of disease
80	Normal activity with effort; some signs or symptoms of disease
70	Cares for self; unable to carry on normal activity or to do active work
60	Requires occasional assistance but is able to care for most personal needs
50	Requires considerable assistance and frequent medical care
40	Disabled; requires special care and assistance
30	Severely disabled; hospitalization is indicated, although death is not imminent
20	Very sick; hospitalization is necessary and active support treatment is necessary
10	Moribund; fatal processes are progressing
0	Dead

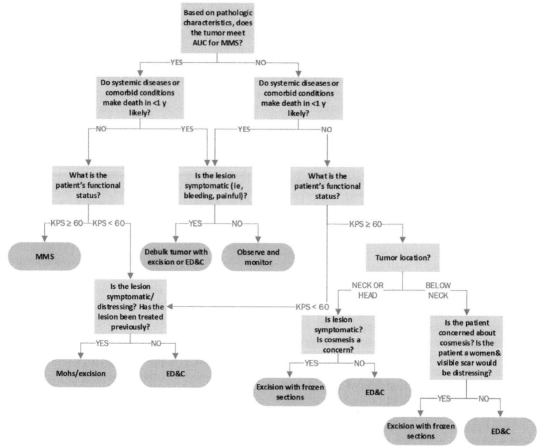

Fig. 1. Algorithm of potential considerations for treatment of NMSC in the elderly. (*Courtesy of* Michael Renzi Jr and Naomi Lawrence.)

estimated to be approximately 20% less expensive than MMS.[20]

Regarding less frequently used treatments, topical imiquimod is often suggested as an effective and less invasive treatment; however, the off-label cost to treat facial NMSCs approaches that of MMS.[10,20] Radiation therapy (RT) is a potential option for patients unable to tolerate surgery, although it is the most expensive treatment with costs as high as $4558 for facial tumors.[20] Balancing cost of care with patient benefit and duration of effect is an important consideration with treatment. However, in a profession wherein patient beneficence and justice are guiding principles, concern for cost should never precede a patient's preference for an appropriate treatment.

MANAGEMENT OF HIGH-MORBIDITY SKIN CANCERS

Malignant melanoma (MM) is the least common type of skin cancer; however, it accounts for the most deaths from cutaneous malignancies. The elderly population, specifically white men older than 65 years old, has the highest risk of developing MM. Mortalities in the elderly have remained stable over the past 3 decades in contrast to the improvement seen among young adults.[21,22] This stable mortality rate is likely due to more aggressive tumor features among the elderly, including thicker tumor depth, higher mitotic rates, and increased likelihood of ulceration.[23] The rising incidence of melanoma in the elderly has created a major economic burden to the health care system resulting in an estimated annual cost of $249 million.[24] The increasing incidence, mortalities, and cost of managing melanoma in the elderly highlight the need for better disease management and prevention.

Choosing a treatment option for melanoma that minimizes both morbidity and mortality but also accounts for life expectancy and impact on QOL can be challenging.[21] When managing geriatric patients with melanoma, there are several key aspects to consider when formulating a treatment plan, including tumor margins, sentinel lymph node biopsy (SLNB), and systemic therapies.

Excision

The treatment of choice for MM of any thickness is surgical excision with histologically negative margins. In 1 international study, elderly patients with melanoma were treated with inadequate surgical margins 16.8% of the time compared with 5% of the younger population.[25] Reported cure rates are predicated on taking appropriate margins; therefore, ensuring tumor margins are adequate based on tumor depth becomes especially important. The current recommendations by the National Comprehensive Cancer Network (NCCN)[26] and American Joint Committee on Cancer[27] for definitive wide local excision of primary cutaneous melanoma are found in **Table 3**.

Sentinel Lymph Node Biopsies

Whether to perform an SLNB on an elderly patient with intermediate MM (1–4 mm in thickness) is another challenging clinical decision. According to the 2018 NCCN guidelines, SLNB should be considered in all patients with melanomas greater than 0.8 mm in thickness.[26] Despite this recommendation, SLNB is less commonly performed in the elderly population likely due to the belief that SLNB is associated with higher lymphatic mapping failure rates, lower rates of node positivity, and poor prognosis in this population.[28,29] However, the rate of successful SLNB has been shown to be up to 98% in individuals greater than 65 years of age.[30] Elderly patients with a positive SLNB are less likely to receive systemic treatment compared with their younger counterparts.[31,32] Many elderly patients may have been undertreated as a result.

The most common complications from SLNB include paresthesias, pain, bruising, lymphedema, and seroma formation.[26] Seroma formation and lymphedema appear to be more common in the elderly, whereas paresthesias occur more often in younger adults.[33] The decision to perform an SLNB in elderly patients with multiple comorbidities and LLE should be carefully considered. Clinicians should weigh the benefits of accurate tumor staging with the risk of significant morbidity from the procedure. However, it is important that clinicians do not rule out SLNB based on age alone particularly now that effective, well-tolerated immunotherapy options are available. An objective measure of functional status, such as the KPS scale (see **Table 2**), is a valuable tool for clinicians when determining whether to perform an SLNB in the elderly population.

Systemic Therapy

Molecular and immune-based systemic therapies have had a significant impact on late-stage melanoma over the past decade. However, even considering their efficacy, the use of systemic therapies has been less common in older patients.[34] Underutilization of these therapies may be attributed to the physician's perception of poor efficacy and tolerance in the elderly; however, this is not supported by the trials on the newer, focused immunologic treatments.

Immune checkpoint inhibitors (ICI) are a novel class of cancer drugs proven to be efficacious in improving progression-free and overall survival in metastatic melanoma as well as many other cancers. In addition, ICI demonstrate better efficacy and fewer adverse effects when compared with traditional cytotoxic drugs.[35] Although there are no elderly-specific trials, preliminary data from phase 3 trials suggest ICI use, specifically nivolumab and ipilimumab, in the elderly is not associated with increased immune-related adverse effects when compared with younger age groups.[36,37]

Half of all melanomas have mutations in the BRAF gene. BRAF inhibitors, vemurafenib, dabrafenib, and encorafenib, have proven to be effective in increasing life expectancy in metastatic melanoma.[38] MEK inhibitors, trametinib, cobimetinib, and binimetinib, are another class of medications used for metastatic melanoma. A combination of MEK and BRAF inhibitors is the most effective approach because it extends the time to resistance and decreases treatment-related adverse effects.[38] The side-effect profile of both therapies is minimal, making these drugs a good choice in treating late-stage MM in the elderly.

Follow-up

There are no evidenced-based guidelines to support a specific follow-up interval in elderly patients with MM. However, the current recommendation is

Table 3
Surgical margins for melanoma

Stage	Tumor Thickness (mm)	Clinically Measured Surgical Margins (cm)
Tis	In situ	0.5–1.0
T1	≤1.00	1.0
T2	>1.0–2.0	1.0–2.0
T3	2.01–4.00	2.0
T4	>4.00	2.0

Data from NCCN Clinical Practice Guidelines in Oncology, Melanoma version 2. 2016, pages 450–73; and American Joint Committee on Cancer. Melanoma of the skin. In: AJCC Cancer Staging Manual. 2010, pages 325–44.

an annual history and physical examination as well as interval self-examinations.[39] In addition, the use of surveillance laboratory tests and imaging studies in asymptomatic patients is not recommended.[40] Clinicians should keep in mind that early detection of asymptomatic distant metastatic disease does not necessarily improve overall survival.[40]

Merkel Cell Carcinoma

Merkel cell carcinoma (MCC) is a very rare and aggressive neuroendocrine tumor occurring predominantly in the elderly, with a mean age of 75 at diagnosis. The incidence of MCC has increased significantly over the last few decades; 1 theory attributes this increase to more specific coding terminology adopted in 1986.[41] MCC is an aggressive tumor with an estimated overall 5-year survival rate of approximately 40%.[42]

Selecting the optimal treatment is the most challenging aspect of treating MCC in the elderly. Surgical excision is the mainstay of treatment for localized disease and should be strongly considered in any patient regardless of age, because the 5-year survival rates for stage I and II disease are between 50% and 80%.[43] SLNB is a frequently used procedure for staging MCC.[44] It is recommended for all patients fit for surgery, regardless of clinical lymph node status.[45] Its impact on overall survival is unclear; however, SLNB remains useful among the elderly, because it is a good prognostic indicator that can influence the decision of whether to perform a complete lymphadenectomy or use adjuvant RT.

The 2018 NCCN recommendations suggest observation is reasonable for patients with small primary tumors (<1 cm) with no risk factors for recurrence or progression, such as lymphovascular invasion or immunosuppression.[45] For larger tumors (≥1 cm) in patients without adverse risk factors, adjuvant RT is generally recommended regardless of age. Patients with a positive SLNB should receive RT to the draining nodal basin. However, those who are SLN negative should also be considered for RT in the case of profound immunosuppression or concern for false-negative SLNB.[45]

Chemotherapy, particularly combination carboplatin or cisplatin with etoposide, was the primary treatment for metastatic disease; however, associated toxicity, especially myelosuppression, was a major concern in the elderly population.[46] Preliminary results from nonrandomized trials have shown improved durable response with the use of PD-1/PDL-1 inhibitors, such as Avelumab and Prembrolizumab, when compared with chemotherapy.[45] As a result, immunotherapy is now the preferred treatment for disseminated disease.

SUMMARY

When managing skin cancer in the elderly, clinicians should use a comprehensive approach that considers patient functional status, QOL, cost, and treatment-related adverse outcomes. This method is applicable in the management of both high- and low-morbidity cancers. Tools for measuring patient functional status, such as the KPS scale, provide clinicians with a consistent and objective value that can be used when formulating a treatment plan. Ultimately, clinicians must not forget that the management of malignancy is a shared decision in which the best interest of the patients must be considered alongside each patient's individual treatment goals.

REFERENCES

1. Ortman JM, Velkoff VA, Hogan H. An aging nation: the older population in the United States current population reports, P25-1140. Washington, DC: US Census Bureau; 2014.
2. Siegel RL, Miller KD, Jemal A. Cancer statistics, 2017. CA Cancer J Clin 2017;67(1):7–30.
3. Wang DM, Morgan FC, Besaw RJ, et al. An ecological study of skin biopsies and skin cancer treatment procedures in the United States Medicare population, 2000 to 2015. J Am Acad Dermatol 2018; 78(1):47–53.
4. Linos E, Parvataneni R, Stuart SE, et al. Treatment of nonfatal conditions at the end of life. JAMA Intern Med 2013;173(11):1006–12.
5. Delaney A, Shimizu I, Goldber LH, et al. Life expectance after Mohs micrographic surgery in patients aged 90 years and older. J Am Acad Dermatol 2013;68(2):296–300.
6. Rogers EM, Connolly KL, Nehal kS, et al. Comorbidity scores associated with limited life. J Am Acad Dermatol 2018;78(6):1119–24.
7. Chauhan R, Munger BN, Chu MW, et al. Age at diagnosis as a relative contraindication for intervention in facial nonmelanoma skin cancer. JAMA Surg 2018; 153(4):390–2.
8. Conolly SM, Baker DR, Coldiron BM, et al. AAD/ACMS/ASDSA/ASMS 2012 appropriate use criteria for Mohs micrographic surgery: a report of the American Academy of Dermatology, American College of Mohs Surgery, American Society for Dermatologic Surgery Association, and the American Society for Mohs Surgery. J Am Acad Dermatol 2012;67(4): 531–50.

9. Garcovich S, Colloca G, Sollena P, et al. Skin cancer epidemics in the elderly as an emerging issue in geriatric oncology. Aging Dis 2017;8(5):643–61.

10. Lee EH, Brewer JD, MacFarlane DF. Optimizing informed decision making for basal cell carcinoma in patients 85 years or older. JAMA Dermatol 2015; 151(8):817–8.

11. Yourman LC, Lee SJ, Schonberg MA, et al. Prognostic indices for older adults: a systematic review. JAMA 2012;307(2):182–92.

12. Yates JW, Chalmer B, McKegney FP. Evaluation of patients with advanced cancer using the Karnofsky performance status. Cancer 1980;45:2220–4.

13. Péus D, Newcomb N, Hofer S. Appraisal of the Karnofsky Performance Status and proposal of a simple algorithmic system for its evaluation. BMC Med Inform Decis Mak 2013;13:72.

14. Regula C, Alam M, Behshad R, et al. Functionality of patients 75 years and older undergoing mohs micrographic surgery: a multi-center study. Dermatol Surg 2017;3(7):904–10.

15. Renzi M, Belcher M, Brod B, et al. Assessment of functionality in elderly patients when determining appropriate treatment for nonmelanoma skin cancers. Dermatol surg, in press.

16. Keeler E, Guralnik JM, Tian H, et al. The impact of functional status on life expectancy in older persons. J Gerontol A Biol Sci Med Sci 2010;65(7): 727–33.

17. Hwang S, Scott CB, Chang VT, et al. Prediction of survival for advanced cancer patients by recursive partitioning analysis: role of Karnofsky performance status quality of life, and symptom distress. Cancer Invest 2004;22(5):678–87.

18. Chren MM, Sahay AP, Bertenthal DS, et al. Quality-of-life outcomes of treatments for cutaneous basal cell carcinoma and squamous cell carcinoma. J Invest Dermatol 2007;127(6):1351–7.

19. Yoon J, Phibbs CS, Chow A, et al. Impact of topical fluorouracil cream on costs of treating keratinocyte carcinoma (nonmelanoma skin cancer) and actinic keratosis. J Am Acad Dermatol 2018;79(3):501–7.

20. Ravitskiy L, Brodland DG, Zitelli JA. Cost analysis: Moh micrographic surgery. Dermatol Surg 2012; 38(4):585–94.

21. Johnson R, Butala N, Murad A, et al. A retrospective case-matched cost comparison of surgical treatment of melanoma and nonmelanoma skin cancer in the outpatient versus operating room setting. Dermatol Surg 2017;43(7):897–901.

22. Leiter U, Eigentler T, Garbe C. Epidemiology of skin cancer. Adv Exp Med Biol 2014;810:120–40.

23. Balch CM, Soong S-J, Gershenwald JE, et al. Prognostic factors analysis of 17,600 melanoma patients: validation of the American Joint Committee on cancer melanoma staging system. J Clin Oncol 2001; 19(16):3622–34.

24. Seidler AM, Pennie ML, Veledar E, et al. Economic burden of melanoma in the elderly population: population-based analysis of the Surveillance, Epidemiology, and End Results (SEER)–Medicare data. Arch Dermatol 2010;146(3):249–56.

25. Ciocan D, Barbe C, Aubin F, et al. Distinctive features of melanoma and its management in elderly patients. JAMA Dermatol 2013;149(10):1150.

26. Coit DG, Thompson JA, Algazi A, et al. Melanoma, version 2.2016, NCCN clinical practice guidelines in oncology. J Natl Compr Canc Netw 2016;14(4): 450–73.

27. American Joint Committee on Cancer. Melanoma of the skin. In: Edge SB, editor. AJCC Cancer Staging Manual. New York: Springer; 2010. p. 325–44.

28. Sener SF, Winchester DJ, Brinkmann E, et al. Failure of sentinel lymph node mapping in patients with breast cancer. J Am Coll Surg 2004;198(5):732–6.

29. Cox CE, Dupont E, Whitehead GF, et al. Age and body mass index may increase the chance of failure in sentinel lymph node biopsy for women with breast cancer. Breast J 2002;8(2):88–91.

30. Grotz TE, Puig CA, Perkins S, et al. Management of regional lymph nodes in the elderly melanoma patient: patient selection, accuracy and prognostic implications. Eur J Surg Oncol 2015;41(1):157–64.

31. Bilimoria KY, Balch CM, Bentrem DJ, et al. Complete lymph node dissection for sentinel node-positive melanoma: assessment of practice patterns in the United States. Ann Surg Oncol 2008;15(6):1566–77.

32. Shah DR, Yang AD, Maverakis E, et al. Age-related disparities in use of completion lymphadenectomy for melanoma sentinel lymph node metastasis. J Surg Res 2013;185:240–4.

33. Wilke LG, McCall LM, Posther KE, et al. Surgical complications associated with sentinel lymph node biopsy: results from a prospective international cooperative group trial. Ann Surg Oncol 2006; 13(4):491–500.

34. Bhatt VR, Shrestha R, Krishnamurthy J, et al. Clinicopathologic characteristics and management trends of cutaneous invasive and in situ melanoma in older patients: a retrospective analysis of the National Cancer Data Base. Ther Adv Med Oncol 2015; 7(1):4–11.

35. Elias R, Morales J, Rehman Y, et al. Immune checkpoint inhibitors in older adults. Curr Oncol Rep 2016; 18(8).

36. Chiarion Sileni V, Pigozzo J, Ascierto P, et al. Efficacy and safety of ipilimumab in elderly patients with pretreated advanced melanoma treated at Italian centres through the expanded access programme. J Exp Clin Cancer Res 2014;33(1):30.

37. Freeman M, Weber J. Subset analysis of the safety and efficacy of nivolumab in elderly patients with metastatic melanoma. J Immunother Cancer 2015; 3(2):133.

38. Mackiewicz J, Mackiewicz A. BRAF and MEK inhibitors in the era of immunotherapy in melanoma patients. Contemp Oncol (Pozn) 2018;22(1A):68–72.

39. Swetter SM, Tsao H, Bichakjian CK, et al. Guidelines of care for the management of primary cutaneous melanoma. J Acad Dermatol 2019;80(1):208–50.

40. Trotter SC, Sroa N, Winkelmann RR, et al. A global review of melanoma follow-up guidelines. J Clin Aesthet Dermatol 2013;6(9):18–26.

41. Fitzgerald TL, Dennis S, Kachare SD, et al. Dramatic increase in the incidence and mortality from merkel cell carcinoma in the United States. Am Surg 2015; 81(8):802–6.

42. Survival Rates for Merkel Cell Carcinoma by Stage. American Cancer Society 2018. Available at: https:// www.cancer.org/cancer/merkel-cell-skin-cancer/detection-diagnosis-staging/survival-rates.html.

43. Duprat JP, Landman G, Salvajoli JV, et al. A review of the epidemiology and treatment of Merkel cell carcinoma. Clinics (Sau Paulo) 2011;66(10): 1817–23.

44. Desch L, Kunstfeld R. Merkel cell carcinoma: chemotherapy and emerging new therapeutic options. J Skin Cancer 2013;2013:327150.

45. Bichakjian CK, Fisher K, Nghiem P, et al. Merkel cell carcinoma, version 1.2018, NCCN clinical practice guidelines in oncology. J Natl Compr Canc Netw 2018;16(6):742–74.

46. Balducci L. Myelosuppression and its consequences in elderly patients with cancer. Oncology 2003;17:27–32.

Topical and Systemic Modalities for Chemoprevention of Nonmelanoma Skin Cancer

Kathleen M. Nemer, MD[1], M. Laurin Council, MD*

KEYWORDS

- Chemoprevention • Nonmelanoma skin cancer • Actinic keratosis • Basal cell carcinoma
- Squamous cell carcinoma in situ • Squamous cell carcinoma • Immunosuppression
- Organ transplant recipient

KEY POINTS

- Chemoprevention of nonmelanoma skin cancer (NMSC) should be considered in patients at high risk of developing numerous NMSCs.
- Organ transplant recipients are most likely to develop high-risk squamous cell carcinomas and may benefit from chemoprevention.
- Topical and systemic chemopreventive agents include photodynamic therapy, 5-fluorouracil, 5-fluorouracil plus chemowraps, 5-fluorouracil plus calcipotriol, imiquimod, diclofenac sodium, ingenol mebutate, retinoids, nicotinamide, and cyclooxygenase inhibitors.
- Further research is needed to evaluate the efficacy of novel agents in the chemoprevention of NMSC.

INTRODUCTION

Nonmelanoma skin cancer (NMSC) is the most common malignancy in the United States.[1] The overall lifetime risk of developing NMSC is 1 in 5,[2] with an estimated 5.4 million cases diagnosed each year in the United States.[1] Most skin cancers are either basal cell carcinomas (BCCs) or squamous cell carcinomas (SCCs). Although BCC accounts for approximately 80% of NMSCs, SCC is more likely to invade and metastasize, and accounts for most of the NMSC-related mortality.[3,4] Nonmelanoma skin cancer is associated with substantial morbidity and cost,[5] and the incidence continues to increase,[1,3] increasing the need for primary and secondary skin cancer prevention strategies.

Primary prevention reduces risk factors using environmental and behavioral modifications, such as decreasing UV light exposure; secondary prevention detects and controls precancerous and/or cancerous processes at an early stage.[5] Chemoprevention is a secondary prevention strategy for patients at high risk of developing numerous NMSCs.[6–8] This article reviews topical and systemic chemoprevention strategies for NMSC in immunocompetent and immunosuppressed individuals.

INDICATIONS FOR CHEMOPREVENTION OF NONMELANOMA SKIN CANCER

Chemoprevention should be considered in patients with extensive actinic damage, a history of

Disclosure Statement: The authors have no commercial/financial conflicts of interest or funding sources.
Division of Dermatology, Department of Medicine, Washington University School of Medicine, St Louis, MO, USA
[1] Present address: 969 North Mason Road, Suite 200, Creve Coeur, MO 63141.
* Corresponding author. Center for Dermatologic and Cosmetic Surgery, 969 North Mason Road, Suite 200, Creve Coeur, MO 63141.
E-mail address: mcouncil@wustl.edu

Dermatol Clin 37 (2019) 287–295
https://doi.org/10.1016/j.det.2019.02.004
0733-8635/19/© 2019 Elsevier Inc. All rights reserved.

derm.theclinics.com

NMSC, and those at risk of developing numerous, invasive, and/or metastatic SCCs.[9–11] **Box 1** details ideal candidates for chemoprevention. Among these, solid organ transplant recipients (OTRs) may benefit most from chemoprevention, given their increased risk of developing numerous and aggressive NMSCs.[10,12] In addition, patients with numerous actinic keratoses (AKs) may also benefit. The estimated transformation of AK to primary SCC (invasive or in situ) is 0.6% at 1 year and 2.57% at 4 years[13]; field-directed therapy for AKs may therefore reduce the risk of SCC.

TOPICAL MODALITIES FOR CHEMOPREVENTION
Photodynamic Therapy

Photodynamic therapy (PDT) combines the use of a photosensitizer and a light source to selectively destroy precancerous skin cells. There are a wide range of photosensitizers and light sources; however, the 2 most commonly used commercial systems are 5-aminolevulinic acid (ALA) plus blue or red light and methyl-esterified ALA (MAL) plus red light.[14] 5-Aminolevulinic acid and MAL are precursors of the endogenous photosensitizer, protoporphyrin IX, which is a natural fluorophore that preferentially accumulates in dysplastic cells. Topical application of ALA or MAL, followed by exposure to blue or red light, leads to the selective production of reactive oxygen species and death of precancerous cells.[14] Based on numerous studies, ALA-PDT and MAL-PDT are equally efficacious in the treatment of AKs.[15,16] Methyl-esterified ALA is more lipophilic than ALA, allowing for deeper skin penetration and a theoretically higher intracellular accumulation of protoporphyrin IX. Methyl-esterified ALA-PDT has thus been rigorously studied as a treatment of NMSC.[15]

5-Aminolevulinic acid is US Food and Drug Administration (FDA) approved for use with blue light as Levulan Kerastick for treatment of AKs. In the United States, ALA is commercially available in a 20% topical hydroalcoholic solution that is freshly prepared before application. The FDA-approved incubation time is 14 to 18 hours without occlusion before illumination with BLU-U fluorescent light (400–450 nm, 10 J/cm^2).[14,17] In clinical practice, this time is often shortened to 1 to 4 hours with retention of efficacy and less phototoxicity.[18] According to the FDA-approved protocol, this treatment may be repeated in 8 weeks to any remaining lesions.[17] In 2016, ALA gained approval for use with red light as Ameluz, a new nanoemulsion gel containing 10% aminolaevulinic acid hydrochloride. Ameluz is applied, incubated for 3 hours under occlusion, then illuminated

---

Box 1
Candidates for chemoprevention

1. Excessive UV light exposure
   - Severe photodamage
   - Numerous precancerous skin lesions (actinic keratoses)
2. History of nonmelanoma skin cancer
   - Development of more than 5 to 10 NMSCs per year
   - Accelerating frequency of NMSCs
   - Multiple NMSCs in high-risk locations (head and neck)
   - Metastatic NMSC
   - Eruptive keratoacanthomas
3. Immunosuppression
   - Organ transplant recipients
   - Chronic immunosuppressive therapies
   - Hematologic malignances (chronic lymphocytic leukemia, non-Hodgkin's lymphoma)
   - Human immunodeficiency virus
4. Genetic syndromes
   - Xeroderma pigmentosum
   - Recessive dystrophic epidermolysis bullosa
   - Albinism
   - Nevoid BCC syndrome
   - Epidermodysplasia verruciformis
   - Bazex syndrome
   - Rombo syndrome
5. Other exposures
   - History of treatment with PUVA light
   - Chronic radiation dermatitis
   - Chronic arsenic exposure
   - Trauma and/or extensive burns

Abbreviations: NMSC, nonmelanoma skin cancer; PUVA, psoralen and UV A.

Data from O'Reilly Zwald F, Brown M. Skin cancer in solid organ transplant recipients: advances in therapy and management: part II. Management of skin cancer in solid organ transplant recipients. J Am Acad Dermatol 2011;65(2):263–279; and Otley CC, Stasko T, Tope WD, et al. Chemoprevention of nonmelanoma skin cancer with systemic retinoids: practical dosing and management of adverse effects. Dermatol Surg 2006;32(4):562–568.

---

with the BF-RhodoLED PDT lamp (635 nm, 37 J/cm^2).[14,19] It is FDA approved for lesion-directed and field-directed treatment of mild to moderate AKs on the face and scalp. According to the FDA-approved protocol, this treatment may be repeated in 3 months to any remaining lesions.[19]

Although not currently available on the US market, MAL is FDA approved as Metvix, a 16.8% cream, for treatment of AKs. Metvix is approved in the European Union for treatment of AKs, superficial and nodular BCC, and squamous cell in situ (SCCIS). Approved administration involves a 3-hour application under occlusion, saline wash, and then illumination with Aktilite CL 128 LED narrow-band red light (630 nm, 37 J/cm^2).[14] The European license for MAL-PDT recommends a single treatment, with nonresponders receiving a second treatment at 3 months. Two MAL-PDT treatments spaced 1 week apart are recommended for superficial/nodular BCC and SCCIS.[15,16]

Multiple agents have been studied as coadjuvant treatments with PDT. Depending on patient characteristics, PDT can be combined with immunomodulatory (imiquimod) and chemotherapeutic (5-fluorouracil, methotrexate, diclofenac, or ingenol mebutate) agents, retinoids (tretinoin), inhibitors of molecules implicated in the carcinogenic process (cyclooxygenase-2 or mitogen-activated protein kinase), lasers, or radiotherapy.[20] Although hyperkeratosis is a major barrier to photosensitizer penetration, curettage and/or occlusion with keratolytic agents (such as tretinoin) can be useful techniques to increase efficacy.[20]

Numerous PDT protocols have been studied, and these range in treatment number and time course based on the photosensitizer, light source, and type of lesion/body area to be treated.[15,16] In our clinical practice, PDT is most commonly used to treat AKs on the face, scalp, and ears, followed by the trunk and extremities. Our protocol for Levulan is a 2-hour incubation, followed by illumination with blue light for a total of 2 to 3 treatments spaced 4 to 6 weeks apart. Our protocol for Ameluz is a 1-hour incubation followed by illumination with red light, for a total of 2 treatments spaced 8 weeks apart. These protocols are often modified based on patient tolerance and achievement of the desired clinical effect. Patients should be educated pretreatment and posttreatment, because an informed patient is imperative to a successful treatment. The most prominent adverse effect of PDT is a burning/stinging pain within the treated area. Inflammation is expected and may manifest as erythema, edema, crusting, and/or frank urticaria. Complete healing usually occurs within 2 weeks, but has been reported to take up to 6 weeks.[15] All of our patients are counseled to avoid daylight for 48 hours posttreatment and to perform comfort skin care, including cold compresses, tepid showers, gentle moisturizers, sunscreen, and over-the-counter analgesics as needed (acetaminophen or ibuprofen).

The introduction of PDT with lower-irradiance regimens, such as daylight PDT (DL-PDT), has greatly improved treatment tolerability. Daylight PDT is an emerging strategy for treatment of AKs, which has shown similar short-term efficacy to conventional PDT with significantly less pain.[21,22] Both ALA and MAL have been studied in DL-PDT. Treatment protocols involve the application of a photosensitizing agent without occlusion, subsequent exposure to ambient daylight within 30 minutes, with a total daylight exposure of 1.5 to 2 hours.[21] The evidence for use of DL-PDT beyond AKs is limited. Additional studies are needed to assess the long-term efficacy of DL-PDT.[22]

Chemoprevention of NMSC with PDT has been most rigorously studied in OTRs, and has shown efficacy in the prevention of NMSCs in this population.[23–25] An open-label intrapatient randomized study of 27 renal transplant patients showed that MAL-PDT with a 3-hour incubation and red light increased the mean time to occurrence of combined outcome (AK, SCC, BCC, kertoacanthoma, wart) from 6.8 months in the untreated areas to 9.6 months in the treated areas, and increased the number of skin areas free of lesions over 12 months (62% vs 35%).[23] This study did not differentiate between NMSC and other keratotic skin lesions. Another intrapatient randomized controlled trial with 81 OTRs showed that successive MAL-PDT (2 treatments spaced 1 week apart, then treatments at 3, 9, and 15 months) with a 3-hour incubation and red light significantly reduced the occurrence of skin lesions (mainly AKs) at 3 months.[24] Lastly, an uncontrolled study of 12 patients examined the efficacy of cyclic ALA-PDT with blue light at 4- to 8-week intervals over 2 years in the chemoprevention of new SCCs in OTRs. Compared with baseline before PDT, the median reduction in SCCs was 79% at 12 months and 95% at 24 months.[25] Given its therapeutic effect on decreasing clinical and subclinical dysplasia, PDT is an effective chemopreventive option for those with significant actinic damage and risk of NMSC.

5-Fluorouracil

Topical 5-fluorouracil (5-FU) inhibits thymidylate synthase and induces apoptosis in highly mitotic cells. It is FDA approved for treatment of AKs and is widely used in clinical practice for this purpose. 5-Fluorouracil is supplied as a 2% or 5% solution or a 0.5%, 1%, 4%, or 5% cream. The 5%

cream is also approved for treatment of superficial BCC, applied twice daily for 3 to 6 weeks.[26] A systemic review of 13 randomized controlled trials (RCTs) found that the average reduction of AKs after treatment with 5-FU is 79.5% with 5% cream and 86.1% with 0.5% cream.[27] The standard treatment regimen for AKs with 5% 5-FU cream is twice daily application for 2 to 4 weeks.[26] Some clinicians may prefer to treat once daily for a longer time course (4–6 weeks) to ease the expected local skin irritation, erythema, and scaling that can limit patient tolerability. If multiple areas necessitate treatment, it is often helpful to treat each sequentially for patient comfort. Some patients (especially high-risk OTRs) may require more than 1 treatment and/or maintenance treatments to achieve the desired clinical effect.

The Veterans Affairs Keratinocyte Carcinoma Chemoprevention (VAKCC) trial was a randomized, double-blinded, placebo-controlled trial that showed 5% 5-FU applied twice daily to the face and ears for up to 4 weeks effectively reduces AKs and spot treatments for over 2 years.[28] A follow-up prospective study tracked AK development in a subset of these patients, showing that 5-FU on the face and ears prevents AKs for 24 to 36 months in high-risk individuals, likely by clearing subclinical dysplasia.[29] In 2018, further data were published from the VAKCC trial concluding that a conventional course of 5-FU to the face and ears reduces the risk of SCC requiring surgery by 75% for the first year after treatment, without significantly affecting the corresponding risk for BCC.[30]

5-Fluorouracil Plus Chemowraps

Self-administered application of 5-FU can be difficult, especially over large treatment areas. According to the manufacturer's guidelines, the maximum area to be treated in one application is 500 cm^2.[31] Several studies have described the use of 5-FU under occlusion (chemowraps) as a useful treatment option for patients with large areas of actinic damage and/or SCC.[31–33] Mann and colleagues treated 3 patients with diffuse actinic damage and biopsy-proven SCCs on the legs with weekly 5-FU under Unna wraps for 4 to 20 weeks. A reduction in clinical lesions was shown at 6 weeks and at 3-year follow-up.[32] Tallon and colleagues described a series of 6 patients treated weekly with 20 g of 5-FU and zinc oxide applied under chemowraps to diffuse hypertrophic AKs on the legs and scalp (the head wrap remained in place for 5 days at a time). Wraps were continued for 4 to 8 weeks, with excellent patient tolerability and a reduction in number and

thickness of AKs, maintained between 6 months and 2 years follow-up. Lastly, Goon and colleagues treated 5 patients with 20 g of 5-FU (legs) and 10 g of 5-FU (arms) and zinc oxide under weekly chemowraps for 12 to 14 weeks.[31] Substantial clinical improvement was noted, with a decrease in the size and/or number of AKs. There were no serious adverse events secondary to 5-FU in any of the above studies.[31–33] The increased compliance, ability for compression, and occlusive environment, whereby a large amount of drug can be safely delivered, make this off-label use of 5-FU a valuable treatment alternative for patients with significant actinic damage.

5-Fluorouracil Plus Calcipotriol

Recently, researchers found a synergistic effect between 5-FU and calcipotriol in the treatment of AKs.[34] Topical calcipotriol blocks carcinogenesis by inducing thymic stromal lymphopoietin expression, an epithelium-derived cytokine that prevents skin carcinogenesis. Four-day, twice daily application of calcipotriol plus 5% 5-FU versus Vaseline plus 5% 5-FU led to an 87.8% versus 26.3% mean reduction of AKs.[34] Importantly, calcipotriol plus 5-FU induced thymic stromal lymphopoietin with minimal pain, crusting, or ulceration. The short treatment duration and minimal side-effect profile make calcipotriol plus 5-FU a promising chemopreventive modality.

Imiquimod

Imiquimod is an immunomodulator that binds to Toll-like receptors 7 and 8 and activates nuclear factor-kappa B. This cascade induces proinflammatory cytokines, activates the innate and adaptive immune systems, and induces apoptosis of tumor cells.[35] Imiquimod is FDA approved for treatment of AKs, superficial BCC, and genital warts. It is supplied as a 2.5%, 3.75%, or 5% cream. The 5% cream is supplied in single-use packets (24 per box), each of which contains 250 mg of cream, equivalent to 12.5 mg of imiquimod. Recommended administration for treatment of AKs is 2 times per week for 16 weeks and for treatment of superficial BCC is 5 times per week for 6 weeks. The treatment area for AKs is defined as one contiguous area measuring 25 cm^2 on the face or scalp. When treating AKs, no more than 1 packet should be applied to the contiguous treatment area at each application.[36] The manufacturer recommends application of imiquimod before bedtime for a duration of 8 hours, after which the cream should be removed with soap and water. Patients should wash their hands before and after each application. The most common adverse reactions are local erythema, edema, scaling, and ulceration, which may limit treatment.

In 2 placebo-controlled studies, daily application of imiquimod 2.5% and 3.75% creams to AKs (with a median baseline of 9–10) on the face and balding scalp for two 3-week cycles led to an 80% median reduction in AKs compared with 23.6% in the placebo group.[35] In addition, 2 phase 3 randomized, double-blind, parallel-group, vehicle-controlled studies showed that imiquimod 5% cream applied 3 times weekly for 16 weeks is a safe and effective treatment of AKs.[37] Imiquimod has also been used to treat SCCIS off-label. In a randomized, placebo-controlled trial of 31 patients with SCCIS, imiquimod 5% cream lead to resolution of SCCIS in 73% of cases with no recurrence at 9-month follow-up.[38]

Diclofenac Sodium

Topical 3% diclofenac sodium in 2.5% hyaluronic acid gel is a nonsteroidal antiinflammatory drug (NSAID) that inhibits cyclooxygenase-2 (COX-2) and, to a lesser degree, COX-1. It is thought to induce apoptosis, alter cellular proliferation, and inhibit angiogenesis.[39] It is FDA approved for treatment of AKs and has been shown to be safe and effective in immunocompetent and immunosuppressed patients.[39–42] It is generally well tolerated; irritant contact dermatitis is the most common side effect. In 2012, Martin and Stockfleth provided a comprehensive update on the clinical data supporting diclofenac 3% gel for treatment of AKs.[39] A phase 4 open-label study showed that 58% of patients achieved complete clearance of AKs at 30 days posttreatment, an effect that was sustained at 1-year follow-up. Active comparator studies demonstrated comparable efficacy of diclofenac 3% gel with 5% 5-FU and imiquimod 5% creams.[39] In addition, in a randomized vehicle-controlled study of OTRs, twice daily application of diclofenac 3% gel to AKs on the face, hands, and balding scalp for 16 weeks showed complete clearance of AKs in 41% of patients compared with 0% in the vehicle group.[42] No invasive SCC was seen in treated areas at 24 months follow-up, suggesting that diclofenac 3% gel may delay development of invasive SCC in high-risk patients.[42]

Ingenol Mebutate

Ingenol mebutate gained FDA approval for topical treatment of AKs in January 2012. It is a macrocyclic diterpene ester, occurring naturally in the sap of *Euphorbia peplus*. It causes cell death and proinflammatory immune responses mediated by protein kinase C delta.[43] In 4 multicenter, randomized, double-blind studies, application of ingenol mebutate gel once daily to a 25-cm^2 contiguous area on the face or scalp (0.015% for 3 days) and to the trunk or extremities (0.05% for 2 days) led to an 83% and 75% median reduction, respectively, in the number of AKs after 57 days of treatment.[44] The most common application-site reactions were pain, pruritus, and irritation. The advantage of ingenol mebutate over other topical AK treatments may be its short application time and quicker resolution of local reactions, theoretically increasing adherence to therapy. However, local reactions limited the blinding of the study, and treatments were only limited to target areas of 25 cm^2.[44]

SYSTEMIC MODALITIES FOR CHEMOPREVENTION
Retinoids

Retinoids are natural and synthetic derivatives of vitamin A that regulate epithelial maturation, cellular differentiation, growth arrest, and apoptosis by activating nuclear retinoid receptors. Oral retinoids for chemoprevention of SCC have been most rigorously studied in the OTR population,[45–47] and current guidelines strongly support their use for those at risk of developing multiple, invasive, or metastatic SCCs.[9–12] The 2 oral retinoids available in the United States are isotretinoin and acitretin. Acitretin is usually the drug of choice, as there are more long-term data in OTRs. However, isotretinoin is preferred in women of childbearing age because of its shorter half-life.[11] Oral retinoids are pregnancy category X and are contraindicated in pregnancy.

A double-blind placebo-controlled RCT evaluated the chemoprophylactic effects of 30 mg/d of acitretin in 44 renal transplant recipients with ≥10 AKs.[45] Following 6 months of treatment, there was a statistically significant difference in the number of new SCCs between treatment and placebo arms.[45] In a second study, 23 renal transplant recipients with a history of NMSC received 25 mg/d of acitretin (or dose modification based on tolerability, up to 50 mg/d) for 12 months in an open-label randomized crossover trial.[46] Significantly fewer SCCs were observed in patients taking acitretin compared with those in the acitretin-free period.[46] A third study of renal transplant recipients compared the effect of 2 different doses of acitretin (0.4 mg/kg/d for 1 year vs 0.4 mg/kg/d for 3 months, followed by 0.2 mg/kg/d for the remaining 9 months).[47] In both groups, the number of AKs decreased by nearly 50%; however, there was no effect on the incidence of new skin malignancies in either group. There was a high incidence of mucocutaneous side effects; however patient contentment with their skin increased significantly.[47] Acitretin had no adverse effects on renal function in any of these studies.[45–47]

Acitretin therapy should be tailored based on patient characteristics, risk for NMSC, and comorbid conditions. Efficacy and side effects of oral retinoids are dose dependent; side effects include mucocutaneous dryness/irritation, hypercholesterolemia, hypertriglyceridemia, liver toxicity, arthralgias/myalgias, increased intracranial pressure, hair loss, and, with long-term use, skeletal demineralization/hyperostosis.[9] To minimize side effects, patients should start at a low dose of 10 mg/d and increase by 10-mg increments at 2- to 4-week intervals.[11] The target dose is 20 to 25 mg/d, because most patients will experience mucocutaneous side effects by 20 mg/d.[11] The goal is to decrease NMSC numbers to a manageable level, because complete elimination would require high-dose retinoids with intolerable side effects. If retinoids are discontinued, a rebound effect occurs that is often difficult to control.[48]

Organ transplant recipients with aggressive SCC or those developing multiple NMSCs per year may benefit from reduction in immunosuppression to the lowest level consistent with stable graft function.[12,49] This should be done in collaboration with the patient's transplant team as an adjuvant-management strategy. Proposed guidelines are detailed in an expert census convened by Otley and colleagues.[49] An alternate approach is conversion from calcineurin inhibitor-based immunosuppression (tacrolimus) to a mammalian target of rapamycin inhibitor (sirolimus or everolimus).[10]

Nicotinamide

Nicotinamide is a water-soluble form of vitamin B_3 (niacin) and the precursor of nicotinamide adenine dinucleotide, an essential cofactor for adenosine triphosphate production.[50] It has recently been shown to be safe and effective in reducing rates of AKs and NMSC. In phase 2, double-blinded RCTs published in 2012, 76 healthy, immunocompetent volunteers with ≥ 4 AKs (face, scalp, and upper limbs) were randomized to 500 mg of nicotinamide or placebo either once or twice daily for 4 months.[51] The primary endpoint was AK count at 4 months, at which point there was a 35% reduction in AKs in those taking 1000 mg/d of nicotinamide ($P = .0006$) and a 29% reduction in AKs in those taking 500 mg/d of nicotinamide ($P = .005$) compared with placebo. During the

study, 20 new NMSCs were diagnosed in the placebo group, and only 4 new NMSCs were diagnosed in both nicotinamide groups. The odds of developing at least 1 skin cancer were significantly lower with nicotinamide (odds ratio = 0.14; 95% confidence interval, 0.03–0.73; $P = .019$) with no significant side effects reported.[51]

In 2015, a phase 3, double-blind RCT was published showing that patients with ≥ 2 NMSCs may benefit from 500 mg twice daily of nicotinamide.[52] At 12 months, the rate of new NMSCs was 23% lower ($P = .02$), and the number of new AKs was 13% lower ($P = .001$) in the nicotinamide group compared with placebo. Adverse events were similar; however, after discontinuation of nicotinamide, there was no evidence of lasting benefit.[52] In conclusion, nicotinamide is well tolerated and costs $5–$10 per month at the doses described.[51] These results suggest that nicotinamide may protect against the development of AKs and NMSC.

Cyclooxygenase Inhibitors

Cyclooxygenase-2 is an enzyme that stimulates prostaglandin synthesis, leading to inflammation, cellular proliferation, and immunosuppression.[53] UV radiation is a potent stimulus for the production of COX-2, and whereas only trace amounts are expressed in normal skin, large amounts are found in UV-induced AKs and SCCs.[54] Nonsteroidal anti-inflammatory drugs inhibit COX-2, and have thus been suggested as potential chemopreventive agents for NMSC. Experimental studies have shown suppression of NMSC with COX-2 inhibition;[54,55] however, studies on the relationship between NSAIDs and NMSC have shown inconsistent results,[56–61] and the known cardiovascular side effects of NSAIDs such as celecoxib may limit their widespread use.

Novel Agents

Several novel agents have been proposed for chemoprevention of NMSC. Further studies are needed to support their use. These include:

- Capecitabine: a prodrug of 5-FU that causes inflamed AKs in patients with metastatic breast or colorectal cancers, and has thus been studied orally for reduction of AKs and NMSC in high-risk patients.[11] In 2009, Endrizzi and Lee published a case series of 3 OTRs initiated on capecitabine as monotherapy to halt the progression of AKs and NMSC.[62] Six months before therapy, each patient had developed an average of 1 or more cutaneous carcinomas per month (most were SCCs). Capecitabine was administered on a dosing regimen of 14 days on, 7 days off, with cycles repeated every 21 days. Each patient received 1000 to 1500 mg/m^2/d, a lower dose compared with the protocol for colorectal cancer (2500 mg/m^2/d, 14 days on, 7 days off, with cycles repeated every 21 days for 6 months). Over a 6-month period, capecitabine halted the rate of tumor development, with lesions decreasing in size, erythema, tenderness, and induration. Most precancerous lesions became inflamed and subsequently improved. The process parallels AK treatment with topical 5-FU, but over an extended period with less inflammation. All patients experienced some degree of hand-foot syndrome; however, dose-limiting toxicities were not seen.[62] Of note, capecitabine is contraindicated in patients with dihydropyrimidine dehydrogenase deficiency, an enzyme involved in uracil and thymine metabolism (exposure could lead to severe toxicity). The authors published a follow-up study in 2013 of 10 OTRs treated with capecitabine as adjuvant prevention for high-incidence NMSC with a similar dosing regimen to their previous study (500–1500 mg/m^2/d for days 1–14 of a 21-day treatment cycle). Organ transplant recipients experienced a clinically and statistically significant decline in incident SCCs over 12 months, with varying degrees of side effects.[63] Although capecitabine is a promising adjuvant treatment of NMSC in OTRs, randomized trials are needed to further delineate its role in chemoprevention.

- T4 endonuclease V: a bacterial-derived polypeptide capable of repairing UV-induced cyclobutene pyrimidine dimers in DNA, studied topically in patients with xeroderma pigmentosum.[6–8]
- Photolyase: a monomeric DNA repair enzyme derived from algae and capable of repairing UV-induced cyclobutene pyrimidine dimers in DNA, studied topically as an additive to sunscreen.[6,8]
- Difluoromethylornithine: an inhibitor of ornithine decarboxylase that protects against UV radiation, studied topically for AKs and orally for NMSC.[6–8]
- Nutritional factors: genistein, lycopene, green tea polyphenols, perillyl alcohol (citrus peels), caffeine, a low-fat diet.[6,7]

REFERENCES

1. Rogers HW, Weinstock MA, Feldman SR, et al. Incidence estimate of nonmelanoma skin cancer (keratinocyte carcinomas) in the U.S. population, 2012. JAMA Dermatol 2015;151(10):1081–6.
2. Rigel DS, Friedman RJ, Kopf AW. Lifetime risk for development of skin cancer in the U.S. population: current estimate is now 1 in 5. J Am Acad Dermatol 1996;35(6):1012–3.
3. Diepgen TL, Mahler V. The epidemiology of skin cancer. Br J Dermatol 2002;146(Suppl 61):1–6.
4. Brougham ND, Dennett ER, Cameron R, et al. The incidence of metastasis from cutaneous squamous cell carcinoma and the impact of its risk factors. J Surg Oncol 2012;106(7):811–5.
5. Apalla Z, Lallas A, Sotiriou E, et al. Epidemiological trends in skin cancer. Dermatol Pract Concept 2017;7(2):1–6.
6. Camp WL, Turnham JW, Athar M, et al. New agents for prevention of ultraviolet-induced nonmelanoma skin cancer. Semin Cutan Med Surg 2011;30(1):6–13.
7. Soltani-Arabshahi R, Tristani-Firouzi P. Chemoprevention of nonmelanoma skin cancer. Facial Plast Surg 2013;29(5):373–83.
8. Lopez AT, Carvajal RD, Geskin L. Secondary prevention strategies for nonmelanoma skin cancer. Oncology (Williston Park) 2018;32(4):195–200.
9. Otley CC, Stasko T, Tope WD, et al. Chemoprevention of nonmelanoma skin cancer with systemic retinoids: practical dosing and management of adverse effects. Dermatol Surg 2006;32(4):562–8.
10. O'Reilly Zwald F, Brown M. Skin cancer in solid organ transplant recipients: advances in therapy and management: part I. Epidemiology of skin cancer in solid organ transplant recipients. J Am Acad Dermatol 2011;65(2):253–61.
11. O'Reilly Zwald F, Brown M. Skin cancer in solid organ transplant recipients: advances in therapy and management: part II. Management of skin cancer in solid organ transplant recipients. J Am Acad Dermatol 2011;65(2):263–79.
12. Berg D, Otley CC. Skin cancer in organ transplant recipients: epidemiology, pathogenesis, and management. J Am Acad Dermatol 2002;47(1):1–17 [quiz: 18–20].
13. Criscione VD, Weinstock MA, Naylor MF, et al. Actinic keratoses: natural history and risk of malignant transformation in the Veterans Affairs Topical Tretinoin Chemoprevention Trial. Cancer 2009; 115(11):2523–30.
14. Cohen DK, Lee PK. Photodynamic therapy for nonmelanoma skin cancers. Cancers (Basel) 2016; 8(10) [pii:E90].
15. Morton CA, McKenna KE, Rhodes LE, et al. Guidelines for topical photodynamic therapy: update. Br J Dermatol 2008;159(6):1245–66.
16. Wong TH, Morton CA, Collier N, et al. British Association of Dermatologists and British Photodermatology Group guidelines for topical photodynamic therapy 2018. Br J Dermatol 2018.

17. Levulan® Kerastick® (aminolevulinic acid hcl) for topical solution, 20%. Highlights of prescribing information. Wilmington (MA): DUSA Pharmaceuticals, Inc.; 2018. Available at: https://www.accessdata.fda.gov/drugsatfda_docs/label/2018/020965s015lbl.pdf. Accessed October 1, 2018.

18. Pariser DM, Houlihan A, Ferdon MB, et al. Randomized vehicle-controlled study of short drug incubation aminolevulinic acid photodynamic therapy for actinic keratoses of the face or scalp. Dermatol Surg 2016;42(3):296–304.

19. Ameluz® (aminolevulinic acid hydrochloride) gel, 10%. highlights of prescribing information. Wakefield (MA): Biofrontera Inc.; 2016. Available at: https://www.accessdata.fda.gov/drugsatfda_docs/label/2016/208081s000lbl.pdf. Accessed October 1, 2018.

20. Lucena SR, Salazar N, Gracia-Cazaña T, et al. Combined treatments with photodynamic therapy for non-melanoma skin cancer. Int J Mol Sci 2015; 16(10):25912–33.

21. Morton CA, Braathen LR. Daylight photodynamic therapy for actinic keratoses. Am J Clin Dermatol 2018;19(5):647–56.

22. Gutiérrez García-Rodrigo C, Pellegrini C, Piccioni A, et al. Long-term efficacy data for daylight-PDT. G Ital Dermatol Venereol 2018;153(6):800–5.

23. Wulf HC, Pavel S, Stender I, et al. Topical photodynamic therapy for prevention of new skin lesions in renal transplant recipients. Acta Derm Venereol 2006;86(1):25–8.

24. Wennberg AM, Stenquist B, Stockfleth E, et al. Photodynamic therapy with methyl aminolevulinate for prevention of new skin lesions in transplant recipients: a randomized study. Transplantation 2008; 86(3):423–9.

25. Willey A, Mehta S, Lee PK. Reduction in the incidence of squamous cell carcinoma in solid organ transplant recipients treated with cyclic photodynamic therapy. Dermatol Surg 2010;36(5):652–8.

26. Efudex® (fluorouracil) topical solutions and cream. Costa Mesa (CA): ICN Pharmaceuticals, Inc.; 2004. Available at: https://www.accessdata.fda.gov/drugsatfda_docs/label/2004/16831slr047_efudex_lbl.pdf. Accessed January 21, 2019.

27. Askew DA, Mickan SM, Soyer HP, et al. Effectiveness of 5-fluorouracil treatment for actinic keratosis–a systematic review of randomized controlled trials. Int J Dermatol 2009;48(5):453–63.

28. Pomerantz H, Hogan D, Eilers D, et al. Long-term efficacy of topical fluorouracil cream, 5%, for treating actinic keratosis: a randomized clinical trial. JAMA Dermatol 2015;151(9):952–60.

29. Walker JL, Siegel JA, Sachar M, et al. 5-Fluorouracil for actinic keratosis treatment and chemoprevention: a randomized controlled trial. J Invest Dermatol 2017;137(6):1367–70.

30. Weinstock MA, Thwin SS, Siegel JA, et al. Chemoprevention of basal and squamous cell carcinoma with a single course of fluorouracil, 5%, cream: a randomized clinical trial. JAMA Dermatol 2018; 154(2):167–74.

31. Goon PK, Clegg R, Yong AS, et al. 5-Fluorouracil "chemowraps" in the treatment of multiple actinic keratoses: a Norwich experience. Dermatol Ther (Heidelb) 2015;5(3):201–5.

32. Mann M, Berk DR, Petersen J. Chemowraps as an adjuvant to surgery for patients with diffuse squamous cell carcinoma of the extremities. J Drugs Dermatol 2008;7(7):685–8.

33. Tallon B, Turnbull N. 5% Fluorouracil chemowraps in the management of widespread lower leg solar keratoses and squamous cell carcinoma. Australas J Dermatol 2013;54(4):313–6.

34. Cunningham TJ, Tabacchi M, Eliane JP, et al. Randomized trial of calcipotriol combined with 5-fluorouracil for skin cancer precursor immunotherapy. J Clin Invest 2017;127(1):106–16.

35. Hanke CW, Beer KR, Stockfleth E, et al. Imiquimod 2.5% and 3.75% for the treatment of actinic keratoses: results of two placebo-controlled studies of daily application to the face and balding scalp for two 3-week cycles. J Am Acad Dermatol 2010; 62(4):573–81.

36. Aldara® (imiquimod) cream, 5%. Highlights of prescribing information. Bristol (TN): Graceway Pharmaceuticals, LLC; 2010. Available at: https://www.accessdata.fda.gov/drugsatfda_docs/label/2010/020723s022lbl.pdf. Accessed January 21, 2019.

37. Korman N, Moy R, Ling M, et al. Dosing with 5% imiquimod cream 3 times per week for the treatment of actinic keratosis: results of two phase 3, randomized, double-blind, parallel-group, vehicle-controlled trials. Arch Dermatol 2005;141(4):467–73.

38. Patel GK, Goodwin R, Chawla M, et al. Imiquimod 5% cream monotherapy for cutaneous squamous cell carcinoma in situ (Bowen's disease): a randomized, double-blind, placebo-controlled trial. J Am Acad Dermatol 2006;54(6):1025–32.

39. Martin GM, Stockfleth E. Diclofenac sodium 3% gel for the management of actinic keratosis: 10+ years of cumulative evidence of efficacy and safety. J Drugs Dermatol 2012;11(5):600–8.

40. Rivers JK, McLean DI. An open study to assess the efficacy and safety of topical 3% diclofenac in a 2.5% hyaluronic acid gel for the treatment of actinic keratoses. Arch Dermatol 1997;133(10):1239–42.

41. Rivers JK, Arlette J, Shear N, et al. Topical treatment of actinic keratoses with 3.0% diclofenac in 2.5% hyaluronan gel. Br J Dermatol 2002;146(1): 94–100.

42. Ulrich C, Johannsen A, Röwert-Huber J, et al. Results of a randomized, placebo-controlled safety and efficacy study of topical diclofenac 3% gel in

organ transplant patients with multiple actinic keratoses. Eur J Dermatol 2010;20(4):482–8.

43. Stockfleth E, Bastian M. Pharmacokinetic and pharmacodynamic evaluation of ingenol mebutate for the treatment of actinic keratosis. Expert Opin Drug Metab Toxicol 2018;14(9):911–8.

44. Lebwohl M, Swanson N, Anderson LL, et al. Ingenol mebutate gel for actinic keratosis. N Engl J Med 2012;366(11):1010–9.

45. Bavinck JN, Tieben LM, Van der Woude FJ, et al. Prevention of skin cancer and reduction of keratotic skin lesions during acitretin therapy in renal transplant recipients: a double-blind, placebo-controlled study. J Clin Oncol 1995;13(8):1933–8.

46. George R, Weightman W, Russ GR, et al. Acitretin for chemoprevention of non-melanoma skin cancers in renal transplant recipients. Australas J Dermatol 2002;43(4):269–73.

47. de Sévaux RG, Smit JV, de Jong EM, et al. Acitretin treatment of premalignant and malignant skin disorders in renal transplant recipients: clinical effects of a randomized trial comparing two doses of acitretin. J Am Acad Dermatol 2003;49(3):407–12.

48. Peck GL. Long-term retinoid therapy is needed for maintenance of cancer chemopreventive effect. Dermatologica 1987;175(Suppl 1):138–44.

49. Otley CC, Berg D, Ulrich C, et al. Reduction of immunosuppression for transplant-associated skin cancer: expert consensus survey. Br J Dermatol 2006; 154(3):395–400.

50. Damian DL. Nicotinamide for skin cancer chemoprevention. Australas J Dermatol 2017;58(3):174–80.

51. Surjana D, Halliday GM, Martin AJ, et al. Oral nicotinamide reduces actinic keratoses in phase II double-blinded randomized controlled trials. J Invest Dermatol 2012;132(5):1497–500.

52. Chen AC, Martin AJ, Choy B, et al. A phase 3 randomized trial of nicotinamide for skin-cancer chemoprevention. N Engl J Med 2015;373(17):1618–26.

53. Lee JL, Mukhtar H, Bickers DR, et al. Cyclooxygenases in the skin: pharmacological and toxicological

implications. Toxicol Appl Pharmacol 2003;192(3): 294–306.

54. An KP, Athar M, Tang X, et al. Cyclooxygenase-2 expression in murine and human nonmelanoma skin cancers: implications for therapeutic approaches. Photochem Photobiol 2002;76(1):73–80.

55. Higashi Y, Kanekura T, Kanzaki T. Enhanced expression of cyclooxygenase (COX)-2 in human skin epidermal cancer cells: evidence for growth suppression by inhibiting COX-2 expression. Int J Cancer 2000;86(5):667–71.

56. Johannesdottir SA, Chang ET, Mehnert F, et al. Nonsteroidal anti-inflammatory drugs and the risk of skin cancer: a population-based case-control study. Cancer 2012;118(19):4768–76.

57. Reinau D, Surber C, Jick SS, et al. Nonsteroidal anti-inflammatory drugs and the risk of nonmelanoma skin cancer. Int J Cancer 2015;137(1):144–53.

58. Torti DC, Christensen BC, Storm CA, et al. Analgesic and nonsteroidal anti-inflammatory use in relation to nonmelanoma skin cancer: a population-based case-control study. J Am Acad Dermatol 2011; 65(2):304–12.

59. Butler GJ, Neale R, Green AC, et al. Nonsteroidal anti-inflammatory drugs and the risk of actinic keratoses and squamous cell cancers of the skin. J Am Acad Dermatol 2005;53(6):966–72.

60. Grau MV, Baron JA, Langholz B, et al. Effect of NSAIDs on the recurrence of nonmelanoma skin cancer. Int J Cancer 2006;119(3):682–6.

61. Elmets CA, Viner JL, Pentland AP, et al. Chemoprevention of nonmelanoma skin cancer with celecoxib: a randomized, double-blind, placebo-controlled trial. J Natl Cancer Inst 2010;102(24):1835–44.

62. Endrizzi BT, Lee PK. Management of carcinoma of the skin in solid organ transplant recipients with oral capecitabine. Dermatol Surg 2009;35(10): 1567–72.

63. Endrizzi B, Ahmed RL, Ray T, et al. Capecitabine to reduce nonmelanoma skin carcinoma burden in solid organ transplant recipients. Dermatol Surg 2013;39(4):634–45.

Medications Associated with Increased Risk of Keratinocyte Carcinoma

Lauren D. Crow, MD, MPH, Katherine A. Kaizer-Salk, BA,
Hailey M. Juszczak, BA, Sarah T. Arron, MD, PhD*

KEYWORDS

- Keratinocyte carcinoma • Photosensitization • Carcinogen • Immunosuppression • Medication

KEY POINTS

- A number of medications for short-term and long-term use have been linked to an increased risk for keratinocyte carcinoma (KC), including cutaneous squamous cell carcinoma and basal cell carcinoma.
- Medications that increase KC risk do so through 3 main mechanistic pathways: (1) photosensitivity and exacerbation of UV-mediated damage repair, (2) immunosuppression and loss of tumor surveillance, and (3) direct molecular effects driving keratinocyte proliferation.
- Regardless of mechanism, immunosuppressive medications with an increased risk of KC should be used with caution in patients with other known risk factors.

INTRODUCTION

A number of medications for short-term and long-term use have been linked to an increased risk for keratinocyte carcinoma (KC), including cutaneous squamous cell carcinoma (cSCC) and basal cell carcinoma (BCC). Several mechanisms have been proposed to explain these correlations (**Table 1**). Immunosuppressive medications have been associated with an increased risk for KC and melanoma due to reduction of antitumor immune surveillance,[1–3] and some immunosuppressive agents also directly impact DNA replication and repair.[3–5] Drug-induced photosensitization is another important mechanism, as clinical and epidemiologic studies have shown an increased risk for KC in users of photosensitizing medications.[6,7] This increased risk is thought to be at least partially attributable to increased ultraviolet (UV) absorption by photosensitization. Additional mechanisms include drug-induced modulation of DNA damage repair, enhancement of keratinocyte proliferation, and direct carcinogenic effect.[4,8] Alternatively, some medications have been shown to decrease KC risk.[9] This article reviews the literature on medications associated with KC risk.

CALCINEURIN INHIBITORS

Calcineurin inhibitors (CNIs) are immunosuppressive agents that inhibit nucleotide excision repair, an important mechanism involved in UV-mediated DNA damage repair.[10] CNIs are the first-line treatment for organ transplant recipients (OTR) given their long-term efficacy for graft survival.

Cyclosporine (CsA) has been used in organ transplantation as well as a variety of dermatologic diseases. CsA also increases cellular malignant potential by increasing production of transforming

Disclosure Statement: Dr S.T. Arron is an investigator for Leo Pharma, SunPharma, Menlo Therapeutics, Castle Biosciences, Genentech/Roche, Pfizer, Regeneron, Eli Lilly, and PellePharm. She is a consultant for Enspectra Health, Regeneron, Sanofi-Genzyme, Castle Creek Pharmaceuticals, SunPharma, Pennside Partners, Biossance, Gerson Lehrman Group, and Rakuten Aspyrian.
Department of Dermatology, University of California San Francisco, 1701 Divisadero Street, Box 0316, San Francisco, CA 94143-0316, USA
* Corresponding author.
E-mail address: sarah.arron@ucsf.edu

Dermatol Clin 37 (2019) 297–305
https://doi.org/10.1016/j.det.2019.02.005
0733-8635/19/Published by Elsevier Inc.

Table 1
Medications that influence keratinocyte carcinoma (KC) risk

Medications	Proposed Mechanism of Action
Tacrolimus	Increased KC risk through ultraviolet (UV)-mediated damage of DNA repair pathways
Cyclosporine	Increased KC risk through activation of oncogene ATF3, decreased apoptosis following UVB damage
Azathioprine>>Mycophenolate mofetil	Increased KC risk through photocarcinogenesis
Everolimus, sirolimus	Decreased KC risk through promotion of autophagy and apoptosis of UV-damaged keratinocytes
Thiazide diuretics	Increased KC risk through photosensitization/phototoxicity
Adalimumab, infliximab, etanercept	Increased KC risk through decreased tumor surveillance via CD8/NK cells, decreased KC risk through inhibition of tumor growth and development
Fluoroquinolones, tetracyclines	Increased KC risk through photosensitization/phototoxicity
Simeprevir, sofosbuvir, efavirenz	Increased photosensitivity, no current evidence of increased KC risk
Voriconazole	Increased KC risk through photosensitization/phototoxicity
Vemurafenib, Dabrafenib	Increased KC through promotion of keratinocyte proliferation
Vismodegib	Potentially increased KC through promotion of keratinocyte proliferation

growth factor-beta, potentiating the activation of the oncogene ATF3, decreasing apoptosis following UVB damage, inhibition of mitochondrial permeability transition pore opening during oxidative stress, and interrupting nuclear factor of activated T cells.[4,5,11,12]

Although CsA-induced skin cancers are documented in organ transplant literature, this association has not been substantiated in patients treated for dermatologic indications with time-limited use and low doses, or in healthy patients with no other immunosuppressant use.[13] Within the transplant population, an increase in skin cancer risk with CsA use has been observed across several data sets. Kidney transplant recipients in a Norwegian cohort study receiving cyclosporine, azathioprine, and prednisolone had a 2.8-fold higher risk of cSCC relative to those receiving azathioprine and prednisolone.[1] This association between CsA and cSCC was dose-dependent.[1]

Tacrolimus is another CNI used as first-line immunosuppression for OTR. Data regarding KC risk and tacrolimus have been conflicting. One study demonstrated a decreased KC risk with tacrolimus compared with CsA (relative risk 0.3, 95% confidence interval [CI] 0.1–0.8).[14] However, this was not significant on multivariate analysis. In a retrospective study of 4089 heart transplant patients, neither tacrolimus nor CsA appeared to have a significant effect on post–heart transplant KC risk.[15] A large, US-based retrospective review found that initial immunosuppression using tacrolimus was associated with a 35% lower incidence of skin cancer.[16] However, immunosuppression is tailored to patient risk, so these data should be interpreted cautiously. Conversely, some studies have shown a twofold to fourfold increased risk of KC with tacrolimus.[17–19] Posttransplant KC also develops earlier in patients on tacrolimus.[20]

MAMMALIAN TARGET OF RAPAMYCIN INHIBITORS

Mammalian target of rapamycin inhibitors (mTORi) belong to a family of phosphatidylinositol-3 kinase-related kinases that inhibit T-cell proliferation and proliferative responses induced by several cytokines.[21] Everolimus and sirolimus have been used with increasing frequency for OTR. mTORi are also effective against malignancies including renal cell carcinoma, Kaposi sarcoma, and large B-cell lymphoma through their anti-angiogenic effects.[22,23]

Comparative studies have examined the relationship between conversion from CNIs to mTORi after transplantation. In renal OTR, mTORi lowered the risk of all malignancies by 60% at 2.6 years posttransplantation.[9] A double-blind randomized controlled trial (RCT) reported that renal OTR on sirolimus without CsA have a significantly lower incidence of skin cancer 2 years posttransplantation compared with renal OTR on sirolimus and CsA.[24] In the TUMORAPA multicenter RCT of patients with a history of skin cancer, secondary prevention of SCC through sirolimus conversion significantly reduced the risk of new SCC.[25]

There is still controversy as to whether the benefit of conversion is sustained. One RCT reported that skin cancer development is reduced by 50% in the first year of follow-up, but that this risk equalized in the following year. The authors concluded that sirolimus may delay skin cancer development, rather than reducing overall risk.[26] However, 5-year follow-up from the TUMORAPA trial confirmed an antitumoral effect of conversion from calcineurin inhibitors to sirolimus maintained at 5 years. They observed a significant reduction of SCC (22% vs 59%, $P<.001$), and BCC (20% vs 37.5%, $P<.05$) with sirolimus conversion.[27]

A systematic review of 29 trials examining mTOR conversion in OTR supports a reduction in overall KC risk, as well as improved preservation of renal function, increased risk of acute rejection, and no difference in overall mortality.[28] Despite data showing a long-term overall safety profile for mTORi in the transplant population, they have high rates of adverse effects that make tolerability a limiting factor for patients. These adverse effects include edema, diarrhea, acne, pneumonitis, hyperlipidemia, myelosuppression, and proteinuria, and led to discontinuation rates as high as 20%.[25,28] If tolerated, the greatest clinical benefits for OTR lie in early conversion to mTOR inhibitors from CNIs, reducing the overall dose of CNI.[29]

PURINE SYNTHESIS INHIBITORS

Azathioprine (AZA) is metabolized to 6-thioguanine, a purine analogue that halts DNA and RNA synthesis, inhibiting white blood cell formation and causing immunosuppression.[30] AZA is used to prevent rejection following organ transplantation, and to treat an array of autoimmune diseases, including rheumatoid arthritis (RA), systemic lupus erythematosus, and atopic dermatitis.[30,31] AZA is a known photocarcinogen with both UVA and UVB.[8]

Studies of AZA across disease areas have found an increased risk of KC.[32–34] In the transplant literature, AZA confers an overall estimated SCC risk of 1.56 (95% CI 1.11–2.18).[32] Although most studies have been observational and significant

heterogeneity has limited meta-analyses, a significant effect of AZA is reported.

Mycophenolate mofetil (MMF) is an antimetabolite used for immunosuppression following organ transplantation. MMF has largely replaced AZA to prevent allograft rejection.[35] Although many studies demonstrate a reduced photocarcinogenic potential and associated skin cancer risk with MMF use, conflicting data remain. The relative reduction in KC risk with MMF versus AZA is through selective suppression of cell-mediated immunity. MMF specifically targets lymphocytes without significantly impacting the proliferation of other cell types. MMF also exhibits decreased UV sensitivity, in large part through its antioxidant activity, and reduced tissue damage and inflammation.[35–37]

A prospective, open-label trial in kidney transplant recipients demonstrated that replacing AZA with MMF effectively reversed previously enhanced UV sensitivity and attenuated UV-induced DNA damage, although it was found that the effects of AZA may persist for years after discontinuing treatment.[37] A Dutch study of lung transplant recipients who switched to MMF from AZA demonstrated a 76% decreased risk for developing SCC.[38] MMF was associated with a 70% reduced risk for SCC in heart transplant recipients and an 83% reduced risk in liver transplant who switched from CNIs to MMF.[15,39] A decreased risk for SCC was also observed with MMF in OTRs without a history of prior AZA exposure.[40]

ANTIHYPERTENSIVES

A recent study of the Kaiser Permanente Northern California cohort reported a 17% increased risk for cSCC among users of photosensitizing antihypertensive medications, including common diuretics (loop, potassium-sparing, thiazide, and combination diuretics), angiotensin receptor enzyme inhibitors, and alpha-2 receptors agonists. This was largely driven by combination thiazide diuretics, which conferred a 30% increased risk for cSCC. Subgroup analyses identified a dose-dependent risk for SCC among users of photosensitizing antihypertensives.[41] A US cohort study found that thiazide diuretic use was associated with a four-fold and twofold increased risk for cSCC and BCC, respectively.[42]

Many diuretics are known photosensitizing medications.[43–45] Thiazides, in particular, are associated with the highest risk for photosensitivity among antihypertensive medications.[43,45,46] Numerous studies have linked hydrochlorothiazide (HCTZ) to cSCC.[7,47–52] Kunisada and colleagues[53] reported the biological process by which HCTZ use increases skin cancer risk through enhanced phototoxic effects. The relationship between HCTZ and cSCC risk is dose-dependent, with a reported twofold increased risk for lip SCC with ever-use and up to sevenfold increased risk with 10 or more years of cumulative use.[54] Similar exposure levels also increased BCC risk in a dose-dependent manner, although risk levels were much smaller in comparison.[54,55]

The 2017 hypertension guidelines of the American College of Cardiology and American Heart Association suggest an estimated additional 4.2 million adults in the United States will require antihypertensives.[56] As HCTZ and other diuretics remain first-line, the possible increased risk for SCC is an important public health issue. Patients should be educated and monitored closely, especially those with a prior history of skin cancer.

TUMOR NECROSIS FACTOR-ALPHA INHIBITORS

Tumor necrosis factor-alpha inhibitors (TNF-αi) are used to treat inflammatory conditions such as psoriasis, inflammatory bowel disease (IBD), and RA. Several meta-analyses have shown an increased risk for KC among TNF-αi users compared with nonusers.[57–59] One secondary analysis of KC risk stratified by TNF-α agent revealed a significantly higher risk association with adalimumab and infliximab compared with etanercept, whereas another identified a trend toward increased risk with adalimumab and etanercept compared with infliximab.[60,61] An increased risk for KC was also observed among TNF-αi compared with methotrexate (MTX) therapy, and adding TNF-αi to MTX or thiopurine significantly increased the KC risk in patients with RA or IBD.[62–64]

TNF-αi appears to be more strongly correlated with cSCC than BCC risk. An 80% increased risk for SCC was observed in patients with psoriasis treated with biologic disease-modifying antirheumatic drugs, of which TNF-αi accounted for 97% of tumors.[65] A meta-analysis evaluating the safety of adalimumab for IBD revealed an overall marginal increase in risk for all KC, including BCC, compared with a fivefold increase in SCC.[66]

In contrast, several studies have found no significant association between TNF-αi and skin cancer risk. A meta-analysis including more than 8800 patients with RA did not find an increased risk for KC with TNF-αi.[67] The short average duration of exposure of less than 1 year may limit these findings. Among subjects enrolled in the British Society for Rheumatology Biologics Register, no significant increased risk for KC was observed.[68] Several

recent, small observational studies did not find an increased risk for KC with TNF-αi.[69,70]

Uncertainty pertaining to the long-term risks of TNF-αi and potential risk of malignancy prompted the US Food and Drug Administration (FDA) to issue a black box warning in 2009. The novelty of this biologic therapy limits the amount of data available, and KC is often excluded from cancer data reporting in registries and clinical trials. Endogenous TNF-α has paradoxic effects, including cytostatic antitumorigenicity through promotion of apoptosis and necrosis of tumor cell vasculature, and alternatively induction of other cytokines and angiogenic factors contributing to DNA damage and enhanced growth/survival of tumor cells.[71] Overall, the conflicting data illustrate the complexity of TNF-α inhibition. Patients using TNF-αi should be educated regarding and monitored for potential KC risk.

ANTIBACTERIALS

Various antibacterial medications have been shown to cause photosensitivity reactions, and several studies have found evidence to support an increased risk of KC with use of these medications.

Fluoroquinolones are used to treat respiratory and urinary tract infections. Fluoroquinolones in combination with ultraviolet A (UVA) increased the likelihood of tumor development in studies of hairless mice.[72,73] One murine model showed that mice treated with lomefloxacin and UVA in combination developed a high rate of large, cystic, and invasive SCC, in comparison with other fluoroquinolones, in which tumors were mostly benign.[72] A more recent murine model examined the differing phototoxic potency of various fluoroquinolones via an in vivo photomicronucleus test. The phototoxic potency from this study ranked the fluoroquinolones from highest phototoxic potency to lowest as follows: (1) sparfloxacin; (2) lomefloxacin; (3) ciprofloxacin, levofloxacin, gemifloxacin; and (4) gatifloxacin.[74] Clinically, studies have reported an increased risk of BCC even with short-term ciprofloxacin use.[7]

Tetracyclines are antibiotics often prescribed to treat acne. Multiple studies have demonstrated an increased risk of BCC with long-term tetracycline use, but none have demonstrated increased risk for SCC with tetracyclines.[75] Studies have a reported a 1.3-fold to 2.0-fold risk of overall and early-onset BCC with tetracycline.[6,7] There is also an increased risk of BCC and SCC with short-term use of sulfamethoxazole with trimethoprim.[7]

ANTIVIRALS

No antivirals have been reported to have sufficient evidence to support an increased risk of KC. However, antivirals are associated with phototoxicity, such as simeprevir, sofosbuvir, and efavirenz.[76–78] Additional research is needed in this area.

ANTIFUNGALS

Voriconazole is an antifungal used for prophylaxis and treatment of infections in immunosuppressed patients, particularly bone marrow and lung transplant recipients. Photosensitivity has been reported in 8% to 10% of patients taking voriconazole.[79–81] This adverse event frequency is even higher at 58% in patients with cystic fibrosis.[82] Multiple epidemiologic studies have substantiated the association between voriconazole and cSCC.[82–86] Studies report a higher likelihood that the SCC would be more aggressive than in a patient not on voriconazole, and a duration-dependent relationship between voriconazole and cSCC.[87,88] These data led to a product label change recommending discontinuation of voriconazole in patients with skin cancer.[89] Further investigation is needed to determine the ideal dosing for voriconazole to minimize cSCC risk while providing effective treatment. *Aspergillus* prophylaxis varies across institutions, and other medications used for this indication, from most commonly used to less commonly used, include inhaled amphotericin B, oral itraconazole, oral voriconazole, intravenous voriconazole, echinocandins, and oral posaconazole.[90]

TARGETED MOLECULAR INHIBITORS

BRAF inhibitors (BRAFi) are drugs used to treat various BRAF-mutated cancers, including melanoma and non–small-cell lung cancer. BRAF is a protein in the MAPK pathway that promotes cell growth.

New primary SCC and keratoacanthoma (KA) were reported in patients following the introduction of BRAFi into the market. The median time to SCC or KA presentation in patients on BRAFi is 8 weeks with vemurafenib and 16 weeks with dabrafenib.[91] The incidence of all-grade and high-grade cSCC in patients on BRAFi is 12.5% and 11.6%, respectively.[92]

MEK inhibitors (MEKi), including trametinib and cobimetinib, can be added to BRAFi when treating BRAF-mutated cancers. Dual therapy decreases risk of developing cSCC. The incidence of all-grade and high-grade cSCC with BRAFi/MEKi therapy was 3.0% and 2.8%, respectively. The relative risk of developing all-grade or high-grade SCC in patients with cancer on BRAFi monotherapy compared with BRAFi/MEKi therapy was 4.72 (all-grade) and 4.92 (high-grade). The CoBRIM phase III trial, which compared 247 patients treated with dual therapy (cobimetinib and vemurafenib) with 246 patients treated with monotherapy (vemurafenib), showed lower frequency of SCC (4 vs 12.6%) and KA (1.6 vs 9.3%) in patients receiving dual therapy.[93]

HEDGEHOG PATHWAY INHIBITORS

Vismodegib and sonidegib are hedgehog pathway inhibitors used to treat locally advanced or metastatic BCC. The approval of vismodegib in 2012 coincided with the observation of SCC induction in patients on BRAF inhibition, and initial case reports of SCC in patients on vismodegib raised concern for increased SCC risk in patients on vismodegib.[94–96] As a first-in class agent and the first effective therapy for metastatic BCC, vismodegib gained FDA approval through a pivotal phase 2 trial without a placebo arm. This made it difficult to substantiate incidence of SCC against a placebo-control group.[97] An initial study to explore this issue reported increased risk of BCC in patients treated with vismodegib.[98] However, this study had significant flaws in methodology.[99] A follow-up large retrospective cohort study compared patients on vismodegib with those with BCC treated with other modalities, and found no association of SCC with vismodegib use.[97] These studies focus on the risk of incidental primary SCC in patients on vismodegib, which must be separated from the phenomenon of phenotype shift, in which a BCC treated with vismodegib can develop squamous and keratinizing histology in the context of drug resistance.[100]

SUMMARY

Medications that increase KC risk do so through 3 main mechanistic pathways: (1) photosensitivity and exacerbation of UV-mediated damage repair, (2) immunosuppression and loss of tumor surveillance, and (3) direct molecular effects driving keratinocyte proliferation. Regardless of mechanism, immunosuppressive medications with an increased risk of KC should be used with caution in patients with other known risk factors, such as older age, male sex, fair skin, tendency to sunburn, and a history of high sun exposure. Future research is needed to better elucidate the epidemiologic effects of these and other emerging medications on KC risk.

REFERENCES

1. Jensen P, Hansen S, Møller B, et al. Skin cancer in kidney and heart transplant recipients and different long-term immunosuppressive therapy regimens. J Am Acad Dermatol 1999;40:177–86.
2. Ingvar A, Smedby KE, Lindelöf B, et al. Immunosuppressive treatment after solid organ transplantation and risk of post-transplant cutaneous squamous cell carcinoma. Nephrol Dial Transplant 2010;25:2764–71.
3. Harwood CA, Toland AE, Proby CM, et al. The pathogenesis of cutaneous squamous cell carcinoma in organ transplant recipients. Br J Dermatol 2017; 177:1217–24.
4. Dziunycz PJ, Lefort K, Wu X, et al. The oncogene ATF3 is potentiated by cyclosporine A and ultraviolet light A. J Invest Dermatol 2014;134:1998–2004.
5. Wu X, Nguyen BC, Dziunycz P, et al. Opposing roles for calcineurin and ATF3 in squamous skin cancer. Nature 2010;465:368–72.
6. Robinson SN, Zens MS, Perry AE, et al. Photosensitizing agents and the risk of non-melanoma skin cancer: a population-based case-control study. J Invest Dermatol 2013;133:1950–5.
7. Kaae J, Boyd HA, Hansen AV, et al. Photosensitizing medication use and risk of skin cancer. Cancer Epidemiol Biomarkers Prev 2010;19:2942–9.
8. Guven M, Brem R, Macpherson P, et al. Oxidative damage to RPA limits the nucleotide excision repair capacity of human cells. J Invest Dermatol 2015; 135:2834–41.
9. Kauffman HM, Cherikh WS, Cheng Y, et al. Maintenance immunosuppression with target-of-rapamycin inhibitors is associated with a reduced incidence of de novo malignancies. Transplantation 2005;80:883–9.
10. Yarosh DB, Pena AV, Nay SL, et al. Calcineurin inhibitors decrease DNA repair and apoptosis in human keratinocytes following ultraviolet B irradiation. J Invest Dermatol 2005;125:1020–5.
11. Hojo M, Morimoto T, Maluccio M, et al. Cyclosporine induces cancer progression by a cell-autonomous mechanism. Nature 1999;397:530–4.
12. Norman KG, Canter JA, Shi M, et al. Cyclosporine A suppresses keratinocyte cell death through MPTP inhibition in a model for skin cancer in organ transplant recipients. Mitochondrion 2010;10: 94–101.
13. Muellenhoff MW, Koo JY. Cyclosporine and skin cancer: an international dermatologic perspective over 25 years of experience. A comprehensive review and pursuit to define safe use of cyclosporine in dermatology. J Dermatolog Treat 2012;23: 290–304.
14. Crespo-Leiro MG, Alonso-Pulpón L, Vázquez de Prada JA, et al. Malignancy after heart transplantation: incidence, prognosis and risk factors. Am J Transplant 2008;8:1031–9.
15. Molina BD, Leiro MG, Pulpón LA, et al. Incidence and risk factors for nonmelanoma skin cancer after heart transplantation. Transplant Proc 2010;42: 3001–5.
16. Kasiske BL, Snyder JJ, Gilbertson DT, et al. Cancer after kidney transplantation in the United States. Am J Transplant 2004;4:905–13.
17. Kaufmann RA, Oberholzer PA, Cazzaniga S, et al. Epithelial skin cancers after kidney transplantation: a retrospective single-centre study of 376 recipients. Eur J Dermatol 2016;26:265–70.
18. Navarro MD, López-Andréu M, Rodríguez-Benot A, et al. Cancer incidence and survival in kidney transplant patients. Transplant Proc 2008;40: 2936–40.
19. Krásová M, Sečníková Z, Göpfertová D, et al. Immunosuppressive therapy in the posttransplant period and skin cancer. Dermatol Ther 2016;29: 433–6.
20. Watorek E, Boratynska M, Smolska D, et al. Malignancy after renal transplantation in the new era of immunosuppression. Ann Transplant 2011;16: 14–8.
21. Faivre S, Kroemer G, Raymond E. Current development of mTOR inhibitors as anticancer agents. Nat Rev Drug Discov 2006;5:671–88.
22. Knoll GA, Kokolo MB, Mallick R, et al. Effect of sirolimus on malignancy and survival after kidney transplantation: systematic review and meta-analysis of individual patient data. BMJ 2014;349: g6679.
23. Yuan R, Kay A, Berg WJ, et al. Targeting tumorigenesis: development and use of mTOR inhibitors in cancer therapy. J Hematol Oncol 2009;2:45.
24. Mathew T, Kreis H, Friend P. Two-year incidence of malignancy in sirolimus-treated renal transplant recipients: results from five multicenter studies. Clin Transplant 2004;18:446–9.
25. Euvrard S, Morelon E, Rostaing L, et al. Sirolimus and secondary skin-cancer prevention in kidney transplantation. N Engl J Med 2012;367:329–39.
26. Hoogendijk-van den Akker JM, Harden PN, Hoitsma AJ, et al. Two-year randomized controlled prospective trial converting treatment of stable renal transplant recipients with cutaneous invasive squamous cell carcinomas to sirolimus. J Clin Oncol 2013;31:1317–23.
27. Dantal J, Morelon E, Rostaing L, et al. Sirolimus for secondary prevention of skin cancer in kidney transplant recipients: 5-year results. J Clin Oncol 2018. https://doi.org/10.1200/JCO.2017. 76.6691.
28. Lim WH, Eris J, Kanellis J, et al. A systematic review of conversion from calcineurin inhibitor to mammalian target of rapamycin inhibitors for

maintenance immunosuppression in kidney transplant recipients. Am J Transplant 2014;14:2106–19.

29. de Fijter JW. Cancer and mTOR inhibitors in transplant recipients. Transplantation 2017;101:45–55.

30. Evans WE. Pharmacogenetics of thiopurine S-methyltransferase and thiopurine therapy. Ther Drug Monit 2004;26:186–91.

31. Patel AA, Swerlick RA, McCall CO. Azathioprine in dermatology: the past, the present, and the future. J Am Acad Dermatol 2006;55:369–89.

32. Jiyad Z, Olsen CM, Burke MT, et al. Azathioprine and risk of skin cancer in organ transplant recipients: systematic review and meta-analysis. Am J Transplant 2016;16:3490–503.

33. Hagen JW, Pugliano-Mauro MA. Nonmelanoma skin cancer risk in patients with inflammatory bowel disease undergoing thiopurine therapy: a systematic review of the literature. Dermatol Surg 2018; 44:469–80.

34. Mabrouk D, Gürcan HM, Keskin DB, et al. Association between cancer and immunosuppressive therapy–analysis of selected studies in pemphigus and pemphigoid. Ann Pharmacother 2010;44: 1770–6.

35. Zwerner J, Fiorentino D. Mycophenolate mofetil. Dermatol Ther 2007;20:229–38.

36. Allison AC, Eugui EM. Mycophenolate mofetil and its mechanisms of action. Immunopharmacology 2000;47:85–118.

37. Hofbauer GFL, Attard NR, Harwood CA, et al. Reversal of UVA skin photosensitivity and DNA damage in kidney transplant recipients by replacing azathioprine. Am J Transplant 2012;12:218–25.

38. Vos M, Plasmeijer EI, van Bemmel BC, et al. Azathioprine to mycophenolate mofetil transition and risk of squamous cell carcinoma after lung transplantation. J Heart Lung Transplant 2018;37:853–9.

39. Aguiar D, Martínez-Urbistondo D, D'Avola D, et al. Conversion from calcineurin inhibitor-based immunosuppression to mycophenolate mofetil in monotherapy reduces risk of de novo malignancies after liver transplantation. Ann Transplant 2017; 22:141–7.

40. Coghill AE, Johnson LG, Berg D, et al. Immunosuppressive medications and squamous cell skin carcinoma: nested case-control study within the skin cancer after organ transplant (SCOT) cohort. Am J Transplant 2016;16:565–73.

41. Su KA, Habel LA, Achacoso NS, et al. Photosensitizing antihypertensive drug use and risk of cutaneous squamous cell carcinoma. Br J Dermatol 2018. https://doi.org/10.1111/bjd.16713.

42. Nardone B, Majewski S, Kim AS, et al. Melanoma and non-melanoma skin cancer associated with angiotensin-converting-enzyme inhibitors, angiotensin-receptor blockers and thiazides: a matched cohort study. Drug Saf 2017;40:249–55.

43. Gould JW, Mercurio MG, Elmets CA. Cutaneous photosensitivity diseases induced by exogenous agents. J Am Acad Dermatol 1995;33:551–73.

44. Harber LC, Lashinsky AM, Baer RL. Photosensitivity due to chlorothiazide and hydrochlorothiazide. N Engl J Med 1959;261:1378–81.

45. Moore DE. Drug-induced cutaneous photosensitivity: incidence, mechanism, prevention and management. Drug Saf 2002;25:345–72.

46. Addo HA, Ferguson J, Frain-Bell W. Thiazide-induced photosensitivity: a study of 33 subjects. Br J Dermatol 1987;116:749–60.

47. Friedman GD, Asgari MM, Warton EM, et al. Antihypertensive drugs and lip cancer in non-Hispanic whites. Arch Intern Med 2012;172:1246.

48. Grosse Y, Loomis D, Lauby-Secretan B, et al. Carcinogenicity of some drugs and herbal products. Lancet Oncol 2013;14:807–8.

49. de Vries E, Trakatelli M, Kalabalikis D, et al. Known and potential new risk factors for skin cancer in European populations: a multicentre case-control study. Br J Dermatol 2012;167:1–13.

50. Friedman GD, Udaltsova N, Chan J, et al. Screening pharmaceuticals for possible carcinogenic effects: initial positive results for drugs not previously screened. Cancer Causes Control 2009;20:1821–35.

51. Jensen A ø, Thomsen HF, Engebjerg MC, et al. Use of photosensitising diuretics and risk of skin cancer: a population-based case–control study. Br J Cancer 2008;99:1522–8.

52. Ruiter R, Visser LE, Eijgelsheim M, et al. High-ceiling diuretics are associated with an increased risk of basal cell carcinoma in a population-based follow-up study. Eur J Cancer 2010;46:2467–72.

53. Kunisada M, Masaki T, Ono R, et al. Hydrochlorothiazide enhances UVA-induced DNA damage. Photochem Photobiol 2013;89:649–54.

54. Pottegård A, Hallas J, Olesen M, et al. Hydrochlorothiazide use is strongly associated with risk of lip cancer. J Intern Med 2017;282:322–31.

55. Pedersen SA, Gaist D, Schmidt SAJ, et al. Hydrochlorothiazide use and risk of nonmelanoma skin cancer: a nationwide case-control study from Denmark. J Am Acad Dermatol 2018;78:673–81.e9.

56. Ioannidis JPA. Diagnosis and treatment of hypertension in the 2017 ACC/AHA guidelines and in the real world. JAMA 2018;319:115.

57. Mariette X, Matucci-Cerinic M, Pavelka K, et al. Malignancies associated with tumour necrosis factor inhibitors in registries and prospective observational studies: a systematic review and meta-analysis. Ann Rheum Dis 2011;70:1895–904.

58. Askling J, Fored CM, Brandt L, et al. Risks of solid cancers in patients with rheumatoid arthritis and after treatment with tumour necrosis factor antagonists. Ann Rheum Dis 2005;64:1421–6.

59. Raaschou P, Simard JF, Asker Hagelberg C, et al, ARTIS Study Group. Rheumatoid arthritis, anti-tumour necrosis factor treatment, and risk of squamous cell and basal cell skin cancer: cohort study based on nationwide prospectively recorded data from Sweden. BMJ 2016;352:i262.

60. Askling J, Fahrbach K, Nordstrom B, et al. Cancer risk with tumor necrosis factor alpha (TNF) inhibitors: meta-analysis of randomized controlled trials of adalimumab, etanercept, and infliximab using patient level data. Pharmacoepidemiol Drug Saf 2011;20:119–30.

61. Amari W, Zeringue AL, McDonald JR, et al. Risk of non-melanoma skin cancer in a national cohort of veterans with rheumatoid arthritis. Rheumatology 2011;50:1431–9.

62. McKenna M, Stobaugh D, Deepak P. Melanoma and non-melanoma skin cancer in inflammatory bowel disease patients following tumor necrosis factor-α inhibitor monotherapy and in combination with thiopurines: analysis of the food and drug administration adverse event reporting system. J Gastrointestin Liver Dis 2014;23(3):267–71.

63. Chakravarty EF, Michaud K, Wolfe F. Skin cancer, rheumatoid arthritis, and tumor necrosis factor inhibitors. J Rheumatol 2005;32:2130–5.

64. Scott FI, Mamtani R, Brensinger CM, et al. Risk of nonmelanoma skin cancer associated with the use of immunosuppressant and biologic agents in patients with a history of autoimmune disease and nonmelanoma skin cancer. JAMA Dermatol 2016;152:164.

65. Asgari MM, Ray GT, Geier JL, et al. Malignancy rates in a large cohort of patients with systemically treated psoriasis in a managed care population. J Am Acad Dermatol 2017;76:632–8.

66. Colombel J-F, Sandborn WJ, Panaccione R, et al. Adalimumab safety in global clinical trials of patients with Crohn's disease. Inflamm Bowel Dis 2009;15:1308–19.

67. Leombruno JP, Einarson TR, Keystone EC. The safety of anti-tumour necrosis factor treatments in rheumatoid arthritis: meta and exposure-adjusted pooled analyses of serious adverse events. Ann Rheum Dis 2009;68:1136–45.

68. Mercer LK, Green AC, Galloway JB, et al. The influence of anti-TNF therapy upon incidence of keratinocyte skin cancer in patients with rheumatoid arthritis: longitudinal results from the British Society for Rheumatology Biologics Register. Ann Rheum Dis 2012;71:869–74.

69. Dreyer L, Mellemkjær L, Andersen AR, et al. Incidences of overall and site specific cancers in TNFα inhibitor treated patients with rheumatoid arthritis and other arthritides - a follow-up study from the DANBIO Registry. Ann Rheum Dis 2013;72:79–82.

70. Tseng H-W, Lu LY, Lam HC, et al. The influence of disease-modifying anti-rheumatic drugs and corticosteroids on the association between rheumatoid arthritis and skin cancer: a nationwide retrospective case-control study in Taiwan. Clin Exp Rheumatol 2018;36:471–8.

71. Balkwill F. Tumor necrosis factor or tumor promoting factor? Cytokine Growth Factor Rev 2002;13: 135–41.

72. Mäkinen M, Forbes PD, Stenbäck F. Quinolone antibacterials: a new class of photochemical carcinogens. J Photochem Photobiol B 1997;37:182–7.

73. Klecak G, Urbach F, Urwyler H. Fluoroquinolone antibacterials enhance UVA-induced skin tumors. J Photochem Photobiol B 1997;37:174–81.

74. Reus AA, Usta M, Kenny JD, et al. The in vivo rat skin photomicronucleus assay: phototoxicity and photogenotoxicity evaluation of six fluoroquinolones. Mutagenesis 2012;27:721–9.

75. Li W-Q, Drucker AM, Cho E, et al. Tetracycline use and risk of incident skin cancer: a prospective study. Br J Cancer 2018;118:294–8.

76. Banerjee D, Reddy KR. Review article: safety and tolerability of direct-acting anti-viral agents in the new era of hepatitis C therapy. Aliment Pharmacol Ther 2016;43:674–96.

77. Simpson CL, McCausland D, Chu EY. Photo-distributed lichenoid eruption secondary to direct anti-viral therapy for hepatitis C. J Cutan Pathol 2015;42:769–73.

78. El-Khayat HR, Fouad YM, Maher M, et al. Efficacy and safety of sofosbuvir plus simeprevir therapy in Egyptian patients with chronic hepatitis C: a real-world experience. Gut 2017;66:2008–12.

79. Denning DW, Griffiths CE. Muco-cutaneous retinoid-effects and facial erythema related to the novel triazole antifungal agent voriconazole. Clin Exp Dermatol 2001;26:648–53.

80. Cowen EW, Nguyen JC, Miller DD, et al. Chronic phototoxicity and aggressive squamous cell carcinoma of the skin in children and adults during treatment with voriconazole. J Am Acad Dermatol 2010; 62:31–7.

81. McCarthy KL, Playford EG, Looke DFM, et al. Severe photosensitivity causing multifocal squamous cell carcinomas secondary to prolonged voriconazole therapy. Clin Infect Dis 2007;44: e55–6.

82. Rondeau S, Couderc L, Dominique S, et al. High frequency of voriconazole-related phototoxicity in cystic fibrosis patients. Eur Respir J 2012;39: 782–4.

83. O'Reilly Zwald F, Brown M. Skin cancer in solid organ transplant recipients: advances in therapy and management: part I. Epidemiology of skin cancer in solid organ transplant recipients. J Am Acad Dermatol 2011;65:253–61.

84. Vanacker A, Fabré G, Van Dorpe J, et al. Aggressive cutaneous squamous cell carcinoma associated with prolonged voriconazole therapy in a renal transplant patient. Am J Transplant 2008;8:877–80.

85. Feist A, Lee R, Osborne S, et al. Increased incidence of cutaneous squamous cell carcinoma in lung transplant recipients taking long-term voriconazole. J Heart Lung Transplant 2012;31:1177–81.

86. Vadnerkar A, Nguyen MH, Mitsani D, et al. Voriconazole exposure and geographic location are independent risk factors for squamous cell carcinoma of the skin among lung transplant recipients. J Heart Lung Transplant 2010;29:1240–4.

87. Singer JP, Boker A, Metchnikoff C, et al. High cumulative dose exposure to voriconazole is associated with cutaneous squamous cell carcinoma in lung transplant recipients. J Heart Lung Transplant 2012;31:694–9.

88. Zwald FO, Spratt M, Lemos BD, et al. Duration of voriconazole exposure: an independent risk factor for skin cancer after lung transplantation. Dermatol Surg 2012;38:1369–74.

89. Williams K, Mansh M, Chin-Hong P, et al. Voriconazole-associated cutaneous malignancy: a literature review on photocarcinogenesis in organ transplant recipients. Clin Infect Dis 2014;58:997–1002.

90. He SY, Makhzoumi ZH, Singer JP, et al. Practice variation in *Aspergillus* prophylaxis and treatment among lung transplant centers: a national survey. Transpl Infect Dis 2015;17:14–20.

91. Anforth R, Fernandez-Peñas P, Long GV. Cutaneous toxicities of RAF inhibitors. Lancet Oncol 2013;14:e11–8.

92. Peng L, Wang Y, Hong Y, et al. Incidence and relative risk of cutaneous squamous cell carcinoma with single-agent BRAF inhibitor and dual BRAF/ MEK inhibitors in cancer patients: a meta-analysis. Oncotarget 2017;8:83280–91.

93. Dréno B, Ribas A, Larkin J, et al. Incidence, course, and management of toxicities associated with cobimetinib in combination with vemurafenib in the coBRIM study. Ann Oncol 2017;28:1137–44.

94. Orouji A, Goerdt S, Utikal J, et al. Multiple highly and moderately differentiated squamous cell carcinomas of the skin during vismodegib treatment of inoperable basal cell carcinoma. Br J Dermatol 2014;171:431–3.

95. Poulalhon N, Dalle S, Balme B, et al. Fast-growing cutaneous squamous cell carcinoma in a patient treated with vismodegib. Dermatology 2015;230: 101–4.

96. Iarrobino A, Messina JL, Kudchadkar R, et al. Emergence of a squamous cell carcinoma phenotype following treatment of metastatic basal cell carcinoma with vismodegib. J Am Acad Dermatol 2013;69:e33–4.

97. Bhutani T, Abrouk M, Sima CS, et al. Risk of cutaneous squamous cell carcinoma after treatment of basal cell carcinoma with vismodegib. J Am Acad Dermatol 2017;77:713–8.

98. Mohan SV, Chang J, Li S, et al. Increased risk of cutaneous squamous cell carcinoma after vismodegib therapy for basal cell carcinoma. JAMA Dermatol 2016;152:527–32.

99. Puig S, Sampogna F, Tejera-Vaquerizo A. Study on the risk of cutaneous squamous cell carcinoma after vismodegib therapy for basal cell carcinoma: not a case-control study. JAMA Dermatol 2016; 152:1172–3.

100. Ransohoff KJ, Tang JY, Sarin KY. Squamous change in basal-cell carcinoma with drug resistance. N Engl J Med 2015;373:1079–82.

Cutaneous Surgery in Patients Who Are Pregnant or Breastfeeding

Jeffrey N. Li, BS, BBA[a], Rajiv I. Nijhawan, MD[b],
Divya Srivastava, MD[b],*

KEYWORDS

- Melanoma • Pregnancy • Lactation • Dermatologic surgery • Cutaneous surgery

KEY POINTS

- Cutaneous surgery can be performed safely on pregnant patients with careful planning.
- Anesthesia, antibiotics, antiseptics, and patient positioning should be adjusted.
- Most antibiotic and anesthetic transmission during lactation is minimal.
- Optimal timing for surgery is the second trimester or postpartum period; however, dermatologic surgery can be safely performed in any trimester.

Performing dermatologic surgery in any patient requires a deliberate approach to provide safe and optimal care. Thoughtful planning is especially important in the pregnant or breastfeeding patient because one must consider the safety of the mother and the fetus or infant. Because of theoretic concerns about potential harm and medicolegal risks, dermatologists and dermatologic surgeons may be hesitant to perform any procedure on pregnant or breastfeeding patients. This article reviews the relevant perioperative considerations to provide effective and safe dermatologic surgery in pregnant and breastfeeding patients.

TIMING
Risk to the Fetus

The timing of cutaneous surgery in pregnant patients is the most critical consideration to minimize risk to the fetus with the safest timing being the second trimester (weeks 13–24) or the postpartum period. These timings avoid the risks of

spontaneous abortion in the first trimester, during which key organogenesis and potential teratogenesis occurs, and preterm labor in the third trimester.[1–3] However, timing must be individualized based on patient factors, diagnosis, and indications for surgery.

Risk to the Patient

The timing of surgery is also important for the patient's optimal outcome, including whether there are any risks in delaying treatment. The risks of delaying treatment until second trimester or postpartum for a subcentimeter superficial basal cell carcinoma on the trunk is quite different than delaying treatment for an invasive melanoma. A basal cell carcinoma can also present a dilemma if a patient has an infiltrative and destructive tumor that can result in tissue loss, loss of function, and nerve damage if not treated in a timely manner. These scenarios require a thorough discussion of the risks and benefits to allow patients to make an informed decision.

Disclosure: The authors have no relevant conflicts of interest to disclose. The authors did not receive financial support for this research.
[a] Department of Dermatology, University of Texas Southwestern Medical Center, 5323 Harry Hines Boulevard, Dallas, TX 75390, USA; [b] Department of Dermatology, University of Texas Southwestern Medical Center, 5939 Harry Hines Boulevard, Professional Office Building 2, Suite 400, Dallas, TX 75390, USA
* Corresponding author.
E-mail address: Divya.Srivastava@UTSouthwestern.edu

Dermatol Clin 37 (2019) 307–317
https://doi.org/10.1016/j.det.2019.03.002
0733-8635/19/© 2019 Elsevier Inc. All rights reserved.

Pregnancy-Associated Malignant Melanoma

Malignant melanoma is the most common malignancy reported during pregnancy.[4] The association between pregnancy and melanoma has been controversial over the last 70 years. Initial reports in the 1950s suggested that pregnancy instigated the transformation of nevi into melanoma and the development of metastatic disease.[5,6] These reports led to recommendations for melanoma patients to avoid pregnancy and even pursue surgical sterilization.[5–7] However, these studies were not controlled and did not account for prognostic factors such as tumor depth.[7]

Although early studies suggested melanoma has a poorer prognosis in pregnant patients, recent studies and reviews demonstrate no significant effect on survival in American Joint Cancer Commission stages I and II disease diagnosed before, during, or after pregnancy.[7,8] Pregnant women with stages III or IV disease who underwent therapy did not show a difference in survival compared with nonpregnant patients.[9] In addition, most studies indicate that women diagnosed with melanoma during pregnancy do not have thicker tumors, more frequent ulceration, or prognostically worse anatomic locations.[8,10]

Lens and colleagues[11] used the Swedish National and Regional registries to compare 185 pregnant women diagnosed with melanoma with 5348 age-matched nonpregnant women diagnosed with melanoma, and reported no overall difference in survival. O'Meara and colleagues[12] demonstrated that 412 women diagnosed with melanoma during pregnancy and up to 1 year postpartum had no significant difference in survival from 2451 age-matched nonpregnant women.

Pregnancy-associated malignant melanoma is not associated with planned birth, preterm birth, stillbirth, an increased rate of cesarean deliveries, or other maternal and neonatal complications.[12,13] The likelihood of premature delivery was unrelated to the trimester in which pregnancy-associated malignant melanoma was diagnosed. Patients diagnosed postpartum were also not more likely to have delivered prematurely.[12]

Few studies have examined metastatic disease in pregnant patients versus nonpregnant, but 1 study of 18 infants in mothers with stage III or IV melanoma revealed similar 2-year maternal survival rates of 56% and 17%, respectively.[9] Treatment was the same as nonpregnant patients, except in the first trimester. Stage IV survival at 2 years (17%) was lower than previously reported in nonpregnant patients (28%).[9]

Fetal metastases have been reported in rare cases of placental metastases.[14] Alexander and colleagues[15] reported 6 cases of neonates developing melanoma out of 27 cases of placental metastases. There are 6 additional reported cases of placental metastasis in literature. One infant developed metastatic melanoma of the brain, and the remaining infants were disease free.[15–20] In patients with metastatic disease, the placenta should be checked histologically and grossly and the neonate carefully screened for melanoma.

Treatment of Malignant Melanoma in Pregnancy

Dermatologists should biopsy clinically and dermoscopically concerning pigmented lesions in pregnant patients in any trimester.[21] Growth and corresponding dermoscopic change of existing nevi can occur on the abdomen or breasts owing to normal skin expansion, whereas nevi located on other sites unaffected by skin stretching do not experience growth.[21,22] This growth does not necessarily indicate malignancy.[22] However, recent evidence demonstrates that normal nevi should not undergo significant change including darkening during pregnancy.[22]

Excision of melanoma under local anesthesia during pregnancy is safe in any trimester, and therefore patients should be treated promptly. If sentinel lymph node biopsy (SLNB) is recommended, the patient will undergo general anesthesia and the obstetrician may recommend fetal monitoring.[21] Despite the risk of fetal exposure to radioactive colloid and blue dye, SLNB is considered safe in pregnant patients.[23] The radiation dose is far below the National Council on Radiation Protection and Measurement limits for pregnant women.[24] Isosulfan blue is associated with allergic reaction and anaphylaxis.[25] Methylene blue is contraindicated in the first trimester owing to an association with atresia of the ileum and jejunum.[26] One study demonstrated that SLNB can be successfully performed with radioactive colloid alone, thereby avoiding administration of blue dye.[27] A thorough discussion with patients of all risks and benefits of SLNB is essential.

If the SLNB is positive, the American College of Obstetrics and Gynecology recommends chest radiographs with appropriate shielding, ultrasonound examination, or MRI without gadolinium.[21] A computed tomography scan without contrast and nuclear medicine studies can be performed if necessary because the radiation doses have not been shown to lead to fetal harm.[21]

PLANNING THE PROCEDURE
Preoperative Considerations

A typical medical history should be taken preoperatively, with an emphasis on the pregnancy-specific history, including recent contractions, vaginal bleeding, and increasing edema. Vital signs should be checked, specifically blood pressure to evaluate for occult preeclampsia. If the pregnancy-specific review of systems is positive or the patient is hypertensive, surgery should be rescheduled, and the patient's obstetrician should be consulted for further evaluation.[1]

Intraoperative Considerations

Positioning
Traditional supine positioning in a pregnant patient can lead to aortocaval compression syndrome, which is caused by a decrease in venous return and cardiac output owing to inferior vena cava (IVC) compression by the gravid uterus and typically occurs after week 20 of pregnancy.[28] Patients present with pallor, lightheadedness, nausea, vomiting, diaphoresis, hypotension, and tachycardia. The patient can instead be placed in the left lateral tilt position of 30° using a wedge or pillow under the hip or between the knees to decrease IVC compression.[14,29] Many previous reviews have recommended 15° of lateral tilt to relieve IVC compression.[14,30–32] However, recent studies by Higuchi and colleagues[33] using MRI imaging of the uterus and IVC have demonstrated that obstruction is only significantly relieved by 30° of left tilt. Greater degrees of tilt do not show extra benefit. Equipment may not be able to provide the full 30° left tilt recommended and/or the patient may feel insecure when the tilt is applied in effective amounts; Kinsella[34] has reported women expressing concern at a mean angle of 9°. In addition to lateral tilt, pelvic tilt was one of the original positioning modalities to minimize aortocaval compression. Increasing the pelvic tilt to greater than 10° has been shown to decrease aortic compression and can be combined with lateral tilt.[34]

Joint laxity also increases during pregnancy, resulting in discomfort, muscle cramps, and back pain, which can be relieved by shifting positions.[35–37] Patients should be encouraged to use the bathroom preoperatively, especially if the procedure time is expected to be longer, owing to physiologic changes resulting in urinary frequency and urgency.[38] Gastric reflux can be prevented by elevating the head.[14,38]

US Food and Drug Administration classification
In 2015, the US Food and Drug Administration (FDA) removed the traditional pregnancy categories A, B, C, D, and X from all human prescription drug and biological product labeling to a narrative structure in the Pregnancy and Lactation Labeling Rule.[39] They concluded that the categories did not clearly identify the differences in risk between products and were frequently misinterpreted. Most drugs have not been redesignated as of this publication, so the traditional categories are used in this review. **Table 1** provides definitions of each category.

Antiseptics
Alcohol is considered safe in the pregnant patient, but is typically only used in skin biopsies as opposed to larger procedures. Alcohol has percutaneous absorption but rapid metabolism leading to low serum levels.[40–42] Chlorhexidine is classified as FDA category B and generally recognized as safe,[1,32,43] but should be avoided around the eyes and inner ears because it can cause keratitis, corneal ulcers, and ototoxicity.

Povidone-iodine is generally avoided owing to a single report of neonatal hypothyroidism after mucous membrane exposure.[35,44] However, 1 study demonstrated that povidone-iodine use during Cesarean delivery did not affect neonatal urine iodine levels.[45] Hexachlorophene is contraindicated because it is absorbed through the skin and has been associated with fetal central nervous system toxicity.[35,46]

Local anesthesia
Lidocaine is pregnancy category B. Although it does cross the placenta, lidocaine did not demonstrate fetal harm in animal reproductive studies.[47,48] In humans, no abnormalities are reported from exposure in the first 4 months of pregnancy.[49]

Epinephrine also crosses the placenta and is considered pregnancy category C because 1 study showed an increased risk of malformations in children of mothers exposed to systemic epinephrine during the first trimester.[48] Although epinephrine can decrease blood flow within the uterus and is concerning for uterine artery spasms, local dilute administration is unlikely to pose serious risks and is considered safe for dermatologic use.[29,32,35,48–51] In fact, endogenous epinephrine produced during states of emotional stress are higher than those produced by injection (28 g/min vs <1 g/min).[52] The use of epinephrine decreases systemic absorption, and, thus, placental transfer of lidocaine through local vasoconstriction, which may decrease the overall dose of lidocaine administered.[51,53] Per recent American Academy of Dermatology evidence-based consensus guidelines, small controlled amounts of lidocaine with epinephrine

Table 1
Classification and description for the FDA's previous pregnancy category system for prescription drugs and biological products

FDA Pregnancy Category	Definition
A	Adequate and well-controlled studies have failed to demonstrate a risk to the fetus in the first trimester of pregnancy (and there is no evidence of risk in later trimesters).
B	Animal reproduction studies have failed to demonstrate a risk to the fetus, and there are no adequate and well-controlled studies in pregnant women.
C	Animal reproduction studies have shown an adverse effect on the fetus and there are no adequate and well-controlled studies in humans, but potential benefits may warrant use of the drug in pregnant women despite potential risks.
D	There is positive evidence of human fetal risk based on adverse reaction data from investigational or marketing experience or studies in humans, but potential benefits may warrant use of the drug in pregnant women despite potential risks.
X	Studies in animals or humans have demonstrated fetal abnormalities and/or there is positive evidence of human fetal risk based on adverse reaction data from investigational or marketing experience, and the risks involved in use of the drug in pregnant women clearly outweigh potential benefits.

Data from Content and format of labeling for human prescription drug and biological products; requirements for pregnancy and lactation labeling. *Fed Reg* 2008;73(104).

do seem to be safe for local anesthesia in pregnant women.[54]

Lidocaine toxicity can present similarly to aortocaval compression syndrome with lightheadedness and tachycardia. Therefore, it is important to record doses and position the patient properly. Lidocaine toxicity is possible at high total doses or if an intravascular injection occurs. If cardiac arrest develops, standard American Advanced Cardiac Life Support protocol will not result in successful resuscitation. The administration of intravenous lipid infusion is key to preventing mortality.[55,56] Bupivacaine and mepivacaine are not recommended because they are FDA category C and associated with the inhibition of cardiac conduction, congenital abnormalities, and fetal bradycardia.[49,53,57]

Topical anesthesia

There is a lack of data on the use of topical anesthesia in pregnant patients. However, given the safety of infiltrated lidocaine and the low serum concentrations of lidocaine after topical application, the Academy of Dermatology guidelines support the topical application of lidocaine during pregnancy and breastfeeding.[35,58,59] Owing to a lack of data on other topical anesthetics, the Academy of Dermatology does not recommend their use in pregnancy and lactation. Rare cases of methemoglobinemia from high doses of prilocaine have been reported.[29] Fetal red blood cells have low levels of erythrocyte methemoglobin reductase and are more susceptible to oxidative stressors.

Electrocautery

The use of electrocautery in the pregnant patient during cutaneous surgery is safe. There have been no adverse effects noted even in intrauterine fetal surgery in which high-voltage electric currents are used for up to 30 minutes.[60]

Design and suture choice

Excisions and closures should be designed with basic surgical principles in mind with the goal to decrease wound tension and orient closures within relaxed skin tension lines. Repair design may be more challenging on the abdomen and chest given the potentially higher wound tension. Longer lasting absorbing sutures such as polydiaxanone may minimize dehiscence or scar spread.

Postoperative Considerations

Analgesia

Acetaminophen, a selective cyclooxygenase-2 inhibitor, is FDA category B and generally considered safe.[32,35,61] One should not exceed the maximum recommended daily dose of 3 g, because a case of acetaminophen poisoning was reported in a pregnant patient taking 9 g/d for 2 weeks resulting in in fulminant hepatotoxicity and fetal demise.[62]

Opioid narcotics are FDA category C owing to the risk of neonatal respiratory depression from perinatal high doses and the risk of neonatal withdrawal from chronic maternal use.[2,63] If they are necessary to achieve adequate pain control, the lowest dose for the shortest duration is recommended.

Nonsteroidal antiinflammatory drugs (NSAIDs) and salicylates are typically not recommended during pregnancy, especially in the third trimester.[64] NSAIDs interfere with platelet function and can caused increased bleeding, as well as block prostaglandin synthesis.[64,65] NSAID use in the second trimester is reasonably safe, but has been associated with rare cases of fetal cryptorchidism, low birthweight, and asthma.[64,65] The FDA advises women to discontinue NSAIDs and aspirin in the last 3 months of pregnancy owing to risks of renal injury, oligohydramnios, and premature closure of the ductus arteriosus.[35,64] One study demonstrated that 1117 women exposed to NSAIDs in the first trimester did not have increased spontaneous abortion, increased birth defects, or pattern of major birth defects compared with 2229 nonexposed women.[66]

Antibiotics

The most commonly prescribed perioperative antibiotics in cutaneous surgery are penicillin-based derivatives and cephalosporins, which are FDA category B and deemed safe in pregnancy by the American Academy of Pediatrics. If needed, erythromycin, clindamycin, and sulfonamides are safe alternatives.[49,67–70] **Table 2** summarizes safe timings and risks.

Erythromycin (category B) is considered safe in pregnancy. However, prolonged use of the estolate form is associated with hepatotoxicity.[1,2,71] Although there is much safety data supporting its safety in the first trimester, 2 studies have indicated an increase in atrial ventricular septal defects (1.8%) and pyloric stenosis (0.2%) when used early in pregnancy.[2,72]

Although sulfonamides and nitrofurantoin have mixed evidence regarding association with birth defects, College of Obstetrics and Gynecology released a 2017 Committee Opinion stating sulfonamides and nitrofurantoin may continue to be used as first-line agents in treatment of urinary tract infections and other infections caused by susceptible organisms.[70] First trimester use is still acceptable when no other alternatives are available. Vancomycin is safe, even in the second and third trimesters.[68] Clindamycin and rifampin are also safe.

Most aminoglycosides can be used in short courses if required, but streptomycin should specifically be avoided owing to irreversible bilateral congenital deafness.[68,73] There is 1 report of gentamicin causing congenital defects, but the overall human data suggest a low risk.[68] Fluoroquinolones should also be avoided owing to classic

associations with bone and cartilage damage, renal toxicity, and cardiac defects.[68,73,74] Tetracyclines are category D and are contraindicated after the 15th week because they cross the placenta and bind to calcium, causing enamel hypoplasia, yellow discoloration of teeth, and inhibition of bone growth, as well as maternal hepatitis.[49,68,75] Inadvertent tetracycline use in the first trimester has not been associated with congenital malformations.[48,63,76]

Complications

Complications are similar to those in nonpregnant patients, and common issues include bleeding, infection, and scar formation. This article does not review all literature on postoperative complications, but highlights some key aspects to consider in pregnancy.

Hemostasis should be maintained similarly to nonpregnant patients. Postoperative bleeding can be controlled with pressure for 15 minutes, or exploration and cauterization of the wound if bleeding continues. Any hematomas should be evacuated immediately because they are a nidus for infection.

Dermatologic surgeons should continue to follow standard antiseptic procedures using the previously mentioned safe antiseptic agents. Antibiotic use for infection or prophylaxis should follow the guidelines in **Tables 2** and **3**. Regardless, pregnant women should never have appropriate antibiotic treatment withheld because untreated infections can lead to worse maternal and fetal complications.

There are no conclusive studies that indicate the best method to close the skin and reduce scarring. Studies in wound closure after cesarean section showed that a running subcuticular stitch provides superior outcome to staples, and buried vertical mattress sutures provide a superior outcome to subcuticular suture alone.[77–79] Use of intralesional triamcinolone, which is FDA category C, to treat hypertrophic scarring in pregnancy has not be specifically studied but intranasal triamcinolone use during pregnancy was not associated with congenital malformations, spontaneous abortion, or small for gestational age.[80] It may be appropriate to treat symptomatic hypertrophic scars.

Lactation

For breastfeeding patients, the anesthetic and antibiotic choices are the primary perioperative issues that can affect the infant through excretion in breastmilk.

Anesthetics

Lidocaine is considered compatible with lactation by the American Association of Pediatrics.[67]

Table 2
Safe times to use and risks of antibiotics in pregnant patients

Antibiotic	FDA Category	Safe Time to Use	Risks
Penicillins[35,46,49,89,97,108]	B	Anytime	Minimal
Cephalosporins/ cephamycins[35,49,68,89–91,97,108]	B	Anytime	Care should be taken at term with ceftriaxone, potential risk of kernicterus
Glycopeptides (vancomycin)[49,68,73,89]	B	Anytime	
Macrolides (azithromycin/ erythromycin)[35,46,49,68,71,72,89,97,109]	B	Anytime	Possible risk of cardiac septal defects and pyloric stenosis in 1st semester
Sulfonamides[49,68,70,89,108]	B	Anytime, when indicated	Mixed evidence, theoretic first trimester risk of folate antagonism when used with trimethoprim
Nitrofurantoin[49,68,70,73,89,108]	B	Anytime, when indicated	Mixed evidence
Clindamycin[49,68,73,89]	B	Anytime	
Rifampin[49,68,89,102]	B	Anytime	
Aminoglycosides (excluding streptomycin)[49,68,73,89,110]	C	Anytime, short courses only, extra care during first trimester	First trimester toxicity
Fluoroquinolones[49,68,73,89]	C	Avoid	Bone and cartilage damage, renal toxicity, cardiac defects
Clarithromycin/ telithromycin[49,68,89,96,109]	C	Avoid	
Streptomycin[49,68,89,110]	D	Avoid	Risk of irreversible bilateral congenital deafness
Tetracyclines[49,68,73,76,89,107]	D	Before the 15th week of gestation	After the 15th week can bind to calcium, causing discoloration of teeth and bones, teratogenic effects

A study of 27 women admitted for cesarean delivery received epidurals with 0.5% bupivacaine and 2% lidocaine. Infants were then breastfed with no adverse effects evident on APGAR scores or 24-hour postdelivery clinical examination.[81] Lidocaine and metabolite concentrations in breast milk are also extremely low.[82,83] The level of plasma lidocaine needed to treat neonatal seizures without adverse effects is much higher than that produced with local anesthetic use.[82–85] Thus, it is safe to breastfeed after lidocaine administration without needing to discard breastmilk.

Epinephrine is excreted in breastmilk but is poorly bioavailable and has a short life. Therefore, it is not likely to affect the infant. However, there is a lack of clear data. Low-dose infusion of epinephrine as part of epidural analgesia does not impair breastfeeding in nursing mothers.[86,87] Tharwat and colleagues[88] compared lidocaine 2% (n = 75) to lidocaine 2% plus epinephrine 1:200,000 (n = 70) after cesarean delivery. Patients who received epinephrine began breastfeeding at 89 minutes after surgery compared with 132 minutes for those receiving lidocaine alone. The difference was statistically significant.

Analgesics
The AAP considers both acetaminophen and ibuprofen compatible with breastfeeding.[67]

Antibiotics
Breastfeeding patients taking antibiotics should be counseled to watch for gastrointestinal distress, gut flora changes, and hypersensitivity reactions

Table 3
Antibiotic safety recommendation and risks during lactation

Antibiotic	FDA Category	Safety Recommendation	Risks
Penicillin	B	Considered safe	
Cephalosporins, first to third generation	B	Considered safe	
Macrolides	B	Considered safe	No published data on clarithromycin and telithromycin to date
Clindamycin	B	Considered safe	
Rifampin	B	Considered safe	
Sulfonamides	B	Considered safe, except in specific cases	Avoid in premature infants, infants with jaundice, and glucose-6-phosphate deficiency
Aminoglycosides	C	Considered safe	
Fluoroquinolones	C	Considered safe but not traditionally used	Theoretic concerns about joint formation, 1 case of infantile pseudomembranous colitis from ciprofloxacin
Tetracyclines	D	Considered safe but not traditionally used	Theoretic risk of tooth staining, but has never been reported in literature to date

in their infants, which may lead to diarrhea and dehydration.[68] **Table 3** summarizes antibiotic safety and risks in lactation.

Penicillin derivates, cephalosporins, macrolides, clindamycin, rifampin, and sulfonamides are considered safe for use during lactation by the AAP.[49,67,68,89–107] Tetracyclines and fluoroquinolones are both considered compatible with lactation by the AAP, although both are traditionally avoided.[67,74] Ciprofloxacin is avoided owing to theoretic concerns about affecting joint development, but studies indicate this is low risk, and concentrations in breast milk are low. There is 1 reported case of an infant developing pseudomembranous colitis after breastfeeding with maternal exposure to ciprofloxacin.[106] Similarly, tetracyclines have theoretic precautions to avoid exposure for fear of tooth staining, but this complication has never been reported in literature.[107]

SUMMARY

Cutaneous surgery can be performed safely and effectively in patients who are pregnant and breastfeeding, as long as proper considerations are given to all aspects of the procedure. To minimize risk factors to the fetus, surgery should be reserved for the second trimester and postpartum period, but can be done during other periods with relatively minor risk. Anesthetic, analgesic, and antibiotic selections should be undertaken thoughtfully with regard to risks and benefits, but selections can be made that will be safe during pregnancy and lactation. Thoughtful preparation and operative planning can result in safe and efficacious outcomes.

REFERENCES

1. Sweeney SM, Maloney ME. Pregnancy and dermatologic surgery. Dermatol Clin 2006;24(2):205–14.
2. Tyler KH, Zirwas MJ. Pregnancy and dermatologic therapy. J Am Acad Dermatol 2013;68(4):663–71.
3. Cunningham F, Leveno K, Bloom S, et al. Placentation, embryogenesis, and fetal development. In: Cunningham F, Leveno KJ, Bloom SL, editors. Williams obstetrics. New York: McGraw-Hill Education; 2014. p. 102. https://doi.org/10.1097/00007611-195710000-00029.
4. Andersson TM-L, Johansson ALV, Fredriksson I, et al. Cancer during pregnancy and the postpartum period: a population-based study. Cancer 2015;121(12):2072–7.
5. Moloney JB, Drury MI. The effect of pregnancy on the natural course of diabetic retinopathy. Am J Ophthalmol 1982;93(6):745–56.
6. Pack GT, Scharnagel IM. The prognosis for malignant melanoma in the pregnant woman. Cancer 1951;4(2):324–34.
7. Todd SP, Driscoll MS. Prognosis for women diagnosed with melanoma during, before, or after pregnancy: weighing the evidence. Int J Womens Dermatol 2017;3(1):26–9.
8. Martires KJ, Stein JA, Grant-Kels JM, et al. Meta-analysis concerning mortality for pregnancy-associated

melanoma. J Eur Acad Dermatol Venereol 2016; 30(10):e107–8.

9. Pagès C, Robert C, Thomas L, et al. Management and outcome of metastatic melanoma during pregnancy. Br J Dermatol 2010;162(2):274–81.

10. Fábián M, Tóth V, Somlai B, et al. Retrospective analysis of clinicopathological characteristics of pregnancy associated melanoma. Pathol Oncol Res 2015;21(4):1265–71.

11. Lens MB, Rosdahl I, Ahlbom A, et al. Effect of pregnancy on survival in women with cutaneous malignant melanoma. J Clin Oncol 2004;22(21): 4369–75.

12. O'Meara AT, Cress R, Xing G, et al. Malignant melanoma in pregnancy: a population-based evaluation. Cancer 2005;103(6):1217–26.

13. Bannister-Tyrrell M, Roberts CL, Hasovits C, et al. Incidence and outcomes of pregnancy-associated melanoma in New South Wales 1994-2008. Aust N Z J Obstet Gynaecol 2015;55(2):116–22.

14. Goldberg D, Maloney M. Dermatologic surgery and cosmetic procedures during pregnancy and the postpartum period. Dermatol Ther 2013;26(4): 321–30.

15. Alexander A, Harris RM, Grossman D, et al. Vulvar melanoma: diffuse melanosis and metastasis to the placenta. J Am Acad Dermatol 2004;50(2):293–8.

16. De Carolis S, Garofalo S, Degennaro VA, et al. Placental and infant metastasis of maternal melanoma: a new case. J Obstet Gynaecol 2015; 35(4):417–8.

17. Uthida-Tanaka AM, Sampaio MCA, Velho PENF, et al. Subcutaneous and cerebral cysticercosis. J Am Acad Dermatol 2004;50(2 Suppl):S14–7.

18. Perret-Court A, Fernandez C, Monestier S, et al. Métastase placentaire de mélanome: un nouveau cas et revue de la littérature. Ann Pathol 2010; 30(2):143–6.

19. Lakshminarayana P, Danson S, Suvarna K, et al. Atrial and placental melanoma metastasis: a case report and literature review. J Med Case Rep 2007;1(1):21.

20. Shuhaila A, Rohaizak M, Phang KS, et al. Maternal melanoma with placental metastasis. Singapore Med J 2008;49(3):e71–2. Available at: http://www.ncbi.nlm.nih.gov/pubmed/18362990. Accessed September 24, 2018.

21. Berk-Krauss J, Liebman TN, Stein JA. Pregnancy and melanoma: recommendations for clinical scenarios. Int J Women's Dermatol 2018;4(2):113–5.

22. Bieber AK, Martires KJ, Driscoll MS, et al. Nevi and pregnancy. J Am Acad Dermatol 2016;75(4): 661–6.

23. Andtbacka RHI, Donaldson MR, Bowles TL, et al. Sentinel lymph node biopsy for melanoma in pregnant women. Ann Surg Oncol 2013;20(2): 689–96.

24. Pandit-Taskar N, Dauer LT, Montgomery L, et al. Organ and fetal absorbed dose estimates from 99mTc-sulfur colloid lymphoscintigraphy and sentinel node localization in breast cancer patients. J Nucl Med 2006;47(7):1202–8. Available at: http://www.ncbi.nlm.nih.gov/pubmed/16818956. Accessed September 24, 2018.

25. Cordeiro CN, Gemignani ML. Breast cancer in pregnancy: avoiding fetal harm when maternal treatment is necessary. Breast J 2017;23(2): 200–5.

26. Toesca A, Gentilini O, Peccatori F, et al. Locoregional treatment of breast cancer during pregnancy. Gynecol Surg 2014;11(4):279–84.

27. Pham Dang N, Cassier S, Mulliez A, et al. Eight years' experience of sentinel lymph node biopsy in melanoma using lymphoscintigraphy and gamma probe detection after radiocolloid mapping. Dermatol Surg 2017;43(2):287–92.

28. Jeejeebhoy FM, Morrison LJ. Maternal cardiac arrest: a practical and comprehensive review. Emerg Med Int 2013;2013:1–8.

29. Lee KC, Korgavkar K, Dufresne RG, et al. Safety of cosmetic dermatologic procedures during pregnancy. Dermatol Surg 2013;39(11):1573–86.

30. Cengiz SB. The pregnant patient: considerations for dental management and drug use. Quintessence Int 2007;38(3):e133–42. Available at: http://www.ncbi.nlm.nih.gov/pubmed/17510722. Accessed September 24, 2018.

31. Cluver C, Novikova N, Hofmeyr GJ, et al. Maternal position during caesarean section for preventing maternal and neonatal complications. Cochrane Database Syst Rev 2013;(3):CD007623.

32. Crisan D, Treiber N, Kull T, et al. Chirurgische Behandlung von Melanomen in der Schwangerschaft: eine praktische Anleitung. J Dtsch Dermatol Ges 2016;14(6):585–94.

33. Higuchi H, Takagi S, Zhang K, et al. Effect of lateral tilt angle on the volume of the abdominal aorta and inferior vena cava in pregnant and nonpregnant women determined by magnetic resonance imaging. Anesthesiology 2015;122(2):286–93.

34. Kinsella SM. Lateral tilt for pregnant women: why 15 degrees? Anaesthesia 2003;58(9):835–7.

35. Richards KA, Stasko T. Dermatologic surgery and the pregnant patient. Dermatol Surg 2002;28(3): 248–56. Available at: http://www.ncbi.nlm.nih.gov/pubmed/11896778. Accessed September 26, 2018.

36. Schauberger CW, Rooney BL, Goldsmith L, et al. Peripheral joint laxity increases in pregnancy but does not correlate with serum relaxin levels. Am J Obstet Gynecol 1996;174(2):667–71.

37. Martin C, Varner MW. Physiologic changes in pregnancy: surgical implications. Clin Obstet Gynecol 1994;37(2):241–55.

38. Hill CC, Pickinpaugh J. Physiologic changes in pregnancy. Surg Clin North Am 2008;88(2):391–401.
39. Food and Drug Administration. Pregnancy and lactation labeling final rule 2014. p. 1–3. Available at: http://www.fda.gov/biologicsbloodvaccines/guidancecomplianceregulatoryinformation/actsrulesregulations/ucm445102.htm. Accessed September 25, 2018.
40. Lachenmeier DW. Safety evaluation of topical applications of ethanol on the skin and inside the oral cavity. J Occup Med Toxicol 2008;3(1):26.
41. Kramer A, Below H, Bieber N, et al. Quantity of ethanol absorption after excessive hand disinfection using three commercially available hand rubs is minimal and below toxic levels for humans. BMC Infect Dis 2007;7(1):117.
42. Garcia-Bournissen F, Finkelstein Y, Rezvani M, et al. Exposure to alcohol-containing medications during pregnancy. Can Fam Physician 2006;52:1067–8.
43. Arifeen SE, Mullany LC, Shah R, et al. The effect of cord cleansing with chlorhexidine on neonatal mortality in rural Bangladesh: a community-based, cluster-randomised trial. Lancet 2012;379(9820):1022–8.
44. Bachrach LK, Burrow GN, Gare DJ. Maternal-fetal absorption of povidone-iodine. J Pediatr 1984;104(1):158–9.
45. Findik RB, Yilmaz G, Celik HT, et al. Effect of povidone iodine on thyroid functions and urine iodine levels in caesarean operations. J Matern Fetal Neonatal Med 2014;27(10):1020–2.
46. Gormley DE. Cutaneous surgery and the pregnant patient. J Am Acad Dermatol 1990;23(2):269–79.
47. Fujinaga M, Mazze RI. Reproductive and teratogenic effects of lidocaine in Sprague-Dawley rats. Anesthesiology 1986;65(6):626–32.
48. Murase JE, Heller MM, Butler DC. Safety of dermatologic medications in pregnancy and lactation: part I. Pregnancy. J Am Acad Dermatol 2014;70(3):401.e1-14 [quiz: 415].
49. Heinonen OP, Sloane D, Shapiro S, editors. Birth defects and drugs in pregnancy. Littleton (CO): Publishing Sciences Group; 1977.
50. Hood DD, Dewan DM, James FM. Maternal and fetal effects of epinephrine in gravid ewes. Anesthesiology 1986;64(5):610–3.
51. Abboud TK, David S, Nagappala S, et al. Maternal, fetal, and neonatal effects of lidocaine with and without epinephrine for epidural anesthesia in obstetrics. Anesth Analg 1984;63(11):973–9. Available at: http://eutils.ncbi.nlm.nih.gov/entrez/eutils/elink.fcgi?dbfrom=pubmed&id=6496982&retmode=ref&cmd=prlinks%5Cnpapers3://publication/uuid/38CC4C7E-833C-4E45-8737-309FD569B8A5.
52. Malamed SF, Orr DL. Medical emergencies in the dental office. 7th edition. St Louis: Mosby; 2014. https://doi.org/10.1016/C2011-0-07159-4.
53. Lee JM, Shin TJ. Use of local anesthetics for dental treatment during pregnancy; safety for parturient. J Dent Anesth Pain Med 2017;17(2):81.
54. Kouba DJ, Lopiccolo MC, Alam M, et al. Guidelines for the use of local anesthesia in office-based dermatologic surgery. J Am Acad Dermatol 2016;74(6):1201–19.
55. Hasan B, Asif T, Hasan M. Lidocaine-induced systemic toxicity: a case report and review of literature. Cureus 2017;9(5):e1275.
56. Neal JM, Mulroy MF, Weinberg GL, American Society of Regional Anesthesia and Pain Medicine. American Society of Regional Anesthesia and pain medicine checklist for managing local anesthetic systemic toxicity: 2012 version. Reg Anesth Pain Med 2012;37. https://doi.org/10.1097/AAP.0b013e31822e0d8a.
57. Moore PA. Selecting drugs for the pregnant dental patient. J Am Dent Assoc 1998;129(9):1281–6.
58. Carruthers JA, Carruthers JDA, Poirier J, et al. Safety of lidocaine 15% and prilocaine 5% topical ointment used as local anesthesia for intense pulsed light treatment. Dermatol Surg 2010;36(7):1130–7.
59. McCleskey PE, Patel SM, Mansalis KA, et al. Serum lidocaine levels and cutaneous side effects after application of 23% lidocaine 7% tetracaine ointment to the face. Dermatol Surg 2013;39(1pt1):82–91.
60. Moreira CM, Amaral E. Use of electrocautery for coagulation and wound complications in Caesarean sections. ScientificWorldJournal 2014;2014:602375.
61. Hinz B, Cheremina O, Brune K. Acetaminophen (paracetamol) is a selective cyclooxygenase-2 inhibitor in man. FASEB J 2007;22(2):383–90.
62. Thornton SL, Minns AB. Unintentional chronic acetaminophen poisoning during pregnancy resulting in liver transplantation. J Med Toxicol 2012;8(2):176–8.
63. Leachman SA, Reed BR. The use of dermatologic drugs in pregnancy and lactation. Dermatol Clin 2006;24(2):167–97.
64. Bloor M, Paech M. Nonsteroidal anti-inflammatory drugs during pregnancy and the initiation of lactation. Anesth Analg 2013;116(5):1063–75.
65. Nezvalová-Henriksen K, Spigset O, Nordeng H. Effects of ibuprofen, diclofenac, naproxen, and piroxicam on the course of pregnancy and pregnancy outcome: a prospective cohort study. BJOG 2013;120(8):948–59.
66. Dathe K, Fietz AK, Pritchard LW, et al. No evidence of adverse pregnancy outcome after exposure to ibuprofen in the first trimester – evaluation of the national Embryotox cohort. Reprod Toxicol 2018;79:32–8.
67. American Academy of Pediatrics Committee on Drugs. Transfer of drugs and other chemicals into human milk. Pediatrics 2001;108(3):776–89.

68. Briggs GG, Freeman RK. Drugs in pregnancy and lactation: a reference guide to fetal and neonatal risk. 10th edition. Philadelphia: Wolters Kluwer Health Adis (ESP); 2014. Available at: https://www.scopus.com/inward/record.uri?eid=2-s2.0-84971450082&partnerID=40&md5=fe29606e1e308c2878d6c9544ef22250.

69. Hernández-Díaz S, Werler MM, Walker AM, et al. Neural tube defects in relation to use of folic acid antagonists during pregnancy. Am J Epidemiol 2001;153(10):961–8. Available at: http://www.ncbi.nlm.nih.gov/pubmed/11384952. Accessed September 26, 2018.

70. Committee on Obstetric Practice. Committee opinion 717: sulfonamides, nitrofurantoin, and risk of birth defects. Obstet Gynecol 2017. https://doi.org/10.1097/aog.0000000000002300.

71. McCormack WM, George H, Donner A, et al. Hepatotoxicity of erythromycin estolate during pregnancy. Antimicrob Agents Chemother 1977;12(5):630–5.

72. Källén B, Danielsson BR. Fetal safety of erythromycin. An update of Swedish data. Eur J Clin Pharmacol 2014;70(3):355–60.

73. Bookstaver PB, Bland CM, Griffin B, et al. A review of antibiotic use in pregnancy. Pharmacotherapy 2015;35(11):1052–62.

74. Kaguelidou F, Turner MA, Choonara I, et al. Ciprofloxacin use in neonates. Pediatr Infect Dis J 2011;30(2):e29–37.

75. Czeizel AE, Rockenbauer M. A population-based case-control teratologic study of oral oxytetracycline treatment during pregnancy. Eur J Obstet Gynecol Reprod Biol 2000;88(1):27–33.

76. Jick H, Slone D. Tetracycline and drug-attributed rises in blood urea nitrogen. A report from the Boston Collaborative drug surveillance program. JAMA 1972;220(3):377–9. Available at: http://www.ncbi.nlm.nih.gov/pubmed/5067108. Accessed September 25, 2018.

77. Frishman GN, Schwartz T, Hogan JW. Closure of Pfannenstiel skin incisions. Staples vs. subcuticular suture. J Reprod Med 1997;42(10):627–30. Available at: http://www.ncbi.nlm.nih.gov/pubmed/9350017. Accessed September 26, 2018.

78. Yang J, Kim KH, Song YJ, et al. Cosmetic outcomes of cesarean section scar; subcuticular suture versus intradermal buried suture. Obstet Gynecol Sci 2018;61(1):79.

79. Buresch AM, Van Arsdale A, Ferzli M, et al. Comparison of subcuticular suture type for skin closure after cesarean delivery: a randomized controlled trial. Obstet Gynecol 2017;130(3):521–6.

80. Bérard A, Sheehy O, Kurzinger ML, et al. Intranasal triamcinolone use during pregnancy and the risk of adverse pregnancy outcomes. J Allergy Clin Immunol 2016;138(1):97–104.e7.

81. Ortega D, Viviand X, Lorec AM, et al. Excretion of lidocaine and bupivacaine in breast milk following epidural anesthesia for cesarean delivery. Acta Anaesthesiol Scand 1999;43(4):394–7.

82. Rey E, Radvanyi-Bouvet MF, Bodiou C, et al. Intravenous lidocaine in the treatment of convulsions in the neonatal period: monitoring plasma levels. Ther Drug Monit 1990;12(4):316–20.

83. Giuliani M, Grossi GB, Pileri M, et al. Could local anesthesia while breast-feeding be harmful to infants? J Pediatr Gastroenterol Nutr 2001;32(2):142–4.

84. Lundqvist M, Ågren J, Hellström-Westas L, et al. Efficacy and safety of lidocaine for treatment of neonatal seizures. Acta Paediatr 2013;102(9):863–7.

85. Dryden RM, Lo MW. Breast milk lidocaine levels in tumescent liposuction. Plast Reconstr Surg 2000;105(6):2267–8.

86. Radzyminski S. The effect of ultra low dose epidural analgesia on newborn breastfeeding behaviors. J Obstet Gynecol Neonatal Nurs 2003;32(3):322–31.

87. Chang ZM, Heaman MI. Epidural analgesia during labor and delivery: effects on the initiation and continuation of effective breastfeeding. J Hum Lact 2005;21(3):305–14.

88. Tharwat AA, Yehia AH, Wahba KA, et al. Efficacy and safety of post-cesarean section incisional infiltration with lidocaine and epinephrine versus lidocaine alone in reducing postoperative pain: a randomized controlled double-blinded clinical trial. J Turk Ger Gynecol Assoc 2016;17(1):1–5.

89. Medicine NL of. Drugs and lactation database (LactMed) | HealthData.Gov. Bethesda (MD): National Library of Medicine; 2018. Available at: https://healthdata.gov/dataset/drugs-and-lactation-database-lactmed.

90. Kafetzis DA, Siafas CA, Georgakopoulos PA, et al. Passage of cephalosporins and amoxicillin into the breast milk. Acta Paediatr Scand 1981;70(3):285–8.

91. Kafetzis DA, Brater DC, Fanourgakis JE, et al. Ceftriaxone distribution between maternal blood and fetal blood and tissues at parturition and between blood and milk postpartum. Antimicrob Agents Chemother 1983;23(6):870–3.

92. Branebjerg PE, Heisterberg L. Blood and milk concentrations of ampicillin in mothers treated with pivampicillin and in their infants. J Perinat Med 1987;15(6):555–8.

93. Matheson I, Samseth M, Sande HA. Ampicillin in breast milk during puerperal infections. Eur J Clin Pharmacol 1988;34(6):657–9.

94. Sørensen HT, Skriver MV, Pedersen L, et al. Risk of infantile hypertrophic pyloric stenosis after maternal postnatal use of macrolides. Scand J Infect Dis 2003;35(2):104–6.

95. Ito S, Blajchman A, Stephenson M, et al. Prospective follow-up of adverse reactions in breast-fed infants exposed to maternal medication. Am J Obstet Gynecol 1993;168(5):1393–9.

96. Goldstein LH, Berlin M, Tsur L, et al. The safety of macrolides during lactation. Breastfeed Med 2009;4(4):197–200.

97. Zhang Y, Zhang Q, Xu Z. Tissue and body fluid distribution of antibacterial agents in pregnant and lactating women. Zhonghua Fu Chan Ke Za Zhi 1997;32(5):288–92 [in Chinese].

98. Steen B, Rane A. Clindamycin passage into human milk. Br J Clin Pharmacol 1982;13(5):661–4.

99. Mann CF. Clindamycin and breast-feeding. Pediatrics 1980;66(6). Available at: http://pediatrics. aappublications.org/content/66/6/1030.3.long. Accessed September 25, 2018.

100. Blumberg HM, Burman WJ, Chaisson RE, et al. American Thoracic Society/Centers for Disease Control and Prevention/Infectious Diseases Society of America: treatment of tuberculosis. Am J Respir Crit Care Med 2003;167(4):603–62.

101. Peters C, Nienhaus A. Fallbericht einer beruflich erworbenen tuberkulose in der schwangerschaft. Pneumologie 2008;62(11):695–8.

102. Keskin N, Yilmaz S. Pregnancy and tuberculosis: to assess tuberculosis cases in pregnancy in a developing region retrospectively and two case reports. Arch Gynecol Obstet 2008;278(5):451–5.

103. Ozturk Z, Tatliparmak A. Leprosy treatment during pregnancy and breastfeeding: a case report and brief review of literature. Dermatol Ther 2017; 30(1):e12414.

104. Gardner DK, Gabbe SG, Harter C. Simultaneous concentrations of ciprofloxacin in breast milk and in serum in mother and breast-fed infant. Clin Pharm 1992;11(4):352–4. Available at: http://www.ncbi.nlm. nih.gov/pubmed/1563233. Accessed September 25, 2018.

105. Chiesa OA, Idowu OR, Heller D, et al. A Holstein cow-calf model for the transfer of ciprofloxacin through milk after a long-term intravenous infusion. J Vet Pharmacol Ther 2013;36(5): 425–33.

106. Harmon T, Burkhart G, Harry A. Perforated pseudomembranous colitis in the breast-fed infant. J Pediatr Surg 1992;27(6):744–6.

107. Konicoff NG, Posner AC, Prigot A. Tetracycline in obstetric infections. Antibiot Annu 1955-1956;3: 345–8. Available at: http://www.ncbi.nlm.nih.gov/ pubmed/13355291. Accessed September 25, 2018.

108. Ailes EC, Gilboa SM, Gill SK, et al. Association between antibiotic use among pregnant women with urinary tract infections in the first trimester and birth defects, National Birth Defects Prevention Study 1997 to 2011. Birth Defects Res A Clin Mol Teratol 2016;106(11):940–9.

109. Bérard A, Sheehy O, Zhao J-P, et al. Use of macrolides during pregnancy and the risk of birth defects: a population-based study. Pharmacoepidemiol Drug Saf 2015;24(12):1241–8.

110. Czeizel AE, Rockenbauer M, Olsen J, et al. A teratological study of aminoglycoside antibiotic treatment during pregnancy. Scand J Infect Dis 2000;32(3):309–13.

Optimizing Patient Safety in Dermatologic Surgery

Cory Smith, BS, Divya Srivastava, MD, Rajiv I. Nijhawan, MD*

KEYWORDS

- Patient safety • Physician safety • Office-based surgery • Dermatologic surgery
- Outpatient surgery • Site identification • Wrong-site surgery prevention • Cutaneous surgery

KEY POINTS

- Dermatologic surgery is low risk overall with low reported rates of complications such as infection and bleeding.
- Strict oversight of the clinic, such as medication administration safety and adherence to sterilization protocols, helps to optimize patient safety in the outpatient setting.
- There are many methods to minimize infection risk, including strict hand hygiene and judicious use of oral antibiotics.
- In general, all blood thinners should be continued perioperatively to minimize the risk of a thromboembolic event because the risk of bleeding can likely be managed without long-term negative outcomes.
- Implementation of photographs within the dermatology clinic, including patient-acquired photographs, can be extremely helpful to reduce the risk for wrong-site surgery.

INTRODUCTION

The publication *To Err is Human: Building a Safer Health System* was the first major attempt to look inward on the medical field and focus on the consequences of medical errors.[1] Dermatology, which involves an abundance of outpatient surgery, has been under scrutiny by both regulators and other surgical-based specialties. Adverse events in dermatologic surgery are overall minimal; however, increased strategies to optimize patient safety should continue to be implemented to maximize patient outcomes.

The annual financial burden of medical errors on the national health system was estimated to be between $17 billion to $29 billion in early studies.[2] One easily overlooked reason for this figure in hospital systems is the opportunity cost for mistakes. Although damaging errors have obvious financial repercussions, there is also considerable cost to mitigating adverse effects before they take place. As an example, an error that negates the results from a laboratory test would need to be recollected and resubmitted at additional costs. Outside of the financial realm, errors result in decreased faith in the medical field, which can last for generations to the detriment of the public's health.

There is still much to be done in discovering and implementing systems to reduce errors and improve patient outcomes in the overall practice of medicine. This article focuses on several ways to optimize patient safety in dermatologic surgery and outpatient-based surgery, such as strict clinic oversight with items like vial safety, management of sharps, infection prevention, and correct surgical site identification.

IMPORTANCE OF STRICT OVERSIGHT IN THE CLINIC

Physicians are viewed as leaders of the medical team, and thus they bear the responsibility of strict oversight of their clinics and staff members. It is

---

Disclosure: The authors have nothing to disclose.
University of Texas Southwestern Medical Center, 5939 Harry Hines Boulevard, Suite 400, Dallas, TX 75390, USA
* Corresponding author.
E-mail address: Rajiv.nijhawan@utsw.edu

Dermatol Clin 37 (2019) 319–328
https://doi.org/10.1016/j.det.2019.02.006

critical for dermatologists to understand all aspects of their practices, because lapses in certain clinical aspects can lead to significant patient safety concerns. Similarly, it is just as important that staff adhere to safe practices to ensure all team members' safety as well.

The Occupational Safety and Health Administration's (OSHA) Bloodborne Pathogens Standard is a guide created to protect workers from needlestick-related disease transmission.[3] Although compliance with these protocols is mandatory, there is concern for adherence by the health care system.[4] In the decade following the publication of OSHA's revised guidelines in 2001, approximately 130,000 patients had been at least potentially exposed to viruses such as hepatitis C (HCV), hepatitis B, and human immunodeficiency virus (HIV) as a result of deviations from guidelines.[4] For workers, the number exposed is estimated to be vastly larger at more than 800,000 annually, with a large portion going unreported.[5] Because of the prevalence of injuries to patients and health care personnel alike, both OSHA and the Centers for Medicare and Medicaid Services (CMS) have increased their unannounced inspections of ambulatory surgery centers, and subsequent fines for those who are noncompliant.[4] Accordingly, medical personnel must ensure their practices are aligned with current standards of practice.

Medication Administration Safety

Dermatologic surgeons administer medications in clinics on a daily basis. Most injectable medications, such as lidocaine with epinephrine, triamcinolone, and neurotoxin, are low risk. Regardless, standardized protocols to safely draw up, label, and administer these medications should be in place in the office.

Errors related to injectable medications have resulted in injury to patients. A 2008 study by Fischer and colleagues[6] traced HCV infection from 3 unrelated patients to a single clinic where they all had received a colonoscopy. These clinics were found to be reusing single-use medication vials between multiple patients, resulting in transmission of HCV.[6] In one survey of provider practices in various clinics and hospitals, 6% admitted to reusing single-use vials on separate patients and 15% reported using the same needle multiple times to withdraw from multiuse vials.[7] In 2012, numerous patients died in the Boston area of fungal meningitis linked to contaminated compounded drugs. These errors have prompted regulatory and accrediting bodies such as the Centers for Disease Control and Prevention (CDC), Food and Drug Administration (FDA), United States Pharmacopeia (USP), and Joint Commission on Accreditation of Healthcare Organizations to establish guidelines for safe administration of in-office medications. Many of these guidelines are pending at the time of publication, and physicians should refer to state and federal regulations to ensure compliance with safety standards.

Proper labeling of medication vials is the first step in tackling medication misuse. According to The Joint Commission (2014) guidelines, this label should include the vial opening date, expiration date, ideal storage conditions, and use type (multiple vs single). Furthermore, to avoid accidental misuse, these vials should not be stored in patient or procedure rooms but in a separate room specific for medications.[8] In the second step, The Joint Commission (2014) included procedural guidelines, which must be followed for both single-use and multiuse vials (**Box 1**).[8] These recommendations are well summarized by The Safe Injection Practices Coalition as "one needle, one syringe, only one time"[9] (see **Box 1**).

Some controversy exists with multiuse vials in dermatology. According to studies, botulinum toxin can be safely reconstituted and then stored for up to 4 weeks without alteration in effectiveness or contamination risk.[10] In addition, it is safe to use vials to treat multiple patients if sterile

---

Box 1
2014 The Joint Commission guidelines on vial safety

- All syringes drawn from multiuse vials should be labeled when prepared. Proper labeling of all vials includes vial opening date, expiration date, ideal storage conditions, and use type (multiple vs single).

- Discard vials that are labeled improperly or found in the incorrect location (eg, in a procedure room), even if unopened.

- Discard single-use vials immediately.

- Each vial must be wiped with 70% alcohol and allowed to dry before every needle puncture.

- Only brand-new syringes are used to withdraw from multiuse vials. After a needle exits a vial, it must not reenter, even to draw additional liquid.

- Syringes should never be reused on another patient. Similarly, multidose delivery pens cannot be used on more than a single patient.

Data from The Joint Commission. Preventing infection from the misuse of vials. *Sentinel Event Alert.* 2014(52):1–6.

technique is used to prepare and administer the medication and there is no cross contamination of needles that are used on patients.[10]

Studies also support safe mixing of lidocaine with sodium bicarbonate for use in office. Pate and colleagues[11] showed that syringes properly prepared with aseptic technique and filled with lidocaine alone, lidocaine with epinephrine, lidocaine with sodium bicarbonate, and lidocaine with both epinephrine and sodium bicarbonate and stored for 4 weeks in controlled cold temperatures are not prone to bacterial or fungal infection. It will be essential for dermatologists to derive safe protocols for in-office medication administration and maintain compliance with state and federal regulations.

Sharps Safety

Sharps injuries are another important aspect of the dermatology clinic with implications to both provider and patient safety. Best-practice recommendations for needle safety have varied over the years. Previous recommendations of recapping every syringe have recently been refuted.[12] Unwala and Jacob[12] (2006) point to the recommendations from OSHA's Bloodborne Pathogens Standard, which recommends needles not be recapped. The authors instead recommend use of more recent safety-engineered syringes.[12] In addition, it is important to track and discard sharps immediately after use and/or procedure completion without any distraction. Easy access to sharps containers without much movement, such as ensuring sharps boxes on both sides of a procedure chair, eases disposal of these sharps. Blade removal systems can help safely remove blades from their handles without risking team member injury.

Maximizing patient safety as it relates to sharps is similarly important. Appropriately labeling sharps and trays with patient identifiers prevents the risk of using them on a different patient. Proper sterilization is imperative, and ensuring that all sterilization machines are appropriately serviced is similarly critical. By following these guidelines, the risk of sharps being left at bedside is minimized, and accidental injury to both patients and practitioners is greatly decreased.

INFECTION PREVENTION

One notable risk for any type of surgery is infection; however, multiple studies within dermatology have shown infection rates to be low. Multiple studies have found office-based clean surgical procedures to have infection rates between 0.07% and 4.25%.[13–15] In an even more recent prospective study of patients undergoing Mohs micrographic surgery (MMS), overall rates were found to be just 0.91%,[16] showing that infection rates remain low even with use of clean surgical technique alone and absence of prophylactic antibiotics. Dermatologists and dermatologic surgeons can still strive to yield even lower infection rates with implementation of best practices, which also may mean dispelling certain myths.

Sterile Versus Nonsterile Gloves

There is variation among dermatologists' preference for using sterile versus nonsterile gloves during procedures. Many assume that the use of nonsterile gloves introduces increased risk of infection to the patient, but there is no significant difference in infection rates. With regard to MMS, studies have shown no difference in infection rates in tumor extirpation between nonsterile and sterile gloves.[17,18] Furthermore, the use of nonsterile gloves serves the added benefit of reducing health care costs, with one study suggesting a $4.03 reduction in cost per case of gloves.[17] Clean, nonsterile gloves have been shown to be noninferior to sterile gloves in infection rates for MMS as well as with reconstruction, and they reduce the time for surgical preparation and operating costs.

Antiseptics

At present, there exists no definitive guideline for antiseptic use in dermatologic surgery. Multiple antiseptics are available for use in cutaneous surgery, including isopropyl alcohol, povidone, and chlorhexidine. Although there are multiple options, each has unique properties. In one Cochrane Review of 7 trials, Edwards and colleagues[19] were unable to find sufficient evidence for the superiority of any antiseptic compared with the others. As such, they recommended choosing antiseptics based on potential side effects and costs. In contrast, other larger studies have found associations between preoperative chlorhexidine use and a lower postoperative infection risk in MMS.[20] Importantly, the benefit shown was minimal. Alam and colleagues[20] estimated the absolute risk reduction of preoperative chlorhexidine use to be between 0.45% and 0.53% and nonadditive with sterile gloves or antibiotic prophylaxis with MMS. This exceptionally small absolute risk reduction puts into question the utility of using these types of preoperative antiseptic scrubs.

Many studies have shown differences in bacterial colonization rates with the use of different antiseptics. One literature review attempted to evaluate the best preoperative regimen and determined iodophor and chlorhexidine alcohols to be more effective than aqueous solutions at decreasing bacterial colonization. However, they ultimately found the evidence of any particular regimen to be weak and recommended selection based on practitioner preference.[21]

Preoperative Decolonization

Up to 30% of the general population are carriers of *Staphylococcus aureus* in their anterior nares, which is commonly thought to cause postoperative nosocomial infections and is thus considered an independent risk factor for surgical site infections (SSIs) in dermatologic surgery.[22–24] In theory, eliminating the bacteria in the nares should decrease nosocomial infections. In one study, the use of topical decolonization with intranasal mupirocin and chlorhexidine body wash was shown to reduce rates of SSI after Mohs for those carriers.[25] Furthermore, topical treatment seems to work better for decolonization compared with oral antibiotics, with less risk.[26] In 1999, CDC guidelines recommended a preoperative shower with chlorhexidine gluconate to reduce bacterial colonization before procedures.[27] However, a more recent Cochrane Review of 7 trials found no definitive evidence for this practice reducing SSIs. Instead, they recommended efforts be spent in areas better proved to reduce poor outcomes.[28]

Data supporting the use of decolonization strategies to reduce SSI risk raise the question of how to advise patients who will be undergoing dermatologic surgery. Options include testing the nares and treating those who are carriers of *S aureus*, or treating patients empirically before their operations.[25] Both options have some benefits and drawbacks, but little research has been done thus far to determine optimal practice guidelines. At present, it is best left to practitioners to determine whether to test and treat, not treat, or do neither based on the patient's risk factors and location of surgery.

Preoperative Hair Removal

Dermatologic surgery often involves hair-bearing skin. However, based on CDC guidelines, preoperative hair removal is not advised, and should only be done if the hair may interfere with the specific procedure. In these instances, certain guidelines are to be adhered to so SSI risk is minimized. Hair should be clipped with as little skin contact as possible to avoid microabrasions, which may allow bacterial entry. Second, hair should not be shaved immediately before the procedure.[21,27]

Strict Hand Hygiene

The CDC considers hand washing to be one of the most important factors to reduce risk of infection (**Box 2**).[29] Proper practice and complete team adherence is essential. Hand washing with soap and water should last for at least 15 seconds, which has been shown to reduce bacterial counts by approximately 90%.[30] Although the CDC overall recommends alcohol-based hand sanitation to be used predominately, there are instances when hand washing with soap and water is still superior, including before eating, after using the restroom, when hands are visibly soiled, and with exposure to *Clostridium difficile*.[31] Alcohol-based hand sanitizers are not effective against spores and lack persistent activity. Another commonly recommended practice is avoidance of artificial fingernails and extenders.[31] It is essential to consider and reevaluate the execution of these guidelines in practice because hand washing is one of the easiest and most basic measures to improve patient outcomes in dermatologic practice (see **Box 2**).

Limit Topical Antibiotics

Although theoretically the use of prophylactic topical antibiotics should reduce risks for SSI, studies have proved otherwise. The American Academy of Dermatology recommends against

---

Box 2
Key recommendations for when hand hygiene should be performed

- Before touching a patient, even if gloves will be worn
- Before exiting patient's room
- After contact with blood or other bodily fluids, such as wound dressings
- Before preparing an aseptic task (eg, preparing an injection)
- If hands will be moving from a contaminated body site (eg, open wound) to a clean body site on same patient
- After gloves are removed

Data from Boyce JM, Pittet D, Healthcare Infection Control Practices Advisory C, Force HSAIHHT. Guideline for Hand Hygiene in Health-Care Settings. Recommendations of the Healthcare Infection Control Practices Advisory Committee and the HICPAC/SHEA/APIC/IDSA Hand Hygiene Task Force. Society for Healthcare Epidemiology of America/Association for Professionals in Infection Control/Infectious Diseases Society of America. *MMWR Recomm Rep.* 2002;51(RR-16):1–45, quiz CE41-44.

this indication in its Choosing Wisely campaigns. Studies have shown that the benefits do not outweigh the risks of these topical antibiotics, especially after clean surgical procedures as performed in dermatologic surgery. A randomized controlled trial showed similar infection rates between topical bacitracin and white petrolatum application.[32] Similarly, in a study of mupirocin ointment applied before dressings, there was no infection rate reduction compared with no ointment.[33] The practice of limiting topical antibiotics minimizes the risk for developing allergic contact dermatitis.

Oral Antibiotics

Judicious use of oral antibiotics is another important component of patient safety (for more information on this topic, see Hillary Johnson-Jahangir and Neha Agrawal's article, "Perioperative Antibiotic Use in Cutaneous Surgery," in this issue). The overall recommendation is to minimize unnecessary administration of oral antibiotics. Overall key points on minimizing infection risk are listed in **Box 3**.

CONTINUE BLOOD THINNERS

Bleeding is another potential risk with dermatologic surgery, but its overall occurrence is low. With an increasing number of patients on

---

anticoagulation and newer anticoagulants on the market, there are often questions about how to manage these medications perioperatively. To continue or discontinue anticoagulation is a balancing act between the risk of perioperative bleeding and the risk of thromboembolic complications.[34] It is estimated that between 25% and 38% of patients undergoing dermatologic surgery take medication that alters hemostatic mechanisms.[34–36] Although there is an increased postoperative bleeding risk in patients taking more than 1 anticoagulant, especially those on both warfarin and clopidogrel, overall risk of continuation remains low.[34–36] Many studies have shown no real increase in major complications with anticoagulation continuation, while showing increases in life-threatening consequences with their discontinuation.[37–39] Even in patients with multiple comorbidities, bleeding and infection risks were negligible compared with risks of discontinuation.[40] However, there is concern for continuing anticoagulation with certain surgical procedures, such as complex staged flaps, in which there may be an increase in serious postoperative bleeding risk.[41]

It is thought that the newer thrombin inhibitors and factor Xa inhibitors, such as dabigatran and rivaroxaban, are similar to traditional anticoagulants in terms of safety in cutaneous surgery.[42,43] One small retrospective study of patients on these newer oral anticoagulants undergoing MMS reported no severe hemorrhagic complications.[42] A separate study on rivaroxaban reported the benefit of continuing antithrombotic therapy with the caveat of a likely increased risk with complex flap closures.[43] A more recent study involving dabigatran, apixaban, and rivaroxaban reported only occasional mild bleeding complications but showed no significant difference in poor outcomes between older and newer anticoagulants.[44] However, many of the recent studies on new oral anticoagulants have small sample sizes, and further evaluation is warranted.

Overall, the risk of thromboembolic events from discontinuing anticoagulants exceeds the minor risk of postoperative bleeding with continuation; consequently, these medications should generally be continued.[34,40,45] In practice, surgeons must consider anatomic location of the surgery, procedure type, and other related factors on a case-by-case basis when deciding whether to continue or stop anticoagulation.[37]

KNOW YOUR ANATOMY

Dermatologic surgeons must also be aware of important anatomic considerations when planning a procedure preoperatively. The major danger

---

> **Box 3**
> **Overall infection prevention strategies**
>
> - Strict hand hygiene is a critical and simple step in minimizing patient infection risk.
> - There is no difference in infection rates with the use of sterile versus nonsterile gloves when used in dermatologic surgery. Nonsterile gloves have an added cost-reduction benefit.
> - In dermatologic surgery, hair trimming should be done only if necessary, and clippers should be used rather than razors to minimize risk of SSI.
> - There is no difference in infection rates when only white petrolatum is applied topically to clean surgical wounds compared with topical antibiotics. In addition, there are lower rates of allergic contact dermatitis with white petrolatum without risking organism resistance.
> - There is limited indicated benefit to oral antibiotic prophylaxis in dermatologic surgery, because there are already low rates of infection with clean surgical procedures. Of note, oral antibiotics have their own inherent risks as well.

zones of the face are named as such because of relative locations of important vessels and nerves. Accidental transection of the temporal branch of the facial nerve can yield unilateral forehead paralysis.[46] Inadvertent intravascular injection of injectable fillers may result in serious side effects, such as necrosis and vision loss.[47] Necrosis is typically caused by accidental injection of filler into the arterial system, resulting in downstream occlusion. Signs of this mistake include pallor, livedo reticularis, slow capillary refill, dusky appearance, and pain.[48] Vision loss is most commonly seen following soft tissue augmentation injections in the periocular/central face area, and avoidance requires awareness and early recognition.[49,50]

TAKE PHOTOGRAPHS

A sometimes-underused tool in dermatology offices is the use of proper photography, which can reduce common errors in cutaneous surgery. Pictures can show patients' baseline asymmetry, can help plan procedures, and are helpful intraoperatively because patients sometimes misgauge the size and/or location of their defects. One of the most beneficial aspects of photography as it relates to patient safety is reducing wrong-site surgery errors.

The Joint Commission classifies wrong site and wrong surgery as sentinel events, and as a result requires the reporting and investigation of these events regardless of their outcomes.[51] With the goal of preventing adverse events in health care, The National Quality Forum created criteria for these serious reportable events, which primarily include wrong site, wrong patient, and wrong procedure.[51] To rectify these errors, they recommend using preprocedure verification, marking the procedure site (ideally with the patient's input), and the use of a time-out before procedure initiation to confirm patient, site, and procedure.[51]

Identifying the correct biopsy site is essential, but there are multiple challenges to achieving this step. When biopsy sites are adjacent to previous biopsy or surgical sites or within a field of extensive actinic damage, both the practitioner and patient may struggle with correctly identifying the proper site before a procedure.[52] These difficulties are amplified when the duration between biopsy and time of procedure is longer, when documentation of the biopsy site is lacking (eg, without adequate photography), and with patients' frequent inability to remember their biopsy site.[52] With clinical examination alone, patients are unable to correctly identify biopsy sites in 16.6% to 29% of cases, whereas dermatologists are unable to correctly identify 5.9% to 12% of times.[53–56]

Self-acquired photographs or selfies can also be helpful to reduce wrong-site surgery, and were shown to significantly improve patients' ability to identify their own biopsy sites.[57] A study of 300 Mohs surgeons reported that 14% of dermatologic malpractice cases were caused by wrong-site surgery,[58] which is perceived as the most serious error among dermatologists.[59] As a result, wrong-site and wrong-procedure errors affect both the patient and the physician, and everything possible must be implemented with clinical practice to ensure correct surgical site identification (**Box 4**).

Self-acquired photographs can also be helpful for triaging postoperative concerns in dermatologic surgery, offering increased convenience to the patients as well as expedited triaging.[61] All patients who sent a photograph when calling with a postoperative issue reported alleviation of their concerns after receiving recommendations via the telephone.[61]

SMOKE PLUME

There is increasing awareness of the potential mutagenic particles released with smoke plume from electrocautery, which can produce measureable amounts of polycyclic aromatic hydrocarbons and can potentially penetrate through medical masks into the respiratory tract.[62–64] Smoke extractors and high-efficiency masks (eg, respiratory masks) may be used to reduce exposure to the smoke plume.[61,65] Because human papilloma virus (HPV) has been isolated in smoke samples,[65] it also begets the question of whether health care

---

Box 4
Tips for correct surgical site identification

- Take photographs: 89% of Mohs surgeons agree this is most helpful to identify biopsy sites
- Wood lamp examination
- Noninvasive imaging, such as dermoscopy or confocal microscopy, if available
- Markings on anatomic diagrams or hand-drawn sketches
- Curettage of suspicious site
- Gauze abrasion of site
- Triangulation measurements from nearby anatomic locations
- Photographs of biopsy sites with smartphones

Data from Refs.[52,53,57,60]

> **Box 5**
> **General patient safety recommendations for the dermatology clinic**
>
> - Good lighting.
> - The clinic should be latex free.
> - Side rails for elderly patients to prevent falls.
> - Ensuring the procedure chair is at its lowest level when practitioner is not in room.
> - All necessary instruments and materials are readily available.
> - Sugar/juice should be available in case patients become hypoglycemic
> - Patients should be reclined even just slightly when receiving injections in case a vasovagal episode occurs. Vasovagal episodes are the most common occurrence, and placing patients in Trendelenburg position, using smelling salts, and ice packs on the neck can all help mitigate these symptoms.
> - For exceedingly rare cases of allergy and/or anaphylaxis, antihistamines and intramuscular epinephrine should be available.[66]
> - In case patients experience signs of cardiac arrest, an automated external defibrillator should be available.[66]
> - Patients should be reclined in cases in which tumor may invade into the calvarium or with bone burring, because air emboli have been reported in seated patients.[67]

workers should be vaccinated with the HPV vaccine.

GENERAL RECOMMENDATIONS

There are also some general practice recommendations to ensure optimal patient safety within the dermatology clinic (**Box 5**).

SUMMARY

With the changing health care climate, there is increasing emphasis on patient safety/outcomes to measure physician success. In the past few decades, office-based surgery has been under increased scrutiny. However, investigations have overall shown complications for all office-based procedures to be rare (<1%) under local anesthesia, with increasing risk with increased sedation.[68] For dermatologists, complications are estimated to be even lower at less than 0.5%.[68] One study of patients undergoing skin cancer excision under local anesthesia reported no lidocaine toxicity, and the minimal adverse events that were reported consisted of minor dizziness

related to epinephrine.[69] Complications from large flaps and grafts performed in the outpatient setting have also been shown to be infrequent and non–life threatening.[70] Dermatologic surgery procedures performed in the outpatient setting have proved to be not only lower risk but also significantly more cost-effective.[71] Dermatologists and dermatologic surgeons must continue to collect and report data from office-based surgeries to highlight the benefits to patients, the general population, and also payers. These data will allow practitioners to identify high-risk practices and better mitigate risk for patients, as well as to create sufficient data to defend the safety of office-based surgery.[68]

REFERENCES

1. Kohn LT, Donaldson MS, Corrigan J. To err is human: building a safer health system. Washington, DC: National Academy Press; 2000.
2. Thomas EJ, Studdert DM, Newhouse JP, et al. Costs of medical injuries in Utah and Colorado. Inquiry 1999;36(3):255–64.
3. Occupational Safety & Health Administration. Revision to OSHA's bloodborne pathogens standard. Washington, DC: United States Department of Labor; 2001.
4. Pyrek KM. Sharps safety and OSHA compliance: staying on the right side of the law. Infection Control Today 2012.
5. Hart PD. Complying with the bloodborne pathogen standard: protecting health care workers and patients. AORN J 2011;94(4):393–9.
6. Fischer GE, Schaefer MK, Labus BJ, et al. Hepatitis C virus infections from unsafe injection practices at an endoscopy clinic in Las Vegas, Nevada, 2007-2008. Clin Infect Dis 2010;51(3):267–73.
7. Pugliese G, Gosnell C, Bartley JM, et al. Injection practices among clinicians in United States health care settings. Am J Infect Control 2010;38(10):789–98.
8. Commission TJ. Preventing infection from the misuse of vials. Sentinel Event Alert 2014;(52):1–6.
9. Safe Injection Practices Coalition. Available at: http://www.oneandonlycampaign.org/content/safe-injection-practices-coalition. Accessed April 2019.
10. Alam M, Bolotin D, Carruthers J, et al. Consensus statement regarding storage and reuse of previously reconstituted neuromodulators. Dermatol Surg 2015;41(3):321–6.
11. Pate DA, Shimizu I, Akin R, et al. Safety of prefilled buffered lidocaine syringes with and without epinephrine. Dermatol Surg 2016;42(3):361–5.
12. Unwala RD, Jacob SE. Needle recapping. J Am Acad Dermatol 2006;55(5):917–8.
13. Messingham MJ, Arpey CJ. Update on the use of antibiotics in cutaneous surgery. Dermatol Surg 2005;31(8 Pt 2):1068–78.

14. Cook JL, Perone JB. A prospective evaluation of the incidence of complications associated with Mohs micrographic surgery. Arch Dermatol 2003;139(2):143–52.

15. Futoryan T, Grande D. Postoperative wound infection rates in dermatologic surgery. Dermatol Surg 1995;21(6):509–14.

16. Rogers HD, Desciak EB, Marcus RP, et al. Prospective study of wound infections in Mohs micrographic surgery using clean surgical technique in the absence of prophylactic antibiotics. J Am Acad Dermatol 2010;63(5):842–51.

17. Rhinehart MB, Murphy MM, Farley MF, et al. Sterile versus nonsterile gloves during Mohs micrographic surgery: infection rate is not affected. Dermatol Surg 2006;32(2):170–6.

18. Mehta D, Chambers N, Adams B, et al. Comparison of the prevalence of surgical site infection with use of sterile versus nonsterile gloves for resection and reconstruction during Mohs surgery. Dermatol Surg 2014;40(3):234–9.

19. Edwards PS, Lipp A, Holmes A. Preoperative skin antiseptics for preventing surgical wound infections after clean surgery. Cochrane Database Syst Rev 2004;(3):CD003949.

20. Alam M, Ibrahim O, Nodzenski M, et al. Adverse events associated with Mohs micrographic surgery: multicenter prospective cohort study of 20,821 cases at 23 centers. JAMA Dermatol 2013;149(12):1378–85.

21. Echols K, Graves M, LeBlanc KG, et al. Role of antiseptics in the prevention of surgical site infections. Dermatol Surg 2015;41(6):667–76.

22. Perl TM, Golub JE. New approaches to reduce Staphylococcus aureus nosocomial infection rates: treating S. aureus nasal carriage. Ann Pharmacother 1998;32(1):S7–16.

23. Perl TM. Prevention of Staphylococcus aureus infections among surgical patients: beyond traditional perioperative prophylaxis. Surgery 2003;134(5 Suppl):S10–7.

24. Kluytmans J, van Belkum A, Verbrugh H. Nasal carriage of Staphylococcus aureus: epidemiology, underlying mechanisms, and associated risks. Clin Microbiol Rev 1997;10(3):505–20.

25. Tai YJ, Borchard KL, Gunson TH, et al. Nasal carriage of Staphylococcus aureus in patients undergoing Mohs micrographic surgery is an important risk factor for postoperative surgical site infection: a prospective randomised study. Australas J Dermatol 2013;54(2):109–14.

26. Cherian P, Gunson T, Borchard K, et al. Oral antibiotics versus topical decolonization to prevent surgical site infection after Mohs micrographic surgery–a randomized, controlled trial. Dermatol Surg 2013;39(10):1486–93.

27. Mangram AJ, Horan TC, Pearson ML, et al. Guideline for Prevention of Surgical Site Infection, 1999. Centers for Disease Control and Prevention (CDC) Hospital Infection Control Practices Advisory Committee. Am J Infect Control 1999;27(2):97–132 [quiz: 133–34]; [discussion: 96].

28. Webster J, Osborne S. Preoperative bathing or showering with skin antiseptics to prevent surgical site infection. Cochrane Database Syst Rev 2012;(9):CD004985.

29. Boyce JM, Pittet D, Healthcare Infection Control Practices Advisory Committee, HICPAC/SHEA/APIC/IDSA Hand Hygiene Task Force. Guideline for Hand Hygiene in Health-Care Settings. Recommendations of the Healthcare Infection Control Practices Advisory Committee and the HICPAC/SHEA/APIC/IDSA Hand Hygiene Task Force. Society for Healthcare Epidemiology of America/Association for Professionals in Infection Control/Infectious Diseases Society of America. MMWR Recomm Rep 2002;51(RR-16):1–45 [quiz: CE41-4].

30. Rotter M. Hand washing and hand disinfection. In: Mayhall CG, editor. Hospital epidemiology and infection control. Philadelphia: Lippincott Williams & Wilkins; 1999.

31. Centers for Disease Control and Prevention. Guide to infection prevention for outpatient settings: minimum expectations for safe care. Atlanta (GA): Centers for Disease Control and Prevention; 2016.

32. Smack DP, Harrington AC, Dunn C, et al. Infection and allergy incidence in ambulatory surgery patients using white petrolatum vs bacitracin ointment. A randomized controlled trial. JAMA 1996;276(12):972–7.

33. Dixon AJ, Dixon MP, Dixon JB. Randomized clinical trial of the effect of applying ointment to surgical wounds before occlusive dressing. Br J Surg 2006;93(8):937–43.

34. Khalifeh MR, Redett RJ. The management of patients on anticoagulants prior to cutaneous surgery: case report of a thromboembolic complication, review of the literature, and evidence-based recommendations. Plast Reconstr Surg 2006;118(5):110e–7e.

35. Shimizu I, Jellinek NJ, Dufresne RG, et al. Multiple antithrombotic agents increase the risk of postoperative hemorrhage in dermatologic surgery. J Am Acad Dermatol 2008;58(5):810–6.

36. Bordeaux JS, Martires KJ, Goldberg D, et al. Prospective evaluation of dermatologic surgery complications including patients on multiple antiplatelet and anticoagulant medications. J Am Acad Dermatol 2011;65(3):576–83.

37. Otley CC. Continuation of medically necessary aspirin and warfarin during cutaneous surgery. Mayo Clin Proc 2003;78(11):1392–6.

38. Stewart LC, Langtry JA. Clopidogrel: mechanisms of action and review of the evidence relating to use

during skin surgery procedures. Clin Exp Dermatol 2010;35(4):341–5.

39. Callahan S, Goldsberry A, Kim G, et al. The management of antithrombotic medication in skin surgery. Dermatol Surg 2012;38(9):1417–26.

40. Arguello-Guerra L, Vargas-Chandomid E, Diaz-Gonzalez JM, et al. Incidence of complications in dermatological surgery of melanoma and non-melanoma skin cancer in patients with multiple co-morbidity and/or antiplatelet-anticoagulants. Five year experience in our Hospital. Cir 2018;86(1):20–8.

41. Correa BJ, Weathers WM, Wolfswinkel EM, et al. The forehead flap: the gold standard of nasal soft tissue reconstruction. Semin Plast Surg 2013;27(2):96–103.

42. Chang TW, Arpey CJ, Baum CL, et al. Complications with new oral anticoagulants dabigatran and rivaroxaban in cutaneous surgery. Dermatol Surg 2015;41(7):784–93.

43. Heard LK, Shanahan C, Maggio KL. Complications with new oral anticoagulants dabigatran and rivaroxaban in cutaneous surgery. Dermatol Surg 2017;43(4):597–9.

44. Antia C, Hone N, Gloster H. Perioperative complications with new oral anticoagulants dabigatran, apixaban, and rivaroxaban in Mohs micrographic surgery: a retrospective study. J Am Acad Dermatol 2017;77(5):967–8.

45. Alam M, Goldberg LH. Serious adverse vascular events associated with perioperative interruption of antiplatelet and anticoagulant therapy. Dermatol Surg 2002;28(11):992–8 [discussion: 998].

46. Flynn TC, Emmanouil P, Limmer B. Unilateral transient forehead paralysis following injury to the temporal branch of the facial nerve. Int J Dermatol 1999;38(6):474–7.

47. Brennan C. Avoiding the "danger zones" when injecting dermal fillers and volume enhancers. Plast Surg Nurs 2014;34(3):108–11 [quiz: 112–3].

48. DeLorenzi C. Complications of injectable fillers, part 2: vascular complications. Aesthet Surg J 2014;34(4):584–600.

49. Carruthers JD, Fagien S, Rohrich RJ, et al. Blindness caused by cosmetic filler injection: a review of cause and therapy. Plast Reconstr Surg 2014;134(6):1197–201.

50. Beleznay K, Carruthers JD, Humphrey S, et al. Avoiding and treating blindness from fillers: a review of the world literature. Dermatol Surg 2015;41(10):1097–117.

51. National Quality Forum. Serious reportable events. Available from: URL: http://www.qualityforum.org/Topics/SREs/Series_Reportable_Events.aspx. Accessed March 19, 2012.

52. Alam M, Lee A, Ibrahimi OA, et al, Cutaneous Surgery Consensus Group. A multistep approach to improving biopsy site identification in dermatology: physician, staff, and patient roles based on a Delphi consensus. JAMA Dermatol 2014;150(5):550–8.

53. Nemeth SA, Lawrence N. Site identification challenges in dermatologic surgery: a physician survey. J Am Acad Dermatol 2012;67(2):262–8.

54. Rossy KM, Lawrence N. Difficulty with surgical site identification: what role does it play in dermatology? J Am Acad Dermatol 2012;67(2):257–61.

55. McGinness JL, Goldstein G. The value of preoperative biopsy-site photography for identifying cutaneous lesions. Dermatol Surg 2010;36(2):194–7.

56. Ke M, Moul D, Camouse M, et al. Where is it? The utility of biopsy-site photography. Dermatol Surg 2010;36(2):198–202.

57. Nijhawan RI, Lee EH, Nehal KS. Biopsy site selfies–a quality improvement pilot study to assist with correct surgical site identification. Dermatol Surg 2015;41(4):499–504.

58. Perlis CS, Campbell RM, Perlis RH, et al. Incidence of and risk factors for medical malpractice lawsuits among Mohs surgeons. Dermatol Surg 2006;32(1):79–83.

59. Watson AJ, Redbord K, Taylor JS, et al. Medical error in dermatology practice: development of a classification system to drive priority setting in patient safety efforts. J Am Acad Dermatol 2013;68(5):729–37.

60. Hussain W. Avoiding wrong site surgery: how language and technology can help. Br J Dermatol 2012;167(5):1186.

61. Jeyamohan SR, Moye MS, Srivastava D, et al. Patient-acquired photographs for the management of postoperative concerns. JAMA Dermatol 2017;153(2):226–8.

62. Tseng HS, Liu SP, Uang SN, et al. Cancer risk of incremental exposure to polycyclic aromatic hydrocarbons in electrocautery smoke for mastectomy personnel. World J Surg Oncol 2014;12:31.

63. Kisch T, Liodaki E, Kraemer R, et al. Electrocautery devices with feedback mode and Teflon-coated blades create less surgical smoke for a quality improvement in the operating theater. Medicine (Baltimore) 2015;94(27):e1104.

64. Naslund Andreasson S, Mahteme H, Sahlberg B, et al. Polycyclic aromatic hydrocarbons in electrocautery smoke during peritonectomy procedures. J Environ Public Health 2012;2012:929053.

65. Georgesen C, Lipner SR. Surgical smoke: risk assessment and mitigation strategies. J Am Acad Dermatol 2018;79(4):746–55.

66. Minkis K, Whittington A, Alam M. Dermatologic surgery emergencies: complications caused by

systemic reactions, high-energy systems, and trauma. J Am Acad Dermatol 2016;75(2):265–84.

67. Minkis K, Whittington A, Alam M. Dermatologic surgery emergencies: complications caused by occlusion and blood pressure. J Am Acad Dermatol 2016;75(2):243–62.

68. Elston DM, Taylor JS, Coldiron B, et al. Patient safety: Part I. Patient safety and the dermatologist. J Am Acad Dermatol 2009;61(2):179–90 [quiz: 191].

69. Alam M, Schaeffer MR, Geisler A, et al. Safety of local intracutaneous lidocaine anesthesia used by dermatologic surgeons for skin cancer excision and postcancer reconstruction: quantification of standard injection volumes and adverse event rates. Dermatol Surg 2016;42(12):1320–4.

70. Schmitt A, DePry J, Tsai S, et al. Retrospective evaluation of the safety of large skin flap, large skin graft, and interpolation flap surgery in the outpatient setting. Dermatol Surg 2018;44(12): 1537–46.

71. Johnson RP, Butala N, Alam M, et al. A retrospective case-matched cost comparison of surgical treatment of melanoma and nonmelanoma skin cancer in the outpatient versus operating room setting. Dermatol Surg 2017;43(7):897–901.

Perioperative Antibiotic Use in Cutaneous Surgery

Hillary Johnson-Jahangir, MD, PhD, MHCDS[a],*, Neha Agrawal, BA[b]

KEYWORDS

- Cutaneous surgery • Dermatologic surgery • Perioperative antibiotics • Preoperative antibiotics
- Postoperative antibiotics • Antibiotic prophylaxis • Postoperative infection • Wound infection

KEY POINTS

- Office-based cutaneous surgical procedures are regarded as safe with low risk of surgical site infections.
- Preoperative antibiotic prophylaxis is indicated for a narrow subset of high-risk patients.
- Antibiotics are selectively indicated for defined populations at high risk for infective endocarditis or hematogenous prosthetic joint infection before invasive procedures at mucosal or infected sites.
- Restricted postoperative prophylactic antibiotic limits the potential for adverse effects, microbiome collateral damage, antibiotic resistance, and health system cost.

INTRODUCTION/BACKGROUND

Perioperative antibiotics in cutaneous surgery are selectively indicated for high-risk situations, and oral antibiotics are not regularly required. Infectious complications associated with clean cutaneous surgical procedures are uncommon. Usual skin preparation of the surgical site, guideline-based hand hygiene, and modified aseptic no-touch surgical techniques reduce the chance of surgical site contamination as a cause of surgical site infections (SSI).[1] Most commonly, microbial causes of SSI are normal skin bacterial flora, such as *Staphylococcus aureus*, that spread to the wound area.[2]

Oral antibiotic prophylaxis for higher-risk populations may be indicated to prevent serious adverse events, such as infectious endocarditis or prosthetic joint infection.[3,4] Bacteremia is a common cause of infectious endocarditis and hematogenous joint infection and can occur following a breach in the mucocutaneous barrier or secondary to SSI.[5]

Infection results when immune system mechanisms fall behind in the body's innate immunity. Antimicrobial therapy is indicated to treat SSI when diagnosed.[3,4] The highest standard for diagnosis of SSI includes the presence of signs and symptoms of infection (purulence, pain, redness, warmth, swelling) in addition to a positive wound culture.[6] Variation in perioperative practices and classification of SSI-positive postoperative wounds is a barrier to identification of generalizable risk factors and preventions strategies. Because SSI occurs in only 1% to 5% of patients after dermatologic surgery, studies tend to lack robust statistical power and generalizability.[7] For these reasons, definitive evidence-based guidelines for oral antibiotic use to prevent SSI are not available. Surgical registries that systematically track complications and outcomes may contribute to future practice-based recommendations if widely adopted and account for prescribing patterns. When measuring infection rates, it is also important to concurrently measure appropriate antibiotic utilization.

Routine provision of antibiotics before or after cutaneous procedures is contraindicated. Overuse may be associated with adverse effects, the spread of multidrug-resistant pathogens, and anaphylaxis.[4] Among the chief concerns of antibiotic use is

Disclosure Statement: The authors have nothing to disclose.
a Dermatology, University of Iowa, 200 Hawkins Drive, Iowa City, IA 52242, USA; b University of Nevada, Reno, School of Medicine, 1664 North Virginia Street, Pennington Medical Education Building, Reno, NV 89557, USA
* Corresponding author.
E-mail address: hillary-johnson@uiowa.edu

Dermatol Clin 37 (2019) 329–340
https://doi.org/10.1016/j.det.2019.03.003
0733-8635/19/© 2019 Elsevier Inc. All rights reserved.

damage to the gut biome, which may induce *Clostridium difficile* infection, selection for antibiotic-resistant microorganisms, and long-term negative effects, such as allergies and obesity. Greater understanding of the role of the skin microbiome for maintaining skin homeostasis limiting overgrowth of normal flora and pathogens is underway.[8–11] The consequences of antibiotic overuse also impact the health care system. Prescribing perioperative antibiotics to patients who may not necessarily need them can increase costs in the health care system.[12] By reducing the amount of indiscriminate antibiotic use, care delivered is higher-value care. Considering these possibilities, perioperative antibiotic does not provide enough of a benefit to outweigh risks in most patients. The right antibiotic targeted to the right patient at the right time, using a personalized approach to care, is safest and most effective.

Perioperative Considerations for Surgical Site Infection

Definition of surgical site infection
SSI diagnosis is defined by the US Centers for Disease Control and Prevention (CDC) as including at least 1 factor in a set of findings at the operative wound site within 30 days of surgery[13]:

- Purulent discharge
- Culture demonstrating infectious organism or oganisms
- One or more signs or symptoms: Tenderness, pain, redness, heat, swelling
- Diagnosis of SSI by the treating surgeon or deliberate opening of the wound

Importance of wound culture and identification of pathogens
Normal postoperative redness and swelling can be easily mistaken as infection (eg, suture granuloma-type inflammatory reactions to absorbable suture

in **Fig. 1** and normal wound healing by second intention in **Fig. 2**). If signs and symptoms are identified, obtaining a culture of the wound before the initiation of antibiotic therapy is a best practice. Wound cultures offer several benefits. Antibiotic therapy is only effective for pathogenic bacterial overgrowth in the wound site. Antibiotic sensitivity testing can confirm appropriate antibiotic selection for culture-proven infections, particularly in the presence of methicillin-resistant *S aureus* (MRSA). The patient presented with symptoms of worsening pain, edema, and erythema on postoperative day 2. Collection of surgical site wound culture samples at surgical sites most often involves use of swab sampling the wound exudate and less commonly tissue biopsy. Testing of the sample includes Gram stain for early results and plating on media for culture growth over time for specificity. Advancements in clinical diagnostic techniques enabling more rapid test results for earlier pathogen identification and sensitivity testing make use of molecular testing or mass spectrometry.[14,15]

Fig. 3 shows a purulent wound on the right cheek. Wound culture swab was performed. A Gram stain revealed many gram-positive cocci and neutrophils. Mass spectrometry permitted early identification of *S aureus* within hours of the sample procurement. After 3 days of growth, the culture sensitivities revealed growth of a combination of methicillin-sensitive *S aureus* and MRSA.

Common causes of SSI include normal commensal organisms, usually beneficial protecting against infection as part of a diverse skin microbiome, but can overgrow or contaminate cutaneous healing wounds. Most SSI are considered to arise from a patient's own mucocutaneous flora, as shown in **Fig. 4**. There are no large population studies examining characteristics of infectious agents in dermatologic surgery.[2]

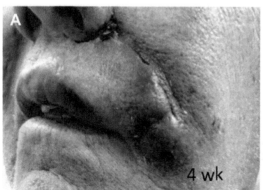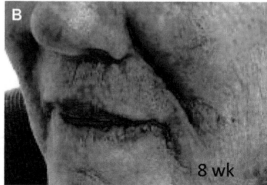

Fig. 1. Postoperative tissue inflammatory response to absorbable suture (polyglactin) following surgical reconstruction on the left nasolabial fold. The inflammatory response is brisk at (*A*) 4 weeks and subsides by (*B*) 8 weeks. (*Courtesy of* Hillary Johnson-Jahangir.)

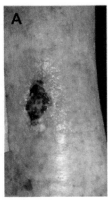
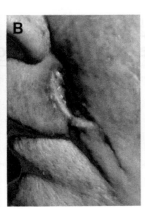
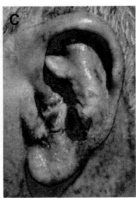
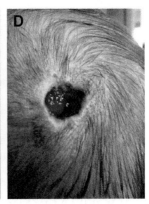

Fig. 2. Granulating superficial skin ulcerations without signs or symptoms of infection. Sites of normal wound healing by second intention (eg, granulation) are present following excisional surgery on the (*A*) left lower leg, (*B*) left upper cutaneous lip, (*C*) left ear antihelix and concha, and (*D*) scalp vertex. (*Courtesy of* Hillary Johnson-Jahangir.)

Common bacterial causes of surgical site infection

- *S aureus*
- *Staphylococcus epidermidis*
- Enterococci
- *Escherichia coli*
- *Pseudomonas aeruginosa*

Use of clean technique in dermatologic surgery

Dermatologic surgery is traditionally practiced using a clean procedural technique with local anesthesia in the office-based environment and is associated with low infection rates. The wounds are classified as nonsterile and clean contaminated. It is well recognized that total skin decontamination removing all microorganisms is technically impossible given commensal skin organisms normally

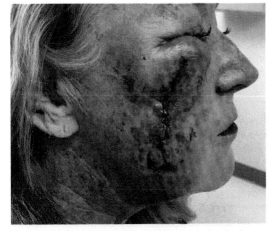

Fig. 3. Culture-proven SSI of the right cheek shown 2 days after MMS with linear reconstruction of the surgical defect. (*Courtesy of* Hillary Johnson-Jahangir.)

present within hair follicles, and oil glands are not eradicated using common preoperative antiseptic skin preparation. Strategies used in clean technique therefore do not focus on sterility, described as free from microorganisms.[16] Rather, the goal is to reduce the number and transfer of pathogens.

Common features of clean technique[6]

- Hand hygiene using hand washing or an alcohol-based hand sanitizer per CDC guidelines
- Preparing a clean field and using clean gloves
- Use of sterile instruments
- Avoidance of direct contamination of materials and persons

Compelling evidence substantiating the impact of clean surgical technique on SSI regards the use of nonsterile gloves. A 2016 meta-analysis published by Brewer and colleagues[17] concluded no difference in rate of postoperative SSI using sterile versus nonsterile gloves for outpatient cutaneous or mucosal procedures. The systematic analysis included 11,071 unique patients who underwent common procedures, such as Mohs micrographic surgery (MMS), laceration repair, standard excisions, and tooth extraction. The combined overall SSI rate was estimated to be 2.1%, and the relative risk for SSI using nonsterile gloves was 1.06 (95% confidence interval, 0.81–1.39). Studies analyzed were several randomized clinical trials, meeting the highest-grade quality of evidence as well as observational studies.

Outside of glove use, there are few robust systematic studies that show a clear role for perioperative and intraoperative conventions typically seen in operating rooms in acute care settings. Most of the published analyses do not feature dermatologic

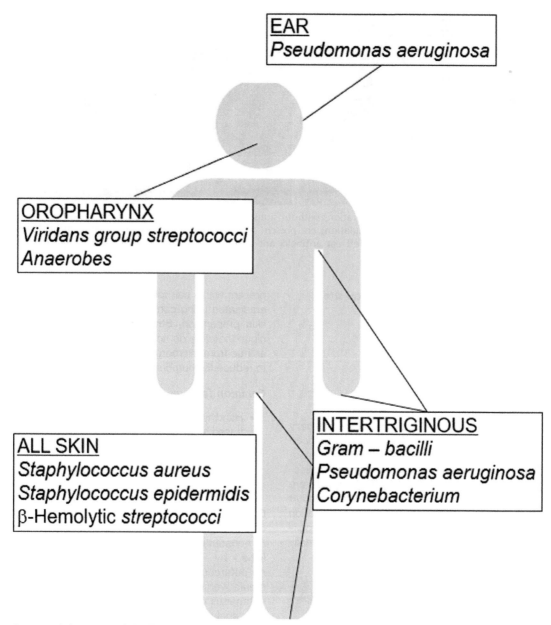

EAR
Pseudomonas aeruginosa

OROPHARYNX
Viridans group streptococci
Anaerobes

INTERTRIGINOUS
Gram – bacilli
Pseudomonas aeruginosa
Corynebacterium

ALL SKIN
Staphylococcus aureus
Staphylococcus epidermidis
β-Hemolytic *streptococci*

Fig. 4. Body locations of skin bacteria. These oftentimes normal floras can be pathogenic, causing wound infections. (*Data from* Lee MR, Paver R. Prophylactic antibiotics in dermatological surgery. Australas J Dermatol 2016;57(2):83–91.)

surgery. Studies of the following items either show no evidence of impact on rate of SSI or lack high quality of evidence overall[16,18,19]:

- Surgical team gowns, hats, shoe covers, masks, nail polish or jewelry, hand antisepsis
- Draping, including plastic adhesive drapes, electrosurgery, antiseptic application
- Patient preoperative hair removal or screening for MRSA
- Postoperative wound dressings

Home wound care and the patient experience
Wound contamination during care at home is a potential cause of SSI. Gastrointestinal or genitourinary floras are isolated from infected wounds.[2] There is no standard for instructing patients on wound care in the home, and wound care recommendations vary per practice or per surgeon.

The aging population may be at higher risk for SSI. Alam and colleagues'[20] multicenter prospective MMS study and smaller retrospective analyses of cutaneous procedures each noted higher rates of SSI in patients older than 70 years compared with younger cohorts. Targeted education and engagement of a care team may be necessary to curtail SSI for this population segment.

Patient preferences for postoperative wound care instructions after dermatologic surgery and the wound care experience are measurable. Patients doing home-based wound care after hospital discharge have highlighted needs to learn new information and develop confidence in the ability to perform the wound care and to communicate about questions or concerns.[21] Recently, focus on incorporation of technology to facilitate home care has examined utility of text messaging, mobile applications, Webinars, and video and electronic chart portals.[22–25] Any 1 approach may not work for all patients, who may have variable health literacy and ability to access or use technology. A personalized approach may be best suited for local populations or procedure types.

Role of topical antibiotics

Topical antibiotics have higher cost and higher risk of contact dermatitis and promote antibiotic resistance. Prospective, randomized studies and meta-analyses have found that topical antibiotics do not offer an advantage for postoperative SSI prophylaxis and are not indicated after dermatologic surgery. Nonetheless, they continue to be used. Petrolatum rather than topical antibiotics serves as an alternative emollient after cutaneous surgery in the outpatient cutaneous setting.[26–28]

Screening and decolonization

Colonization refers to the presence of bacteria on a surface without eliciting a host response, whereas infection suggests a host response to bacteria causing disease. Nasal colonization with S aureus may be associated with greater skin infection risk. Screening for colonizing pathogens to target only the highest-risk patients for antibiotic prophylaxis lacks sufficient evidence.[16] Decolonization interventions may pose an alternative method of preventing infection without selecting for drug-resistant microorganisms. To the authors' knowledge, a cost-benefit analysis for carrier screening and preprocedural decolonization has not been conducted in a wider scale. Highlights of research efforts to screen and treat nasal colonization before MMS are summarized here:

- Intervention for nasal colonization: Topical antibiotic and oral antibiotic: Cordova and colleagues[29] retrospectively evaluated preoperative rapid nasal swab screening. They found 23 MRSA carriers of 963 MMS patients. Before MMS, 22 of the MRSA carriers were treated with preoperative intranasal mupirocin and oral trimethoprim-sulfamethoxazole and did not experience an SSI.[29] Although encouraging, results represent uncontrolled and nonrandomized single-institution retrospective observational study.
- Intervention for nasal colonization: Topical antibiotic and biocide body wash or oral antibiotic: A randomized controlled trial conducted in 2013 showed that patients had fewer SSI when using topical decolonization methods than in patients who received perioperative oral antibiotics.[30] This single-site study found a 25% S aureus nasal carriage rate in the 693 MMS patients over a 30-week time frame. The S aureus carriers were randomized to 1 of 2 options for decolonization: (1) topical intranasal mupirocin twice daily and 4% chlorhexidine body wash daily for the 5 days before surgery versus (2) oral antibiotic dosage 30 to 60 minutes preoperatively and again 6 hours postoperatively. None of the topically treated patients compared with 9% receiving oral antibiotics developed an SSI at 7 days after surgery.

Oral Antibiotic Prophylaxis for Prevention of Bacterial Endocarditis and Hematogenous Joint Infection

Although not specific to dermatologic surgery, recommendations made by the American Heart Association (AHA), American Dental Association (ADA), and American Academy of Orthopedic Surgeons (AAOS) are available to help determine the use of antibiotic prophylaxis in patients at high risk for infective endocarditis (IE) or prosthetic joint infection.

Algorithms can facilitate risk stratification to help identify the highest-risk segments for which antibiotic prophylaxis is called for (**Figs. 5** and **6**). Simply put, antibiotic prophylaxis for IE and prosthetic joint infection may be limited to selected individuals who need procedures performed on infected skin or mucosa.

Prevention of infective endocarditis

IE, although uncommon, has a high risk of morbidity and mortality. The latest AHA guideline update issued in 2007 restricted indications for perioperative antibiotic prophylaxis before dental procedures. Some dental procedures can lead to risk of blood infection by oral commensal bacteria, particularly viridans group streptococci. For dental procedures perforating the oral mucosa or gingival manipulation, antibiotics are only recommended to be given for patients associated with having the highest risk of IE and adverse outcomes.[31,32]

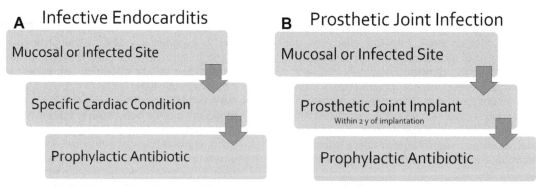

A Infective Endocarditis

Mucosal or Infected Site

Specific Cardiac Condition

Prophylactic Antibiotic

B Prosthetic Joint Infection

Mucosal or Infected Site

Prosthetic Joint Implant
Within 2 y of implantation

Prophylactic Antibiotic

Fig. 5. Algorithms can aid decision making for preoperative prophylactic antibiotic use. Is there an invasive procedure on mucosal or infected skin sites? If yes, decision making for prophylaxis is considered for (A) IE and (B) hematogenous prosthetic joint infection. (*Data from* Infective endocarditis. American Heart Association. Available at: https://www.heart.org/en/health-topics/infective-endocarditis; and Wright TI, Baddour LM, Berbari EF, et al. Antibiotic prophylaxis in dermatologic surgery: advisory statement 2008. J Am Acad Dermatol 2008;59(3):464–73.)

Trends in incidence in infective endocarditis

The epidemiologic trends in incidence in health care–associated IE over decades have been an active area of investigation to track the impact of prescribing and risk. Mandatory reporting of patients hospitalized with endocarditis is required in New York and California.[33] In these 2 states, the standardized rates of IE from 1998 to 2013 were stable. Likewise, the 2002 to 2013 rate of hospitalizations due to IE in the Canadian population was stable.[34] These time spans cover the 2007 AHA guideline update implementation and suggest the prescribing restrictions did not impact rates of IE. Analysis of prescription benefit and claims data from a proprietary data set for US commercial and Medicare patients from 2003 to 2015 showed concern for high-risk populations, in particular.[35] In this data set, higher-risk categorization correlated with underprescribed antibiotic prophylaxis and increased IE incidence. The investigators called for further investigation of prescribing patterns and risk.

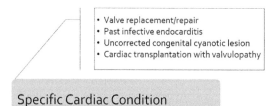

- Valve replacement/repair
- Past infective endocarditis
- Uncorrected congenital cyanotic lesion
- Cardiac transplantation with valvulopathy

Specific Cardiac Condition

Fig. 6. Select high-risk cardiac conditions qualifying for antibiotic prophylaxis. If an invasive procedure on mucosal or infected skin is required, oral antibiotic prophylaxis is indicated to reduce risk of IE. (*Data from* Infective Endocarditis. American Heart Association. Available at: https://www.heart.org/en/health-topics/infective-endocarditis.)

Who are the patients at highest risk for infective endocarditis?

Only a subset of patients with certain following cardiac conditions is deemed eligible for antibiotic prophylaxis[31]:

- Prosthetic heart valve
- Heart valve repaired with prosthetic material
- History of endocarditis
- Heart transplant with abnormal heart valve function
- Congenital heart defects:
  - Cyanotic congenital heart disease that has not been fully repaired
  - Congenital heart defect repaired with prosthetic material
  - Congenital heart defect repaired with a device within 6 months
  - Repaired congenital heart disease with residual defects
  - Repaired congenital heart disease adjacent to a prosthetic patch or prosthetic device

What dermatologic procedures are included?

Although dermatologic procedures were not mentioned in the 2007 AHA guidelines, antibiotic prophylaxis in procedures pertaining to urinary, reproductive, and gastrointestinal tracts was not recommended.[31] Clean dermatologic procedures are very commonly performed and have fewer risk factors for bacteremia compared with dental procedures. Recommendations for antibiotic prophylaxis for high-risk patients are considered reasonable for invasive procedures at mucosal sites or infected skin or skin structures. Procedures are invasive if they breach the mucocutaneous barrier.[3,31,32] Invasive procedures can include not only surgery but also minor procedures like skin biopsy.

In MMS, a clean surgical technique, the rate of bacteremia is low at approximately 2%, and the incidence rate of SSI is also low, between 1% and 3% in most studies.[5] However, despite this low rate of infection, some Mohs surgeons routinely use prophylactic antibiotics for lower-risk patients, such as those with a history of prostheses, those with nonphysiologic heart murmurs, or those with valvular disease.[36]

What is the appropriate oral antibiotic for prophylactic use?

The antibiotic therapy regimen is traditionally provided as a single dose 30 to 60 minutes before the procedure. A postprocedure dose can be given if the prophylactic therapy is accidentally not provided beforehand. **Table 1** features the range of commonly used oral antibiotics for (A) and (B). Cephalexin is the medication of choice for procedures located on infected skin or skin structures, whereas amoxicillin is preferred for mucosal sites. Clindamycin may be considered for immediate hypersensitivity-type penicillin allergy.[31,32]

Prevention of hematogenous prosthetic joint infection

Is it time to revisit prophylactic antibiotic prescribing for patients with prosthetic joints before dermatologic procedures? The 2008 *Journal of the American Academy of Dermatology* (JAAD)

advisory statement was based on the 2003 version ADA guidelines for dental procedures. This 2008 statement suggested antibiotic prophylaxis within 2 years of a prosthetic joint implant was recommended before dermatologic procedures performed on mucosal sites or infected skin.[3] Newer recommendations for antibiotic prophylaxis for patients at higher risk of hematogenous prosthetic joint infection are available for dental but not dermatologic procedures.

American Dental Association 2015 revised guidelines for prophylactic antibiotic use

ADA guidelines have progressed toward reducing antibiotic prescribing before dental procedures in patients with prosthetic joints.[37] The movement away from routine antibiotic prophylaxis started with the 2012 AAOS-ADA Clinical Practice Guidelines. Next, antibiotics were generally not recommended before dental procedures in the 2015 ADA guideline update.[32,38,39] This update reflected the lack of evidence to associate dental procedures and total joint infection. Dental procedures are no longer considered a relevant cause of prosthetic joint infections. Furthermore, no evidence of the clinical effectiveness of antibiotic prophylaxis to prevent prosthetic joint infection could be found that supports routine antibiotic use. Even in patients with prosthetic joint implants, prophylactic antibiotics are not routinely recommended to prevent

---

Table 1
Antibiotic regimen for preprocedural antibiotic prophylaxis (adult only)

Nonoral Infected Site	Antibiotic Agent	Dose
No penicillin allergy	Cephalexin	2 g po
Penicillin allergy	Clindamycin Azithromycin/clarithromycin	600 mg po 500 mg po
Unable to take po	Cefazolin/ceftriaxone	1 g IM/IV
Unable to take po and penicillin allergy	Clindamycin	600 mg IM/IV
Pathogen known	Specific for pathogen	
Oral Site	**Antibiotic Agent**	**Dose**
No penicillin allergy	Amoxicillin	2 g po
Penicillin allergy	Clindamycin Azithromycin/clarithromycin	600 mg po 500 mg po
Unable to take po	Cefazolin/ceftriaxone Ampicillin	1 g IM/IV 2 g IM/IV
Unable to take po and penicillin allergy	Clindamycin	600 mg IM/IV

Antibiotic choice depends on coverage needs for cutaneous vs mucosal locations and the presence of medication allergy. Options are displayed for procedural sites located on the (A) skin and (B) oral mucosa.

Abbreviations: IM, intramuscular; IV, intravenous; po, by mouth.

Data from Infective Endocarditis. American Heart Association. Available at: https://www.heart.org/en/health-topics/infective-endocarditis and Wright TI, Baddour LM, Berbari EF, et al. Antibiotic prophylaxis in dermatologic surgery: advisory statement 2008. J Am Acad Dermatol 2008;59(3):464–73.)

joint infection. Although cutaneous surgeries are not specifically mentioned, a similar approach to antibiotic use could be considered for performing procedures on the oral mucosa. Because oral antibiotics are no longer recommended in the setting of dental procedures, recommendations for mucocutaneous procedures in the setting of dermatologic care merit reconsideration.

Is antibiotic prophylaxis ever indicated before dental procedures?

Prophylactic antibiotics do not prevent hematogenous joint infection and are not generally recommended. In patients who have had joint replacement surgery complications, prophylactic antibiotics might be given on a case-by-case basis.[32,37] In these situations, it is recommended that the antibiotic be prescribed by the orthopedic surgeon. Orthopedic surgeons now have evidence-based decision aids to help determine when prophylactic antibiotics may be best used.

Appropriate use criteria for antibiotic prophylaxis for hematogenous prosthetic joint infection

How do orthopedic surgeons decide when prophylactic antibiotics are useful? The AAOS released Appropriate Use Criteria (AUC) in 2016 regarding prophylactic antibiotic use.[40] It offers a consensus-based decision tool to determine antibiotic prophylactic use in high-risk joint implant patients undergoing dental procedures. The AUC includes the type of planned dental procedure, immunocompromised status, glycemic control, history of joint infection that required operation, and timing since hip or knee joint replacement procedure to help with an orthopedic surgeon's decision making. In addition to these factors used in the AUC, AAOS also states that there is moderate evidence to suggest an increase in SSI in patients with certain underlying conditions like chronic kidney disease, diabetes, tobacco use/smoking, and malnutrition.[41] This guideline also demonstrates the push away from perioperative antibiotic use except in high-risk cases.

Oral Antibiotic Prophylaxis for Surgical Site Infections Prevention

Oral antibiotic use for SSI prevention after dermatologic surgery is controversial. In general, discussion in the literature favors reserving oral antibiotic use for infections after they are detected rather than prescribing them for all surgical patients or based on intuition. A 2012 survey of Mohs surgeons self-reported overuse of oral antibiotics in a wider patient population above and beyond the potentially higher risk.[42] Lack of high-level

evidence and reliance on data from other nondermatologic surgical disciplines have been barriers to development of widespread practice standards. Larger and randomized controlled studies have been called for. The establishment of national clinical data registries may facilitate future data collection and tracking of SSI.[43]

No existing guidelines direct appropriate prescription of antibiotics for postoperative SSI prophylaxis in the context of dermatologic surgery. A published 2008 advisory statement in the JAAD referenced observations that some endogenous patient factors or the anatomic location of the surgery may be associated with higher risk for SSI.[3,44–46] Various procedures and their locations have correlated with increased SSI.

- A 2006 single-site prospective study identified the following surgical locations as higher risk for SSI: lower extremity, groin, wedge excisions of the lip or ear, flaps on the nose, and skin grafts.[46]
- A retrospective review of 1977 procedures in The Netherlands identified larger defects closed with flaps or second intention and ear surgery as higher risk.[47]
- A 2018 randomized controlled trial supported preoperative cephalexin 2 g before delayed reconstructive surgery on the ear or nose after staged excision in 154 patients based in Australia. The cephalexin single dose reduced the infection rate from 11.6% in controls to 1.4% in the interventional group.[48] The investigators postulate that both the nose and the ear contain a high concentration of sebaceous glands compared with other body sites, which, combined with bacterial colonization and complex dermatologic repairs, can lead to higher rates of infection.

The lower extremity: an example of a location labeled "high risk" for surgical site infections

Antibiotic prophylaxis for lower-extremity surgical sites has been suggested because postoperative infection rates were considered higher on the lower legs.[3] Recent data are mixed and less conclusive. A prospective randomized placebo-controlled double-blind trial conducted in Australia revealed that there may be modest risk reduction for SSI by using cephalexin after skin excision.[49] However, this study had a small sample size of 52 patients and was statistically underpowered. Another recent 24-month retrospective study examined the rate of infection in lower-extremity surgical sites of 271 patients and did not reveal a statistically significant difference in infection rates between prophylactic doxycycline-prescribed and control patients.[50,51] Although there needs to be greater study on perioperative antibiotic use for lower-extremity excisions, current evidence does not strongly suggest the use of antibiotics in such surgeries.

Findings from larger, multiple site studies

There are few multi-institutional studies of perioperative antibiotic use during cutaneous surgery. Two short-term registries evaluating SSI in patients after MMS conclude a minimal role for antibiotic prophylaxis. Additional population-level data are needed.

- SSI incidence was low and did not correlate with prophylactic antibiotic use. Registry data collected within this US-based multi-institutional data set detail greater than 800 tumors of which 467 had follow-up.[48] Postoperative wound infections were reported in 3.4% of this population treated by fellowship-trained US-based Mohs surgeons. Infection rates were *higher* in patients who were prescribed prophylactic antibiotics for high-risk situations matching those listed in the 2008 JAAD advisory on antibiotic prophylaxis. Oral antibiotic prescribing appeared in accordance with the 2008 JAAD advisory statement limited to when potential risk for SSI might be high. Investigators suggest the statistical analysis and generalizability be limited by the low rate of infection.
- A large prospective registry examined 20,821 tumors and found an extremely low rate of adverse events of 0.72%. In this 2013 report by Alam and colleagues,[20] the use of chlorhexidine, antibiotic prophylaxis, or sterile gloves during MMS correlated with reduced postoperative infections. The absolute risk reduction for each infection control practice ranges from 0.45% to 0.53%. Because of this low value, the study investigators suggest that the clinical benefit of the reduction in infection rate may not outweigh the risks and increased costs associated with perioperative antibiotic use. Given that the effect of these infection control practices is not additive, using an antiseptic alone may be enough to prevent infection without increasing the risk of antibiotic resistance or adverse effects.

Alternatives to antibiotic prophylaxis for surgical site infections: consideration of dilute acetic acid antisepsis

The use of dilute acetic acid as an inexpensive, nontoxic antiseptic agent is reported after dermatologic surgery.[52–54] It is more commonly used in areas prone to infection, such as the lower extremities and ear, related to its well-established antipseudomonal activity.[55] Sterile 0.25% acetic acid is commercially available as approved as an adjunct to management of pseudomonal wound infections. Home preparation instructions for dilute "vinegar soaks" using store-purchased vinegar mixed into tap water are usually given because there is no evidence using sterile versus tap water for routine cleansing makes a difference.[19] Acetic acid has been used in wound-healing practices for more than 6000 years and is experiencing a rebirth in popularity. An acidic wound environment is important for inhibiting growth of microorganisms.[52] Studies of burn and chronic wounds have demonstrated reduction in biofilm-producing pathogens[54]; however, the contribution of biofilm to SSI after dermatologic surgery is uncertain.[56]

Alternatives to antibiotic prophylaxis for surgical site infections: the case for no prophylactic antibiotics

Indications for usage of oral antibiotics suggest restriction for treatment of skin and skin structure infections only when there is a proven or strongly suspected bacterial infection (**Fig. 7**). Default of no prophylactic antibiotics and use of culture-directed oral antibiotic therapy for SSI are not new, but have been conventional practice by some for several years.

- A prospective study with 1000 patients conducted in 2010 showed an extremely low rate of SSI at 0.91% using clean surgical technique in the absence of prophylactic antibiotics.[55]
- A predictive model generated from 1407 patients to identify SSI risk at a single surgical location featured a need to treat more than 8 patients meeting high-risk criteria to avoid just 1 infection. High-risk criteria referred to the tumor size, location, and closure type (eg, large wound size, tumors on the ear, and reconstruction using flaps). Several

Sign/Symptom → Culture → Antibiotic

Fig. 7. Algorithm for postoperative therapeutic oral antibiotic use to treat SSI. This algorithm may be useful guidance for antibiotic stewardship initiatives intending to restrict perioperative antibiotic prophylaxis. Oral antibiotic prescribing is limited to postoperative SSI after diagnosis. (*Data from* Rogers HD, Desciak EB, Marcus RP, et al. Prospective study of wound infections in Mohs micrographic surgery using clean surgical technique in the absence of prophylactic antibiotics. J Am Acad Dermatol 2010;63(5):842–51.)

unnecessary courses of oral antibiotics would be prescribed in this scenario.[57]

- Studies with a wider lens have identified additional patient risk factors, including geographic location and patient demographics. Interestingly, these factors were more closely correlated with SSI risk than use of prophylactic antibiotics.[58]

Need for antimicrobial stewardship in dermatologic surgical practice

Dermatologic surgeons looking to reduce antibiotic overuse and more appropriately prescribe perioperative antibiotics can be guided by antimicrobial stewardship. Stewardship programs are organized to help set goals and measure adherence with evidence-based prescribing. Any practice can start by measuring patterns of antibiotic use to help identify trends and then establish targets for desired use.[59–61]

Consequences of antibiotic overuse are now recognized as negatively impacting on an individual's microbiome, ultimately increasing risk for chronic disease.[62] Antibiotic overuse also contributes to the established costs of growing antibiotic resistance and potential adverse medication reactions.

SUMMARY

Perioperative antibiotic use in mucocutaneous procedures is controversial due to the lack of large, randomized control trials that link infections to cutaneous surgery practices, risk factors, and interventions. However, growing evidence has led to practice protocol change restricting antibiotic prophylaxis in the context of dermatologic surgery. Certain professional organizational guidelines have been modified to reflect benefits of lesser antibiotic use. Increasing awareness of guidelines and coordinated antibiotic stewardship efforts may help surgical practices revise and reduce perioperative oral antibiotic prescribing.

REFERENCES

1. Haas AF, Grekin RC. Antibiotic prophylaxis in dermatologic surgery. J Am Acad Dermatol 1995; 32(2 Pt 1):155–76.
2. Lee MR, Paver R. Prophylactic antibiotics in dermatological surgery. Australas J Dermatol 2016;57(2): 83–91.
3. Wright TI, Baddour LM, Berbari EF, et al. Antibiotic prophylaxis in dermatologic surgery: advisory statement 2008. J Am Acad Dermatol 2008;59(3):464–73.
4. CDC guidelines for prevention of surgical site infection. Available at: https://www.cdc.gov/infectioncontrol/guidelines/ssi/index.html. Accessed August 8, 2018.
5. Christaki E, Giamarellos-Bourboulis EJ. The complex pathogenesis of bacteremia: from antimicrobial clearance mechanisms to the genetic background of the host. Virulence 2014;5(1):57–65.
6. The Joint Commission. Preventing central line–associated bloodstream infections: useful tools, An International Perspective. Nov 20, 2013. Available at: http://www.jointcommission.org/CLABSIToolkit. Accessed August 8, 2018.
7. Maragh SL, Brown MD. Prospective evaluation of surgical site infection rate among patients with Mohs micrographic surgery without the use of prophylactic antibiotics. J Am Acad Dermatol 2008; 59(2):275–8.
8. Johanesen PA, Mackin KE, Hutton ML, et al. Disruption of the gut microbiome: clostridium difficile infection and the threat of antibiotic resistance. Genes (Basel) 2015;6:1347–60.
9. Belkaid Y, Hand TW. Role of the microbiota in immunity and inflammation. Cell 2014;157(1):121–41.
10. Cox LM, Blaser MJ. Antibiotics in early life and obesity. Nat Rev Endocrinol 2015;11(3):182–90.
11. Blaser MJ. Antibiotic use and its consequences for the normal microbiome. Science 2016;352(6285): 544–5.
12. Müller CS, Hubner W, Thieme-Ruffing S, et al. Pre- and perioperative aspects of dermatosurgery. J Dtsch Dermatol Ges 2017;15(2):117–46.
13. Horan TC, Gaynes RP, Martone WJ, et al. CDC definitions of nosocomial surgical site infections, 1992: a modification of CDC definitions of surgical wound infections. Infect Control Hosp Epidemiol 1992;13: 606–8.
14. Chong YK, Ho CC, Leung SY, et al. Clinical mass spectrometry in the bioinformatics era: a hitchhiker's guide. Comput Struct Biotechnol J 2018;16:316–34.
15. Budding AE, Hoogewerf M, Vandenbroucke-Grauls CM, et al. Automated broad-range molecular detection of bacteria in clinical samples. J Clin Microbiol 2016;54(4):934–43.
16. Saleh K, Schmidtchen A. Surgical site infections in dermatologic surgery: etiology, pathogenesis, and current preventative measures. Dermatol Surg 2015;41(5):537–49.
17. Brewer JD, Gonzalez AB, Baum CL, et al. Comparison of sterile vs nonsterile gloves in cutaneous surgery and common outpatient dental procedures: a systematic review and meta-analysis. JAMA Dermatol 2016;152(9):1008–14.
18. Eisen DB. Surgeon's garb and infection control: what's the evidence? J Am Acad Dermatol 2011; 64(5):960.e1-20.
19. Ploegmakers IB, Olde Damink SW, Breukink SO. Alternatives to antibiotics for prevention of surgical infection. Br J Surg 2017;104(2):e24–33.
20. Alam M, Ibrahim O, Nodzenski M, et al. Adverse events associated with Mohs micrographic surgery

multicenter prospective cohort study of 20 821 cases at 23 centers. JAMA Dermatol 2013;149(12):1378–85.

21. Sanger PC, Hartzler A, Han SM. Patient perspectives on post-discharge surgical site infections: towards a patient-centered mobile health solution. J Drugs Dermatol 2018;17(7):766–71.

22. Newsom E, Lee E, Rossi A, et al. Modernizing the mohs surgery consultation: instituting a video module for improved patient education and satisfaction. Dermatol Surg 2018;44(6):778–84.

23. Hawkins SD, Koch SB, Williford PM, et al. Web App- and text message-based patient education in mohs micrographic surgery-a randomized controlled trial. Dermatol Surg 2018;44(7):924–32.

24. Hawkins SD, Barilla S, Williford PWM, et al. Patient perceptions of text-messages, email, and video in dermatologic surgery patients. Dermatol Online J 2017;23(4) [pii:13030/qt53n342dd].

25. Migden M, Chavez-Frazier A, Nguyen T. The use of high definition video modules for delivery of informed consent and wound care education in the Mohs Surgery Unit. Semin Cutan Med Surg 2008;27(1):89–93.

26. Levender MM, Davis SA, Kwatra SG, et al. Use of topical antibiotics as prophylaxis in clean dermatologic procedures. J Am Acad Dermatol 2012;66:445–51.

27. Dixon AJ, Dixon MP, Dixon JB. Randomised clinical trial of the effect of applying ointment to surgical wounds before occlusive dressing. Br J Surg 2006;93:937–43.

28. Saco M, Howe N, Nathoo R, et al. Topical antibiotic prophylaxis for prevention of surgical wound infections from dermatologic procedures: a systematic review and meta-analysis. J Dermatolog Treat 2015;26(2):151–8.

29. Cordova KB, Grenier N, Chang KH, et al. Preoperative methicillin-resistant Staphylococcus aureus screening in Mohs surgery appears to decrease postoperative infections. Dermatol Surg 2010;36(10):1537–40.

30. Cherian P, Gunson T, Borchard K, et al. Oral antibiotics versus topical decolonization to prevent surgical site infection after Mohs micrographic surgery–a randomized, controlled trial. Dermatol Surg 2013;39(10):1486–93.

31. Infective Endocarditis. American Heart Association. Available at: https://www.heart.org/en/health-topics/infective-endocarditis. Accessed August 8, 2018.

32. Antibiotic Prophylaxis Prior to Dental Procedures. American Dental Association. 2018. Available at: https://www.ada.org/en/member-center/oral-health-topics/antibiotic-prophylaxis. Accessed August 8, 2018.

33. Toyoda N, Chikwe J, Itagaki S, et al. Trends in infective endocarditis in California and New York State, 1998-2013. JAMA 2017;317(16):1652–60.

34. Mackie AS, Liu W, Savu A, et al. Infective endocarditis hospitalizations before and after the 2007 American Heart Association prophylaxis guidelines. Can J Cardiol 2016;32(8):942–8.

35. Thornhill MH, Gibson TB, Cutler E, et al. Antibiotic prophylaxis and incidence of endocarditis before and after the 2007 AHA recommendations. J Am Coll Cardiol 2018;72(20):2443–54.

36. Asgari MM, Olson JM, Alam M. Needs assessment for Mohs micrographic surgery. Dermatol Clin 2012;30(1):167–75.

37. Sollecito TP, Abt E, Lockhart PB, et al. The use of prophylactic antibiotics prior to dental procedures in patients with prosthetic joints: evidence-based clinical practice guideline for dental practitioners–a report of the American Dental Association Council on Scientific Affairs. J Am Dent Assoc 2015;146(1):11–6.e8.

38. Watters W 3rd, Rethman MP, Hanson NB, et al. Prevention of orthopaedic implant infection in patients undergoing dental procedures. J Am Acad Orthop Surg 2013;21(3):180–9.

39. Quinn RH, Murray JN, Pezold R, et al. The American Academy of Orthopaedic Surgeons Appropriate Use Criteria for the management of patients with orthopaedic implants undergoing dental procedures. J Bone Joint Surg Am 2017;99(2):161–3.

40. American Academy of Orthopedic Surgeons. Appropriate use criteria for the management of patients with orthopaedic implants undergoing dental procedures. Rosemont (IL): American Academy of Orthopaedic Surgeons; 2018. Available at: https://www.aaos.org/uploadedFiles/PreProduction/Quality/AUCs_and_Performance_Measures/appropriate_use/auc-patients-with-orthopaedic-implants-dental-procedures.pdf. Accessed August 8, 2018.

41. American Academy of Orthopaedic Surgeons. Systematic literature review on the management of surgical site infections. 2018. Available at: https://www.aaos.org/ssi. Accessed August 8, 2018.

42. Bae-Harboe YS, Liang CA. Perioperative antibiotic use of dermatologic surgeons in 2012. Dermatol Surg 2013;39(11):1592–601.

43. Council ML, Alam M, Gloster HM Jr, et al. Identifying and defining complications of dermatologic surgery to be tracked in the American College of Mohs Surgery (ACMS) Registry. J Am Acad Dermatol 2016;74(4):739–45.

44. Futoryan T, Grande D. Postoperative wound infection rates in dermatologic surgery. Dermatol Surg 1995;21:509–14.

45. Rosengren H, Dixon A. Antibacterial prophylaxis in dermatologic surgery: an evidence-based review. Am J Clin Dermatol 2010;11(1):35–44.

46. Dixon AJ, Dixon MP, Askew DA, et al. Prospective study of wound infections in dermatologic surgery in the absence of prophylactic antibiotics. Dermatol Surg 2006;32:819–26.

47. Liu X, Sprengers M, Nelemans PJ, et al. Risk factors for surgical site infections in dermatological surgery. Acta Derm Venereol 2018;98(2):246–50.

48. Rosengren H, Heal CF, Buttner PG. Effect of a single prophylactic preoperative oral antibiotic dose on surgical site infection following complex dermatological procedures on the nose and ear: a prospective, randomised, controlled, double-blinded trial. BMJ Open 2018;8(4):e020213.

49. Smith SC, Heal CF, Buttner PG. Prevention of surgical site infection in lower limb skin lesion excisions with single dose oral antibiotic prophylaxis: a prospective randomised placebo-controlled double-blind trial. BMJ Open 2014;4(7):e005270.

50. Bari O, Eilers RE Jr, Rubin AG, et al. Clinical characteristics of lower extremity surgical site infections in dermatologic surgery based upon 24-month retrospective review. J Drugs Dermatol 2018;17(7):766–71.

51. Levin EC, Chow C, Makhzoumi Z. Association of postoperative antibiotics with surgical site infection in Mohs micrographic surgery. Dermatol Surg 2019;45(1):52–7.

52. Nagoba BS, Suryawanshi NM, Wadher B, et al. Acidic environment and wound healing: a review. Wounds 2015;27(1):5–11.

53. Kumara DU, Fernando SS, Kottahachchi J, et al. Evaluation of bactericidal effect of three antiseptics on bacteria isolated from wounds. J Wound Care 2015;24(1):5–10.

54. Halstead FD, Rauf M, Moiemen NS, et al. The antibacterial activity of acetic acid against biofilm-producing pathogens of relevance to burns patients. PLoS One 2015;10(9):e0136190.

55. Rogers HD, Desciak EB, Marcus RP, et al. Prospective study of wound infections in Mohs micrographic surgery using clean surgical technique in the absence of prophylactic antibiotics. J Am Acad Dermatol 2010;63(5):842–51.

56. Edmiston CE Jr, McBain AJ, Roberts C, et al. Clinical and microbiological aspects of biofilm-associated surgical site infections. Adv Exp Med Biol 2015; 830:47–67.

57. Liu X, Kelleners-Smeets NWJ, Sprengers M, et al. A clinical prediction model for surgical site on infections in dermatological surgery. Acta Derm Venereol 2018;98(7):683–8.

58. O'Neill JL, Shutty B, Sun Lee Y, et al. Comparing demographic characteristics and adverse event rates at two dermatologic surgery practices. J Cutan Med Surg 2014;18(5):337–40.

59. Gibbons JA, Smith HL, Kumar SC, et al. Antimicrobial stewardship in the treatment of skin and soft tissue infections. Am J Infect Control 2017;45(11): 1203–7.

60. Cooper R, Kirketerp-Møller K. Non-antibiotic antimicrobial interventions and antimicrobial stewardship in wound care. J Wound Care 2018;27(6): 355–77.

61. Roberts CD, Leaper DJ, Assadian O. The role of topical antiseptic agents within antimicrobial stewardship strategies for prevention and treatment of surgical site and chronic open wound infection. Adv Wound Care 2017;6(2):63–71.

62. Lederer AK, Pisarski P, Kousoulas L, et al. Postoperative changes of the microbiome: are surgical complications related to the gut flora? A systematic review. BMC Surg 2017;17(1):125.

Postoperative Pain Management in Dermatologic Surgery
A Systematic Review

Michael Saco, MD*, Nicholas Golda, MD

KEYWORDS

- Acetaminophen • Ibuprofen • Mohs micrographic surgery • Dermatologic surgery • Opioid
- Narcotic • Analgesia • Postoperative pain

KEY POINTS

- A systematic review was performed to analyze postoperative pain management in outpatient dermatologic surgery.
- Mohs micrographic surgery and standard excisions are both associated with low postoperative pain scores overall with 2 studies showing pain being greatest on the day of surgery and gradually decreasing thereafter.
- Studies vary based on whether certain anatomic locations and repair types result in higher postoperative pain scores.
- Acetaminophen and ibuprofen should be emphasized as first-line postoperative analgesia in dermatologic surgery.
- If given, opioids should only be prescribed to last the patient a few days post-operatively.

INTRODUCTION

Postoperative analgesia, whether through over-the-counter or prescription medications, constitutes a critical component of dermatologic surgery. New legislation to combat the current opioid epidemic has placed an emphasis on limiting the amount of opioids prescribed.[1] Multiple studies have indicated that there is significant heterogeneity in opioid-prescribing habits among dermatologic surgeons, and that most patients either take no or only a few of the opioids they are prescribed.[2–5] Accordingly, attempts have been made to limit the amount of opioids prescribed and to find nonopioid alternatives for postoperative analgesia. The objective of this study was to perform a systematic review to answer the following question: what is the strength of evidence supporting current practices for pain control in dermatologic surgery?

METHODS

The literature search for this systematic review was performed by searching PubMed, CINAHL, Embase, and Ovid online databases for relevant English-language scholarly articles from the inception of each database to July 21, 2018. A flowchart detailing the literature search performed to obtain the articles used for this systematic review is presented in **Fig. 1**. For each online database, the following searches were entered: Mohs postoperative pain, pain control Mohs, and pain Mohs. In addition, the following search terms and phrases

Disclosure Statement: The authors report no commercial or financial conflicts of interest or funding sources.
Department of Dermatology, University of Missouri, One Hospital Drive, Room MA111, Columbia, MO 65212, USA
* Corresponding author.
E-mail address: sacom@health.missouri.edu

Dermatol Clin 37 (2019) 341–348
https://doi.org/10.1016/j.det.2019.03.004
0733-8635/19/Published by Elsevier Inc.

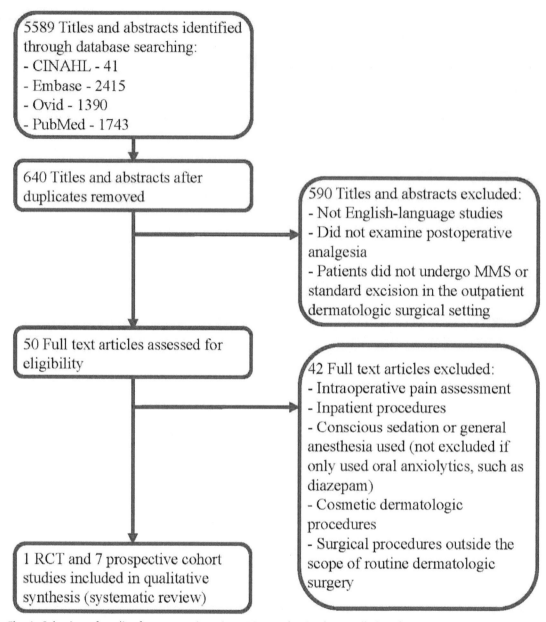

Fig. 1. Selection of studies for systematic review. RCT, randomized controlled trial.

were combined through the Boolean connectors AND and OR and then entered into all 4 databases: postoperative, post-operative, postprocedure, post-procedure, pain, skin, cutaneous, cancer, excision, dermatologic, dermatology, surgery, opioid, opiate, narcotic, hydromorphone, hydrocodone, oxycodone, codeine, tramadol, acetaminophen, aspirin, ibuprofen, NSAID, nonsteroidal anti-inflammatory, nonsteroidal antiinflammatory, pregabalin, gabapentin, fentanyl, fentanil, morphine, and analgesia. The authors will make the exact search expression of terms and phrases

available upon request; it was excluded from publication because of its length (**Fig. 1**).

Inclusion criteria included English-language studies examining postoperative analgesia in patients of any age group undergoing Mohs micrographic surgery (MMS) or standard excision in the outpatient dermatologic surgical setting. Exclusion criteria included studies examining solely intraoperative pain assessment, inpatient procedures, procedures in which conscious sedation or general anesthesia were used, as well as studies solely pertaining to postoperative analgesia for cosmetic dermatologic procedures (eg, laser resurfacing, chemical peeling) and surgical procedures outside the scope of routine dermatologic surgery (eg, abdominoplasty, rhytidectomy). Of note, studies in which patients were given oral anxiolytics, such as diazepam, were not excluded from the systematic review unless the oral anxiolytic given was part of a conscious sedation or general anesthesia regimen. The quality of evidence (high-, limited-, and low-quality) for each study and grade of recommendation (1, 2A, and 2B) were assigned based on the classification system published by Robinson and colleagues.[6] Data were deemed statistically significant either if the P value was less than .05 or if the authors explicitly stated the data were statistically significant.

RESULTS

Multiple studies showed that MMS is associated with minimal postoperative pain (**Table 1**).[7–10] Pain was greatest on the day of surgery and decreased progressively thereafter.[11,12] Studies in which opioids were prescribed for postoperative pain showed that patients often either did not use them or used much fewer pills than the amount prescribed.[2,3]

Although some studies showed a statistically significant increase in postoperative pain experienced by women compared with men,[7,8] other studies demonstrated that the difference was not statistically significant.[11,12] The effect of younger age on higher pain scores was also inconsistent between studies.[8,11,12]

An examination of MMS patients showed that healing by second intention was less painful than repair via flaps, linear closure, and grafts.[11] There were also data indicating that linear closures produced less pain than flap closures, although these data did not reach statistical significance ($P = .052$).[11] No association between postoperative defect size and type of postoperative pain medication used was found.[11] In addition, the average postoperative pain score was found to be the highest for the lip, then the forehead, chest, leg, and nose.[11] No data were available to determine whether these differences in average postoperative pain scores were statistically significant.[11]

A randomized controlled trial studying pain following MMS showed that sites on the lip, nose, and ear were associated with higher levels of postoperative pain than sites on the forehead and cheek.[9] Acetaminophen 1000 mg and ibuprofen 400 mg taken together immediately after surgery and then every 4 hours thereafter for up to 4 doses was associated with better postoperative pain control after MMS compared with the same frequency of administration for either acetaminophen 1000 mg alone or acetaminophen 325 mg plus codeine 30 mg.[9] Overall, 87% of patients were satisfied with the acetaminophen and codeine combination, and 93% of patients were satisfied with either acetaminophen alone or the acetaminophen and ibuprofen combination. The differences between these groups were not statistically significant. It is also notable that there were no statistically significant differences between the 3 aforementioned groups in terms of postoperative bleeding, thus supporting the concept that ibuprofen, although a nonsteroidal anti-inflammatory drug (NSAID), may not predispose to bleeding complications following dermatologic surgery.[9]

The greatest postoperative pain in a prospective cohort study was associated with interpolation flaps and the least postoperative pain with second intention healing.[8] Postoperative pain for linear, random pattern flap, and skin graft repairs was similar. Pain levels after MMS on the genitalia were highest, although only 3 patients in this study had MMS on a genital site. Pain levels from MMS on the lip and nose were also found to be higher than pain level for sites on the trunk, neck, and extremities, albeit to a lesser extent.[8]

Another study,[3] which examined dermatologic surgery patients, found that closures requiring grafts and, to a lesser extent, flaps, resulted in greater postoperative pain scores and prescription opioid use. No associations between postoperative defect size or anatomic location and postoperative use of opioids were found.[3]

Tumors located on the scalp were associated with the greatest amount of postoperative pain in 1 study.[12] In addition, postoperative defect sizes ≥ 3.0 cm were associated with an increased likelihood of patients requiring postoperative opioids.[12]

According to a prospective cohort study,[7] postoperative pain management starts with assessment of pain anxiety preoperatively. Although the study demonstrated that most patients experienced little postoperative pain after MMS, patients with high anxiety toward pain experienced greater postoperative pain to a degree that was statistically significant ($P<.001$). The study also found that lower-extremity MMS surgical sites resulted in increased postoperative pain, whereas second intention healing resulted in less postoperative pain.[7]

DISCUSSION

Although some variation exists among the studies examined in the systematic review, a common

Table 1
Postoperative pain associations relevant to the current study's systematic review

Source, y	Type of Study, Study Sample, and Interventions or Exposures	Associations with Statistical Significance	Associations with No Statistical Significance or Insufficient evidence[a]	Quality of Evidence (A, B, C)
Firoz et al,[11] 2010	• Prospective cohort study of 433 MMS patients; patients used icepacks and acetaminophen as needed, received prescription opioids only if they requested them	• Greater pain in patients younger than 66 y of age • Pain was greatest on the day of the surgery and decreased progressively thereafter • Healing by second intention was less painful than repair via flaps, linear closure, and grafts	• No difference in postoperative pain between men and women • Data indicating that linear closures produced less pain than flap closures did not reach statistical significance ($P = .052$) • No association between postoperative defect size and type of postoperative pain medication consumed • Average postoperative pain score was highest for the lip, then the forehead, chest, leg, and nose; no data were available to determine whether or not these differences in average postoperative pain scores were statistically significant	B
Tschoeke et al,[10] 2010	• 124 MMS patients agreed to participate; 87 patients returned a complete survey; general satisfaction survey	• MMS is associated with minimal postoperative pain	N/A	B
Sniezek et al,[9] 2011	• Randomized, double-blind, controlled study of 208 patients undergoing MMS and surgical reconstruction of head and neck skin cancers; patients were distributed relatively evenly among 3 groups and received acetaminophen 1000 mg, acetaminophen 1000 mg, plus ibuprofen 400 mg taken together, or acetaminophen 325 mg plus codeine 30 mg taken together	• MMS is associated with minimal postoperative pain • Mean pain scores for MMS sites on the lip, nose, and ear were associated with higher levels of postoperative pain than mean pain scores for MMS sites on the forehead and cheek • Combination of acetaminophen and ibuprofen led to better postoperative pain control after MMS compared with either acetaminophen alone or acetaminophen	• Overall, 87% of patients were satisfied with the acetaminophen and codeine combination, and 93% of patients were satisfied with either acetaminophen alone or the acetaminophen and ibuprofen combination; the differences between these groups were not statistically significant • No statistically significant differences between the acetaminophen, acetaminophen plus ibuprofen, and	A

(continued on next page)

Table 1
(continued)

Source, y	Type of Study, Study Sample, and Interventions or Exposures	Associations with Statistical Significance	Associations with No Statistical Significance or Insufficient evidence[a]	Quality of Evidence (A, B, C)
	immediately after surgery was finished and then every 4 h up to 4 doses	plus codeine based on statistically significant differences in multiple postoperative pain scores reported at various intervals throughout the study	acetaminophen plus codeine groups in terms of postoperative bleeding	
Merritt et al,[8] 2012	• Multicenter prospective cohort study of 1550 MMS patients with 1792 tumors, follow-up obtained in 1709 of the 1792 tumors; study examined rates of major and minor complications and postoperative pain	• MMS is associated with minimal postoperative pain • More pain reported in women, younger patients, active smokers, patients requiring more stages • Greatest postoperative pain was with interpolation flaps • Least postoperative pain was with second intention healing • Pain levels from MMS on the lip and nose were found to be higher than pain level for sites on the trunk, neck, and extremities	• Postoperative pain for linear, random pattern flap, and skin graft repairs was similar • Pain levels after MMS on the genitalia were highest, although only 3 patients had MMS on a genital site	B
Harris et al,[3] 2013	• 212 dermatologic surgery patients, prospective observational study examining postoperative opioid use; 72 of the 212 patients were prescribed opioids	• Patients often either did not use postoperative opioids prescribed or used much fewer pills than the amount prescribed • Closures requiring grafts and, to a lesser extent, flaps, resulted in greater postoperative pain scores and prescription opioid use	• No associations between postoperative defect size or anatomic location and postoperative use of opioids were found	B
Limthongkul et al,[12] 2013	• 158 MMS patients, prospective cohort study that examined postoperative pain and factors associated with increased postoperative pain	• Pain was greatest on the day of the surgery and decreased progressively thereafter • Tumors located on the scalp were associated with the greatest amount of postoperative pain • Postoperative defect size ≥ 3.0 cm was associated with an increased likelihood of patients requiring postoperative opioids	• No difference in postoperative pain was found between the age groups examined or gender	B

(continued on next page)

Table 1
(continued)

Source, y	Type of Study, Study Sample, and Interventions or Exposures	Associations with Statistical Significance	Associations with No Statistical Significance or Insufficient evidence[a]	Quality of Evidence (A, B, C)
Harris et al,[2] 2014	• 233 patients from a single institution, 82 of whom received opioid prescriptions; retrospective chart review to examine opioid prescribing patterns among dermatologic surgeons; also e-mail survey of 556 ASDS members	• Patients often either did not use postoperative opioids prescribed or used much fewer pills than the amount prescribed	N/A	B
Chen et al,[7] 2015	• 356 MMS patients from 2 private practices in a prospective cohort study; objective of study was to determine if pain anxiety can predict postoperative pain after MMS	• MMS is associated with minimal postoperative pain • Lower-extremity MMS surgical sites resulted in increased postoperative pain • Second intention healing resulted in less postoperative pain • Increase in postoperative pain experienced by women compared with men • Patients with high anxiety toward pain experienced greater postoperative pain ($P<.001$)	N/A	B

Abbreviations: ASDS, American Society of Dermatologic Surgery; N/A, not applicable.

  [a] Data in this column with insufficient evidence will be specified as having insufficient evidence. Any other data in this column can be assumed to show no statistically significant difference between groups.

theme is that MMS is associated with minimal postoperative pain.[7–10] Overall, insufficient data exist to determine which scenarios can predict the need for postoperative opioid prescriptions over nonopioid alternatives. Accordingly, no recommendations can be made regarding which specific scenarios warrant postoperative opioids. A meta-analysis could not be performed given the significant clinical heterogeneity among the studies included in the systematic review. Studies varied based on whether gender, age, anatomic location of the surgical site, postoperative defect size, and type of repair resulted in higher postoperative pain scores or greater postoperative pain requirements. Multiple studies did show, however, that healing by second intention resulted in less postoperative pain than linear, graft, or flap closures.[8,11] Some studies also indicated that graft[3] and flap[3,11] closures were associated with higher rates of postoperative pain than linear closures. Interestingly, Merritt and colleagues[8] indicated that interpolation flaps were associated with increased postoperative pain scores, but that linear, random pattern flap and skin graft repairs had relatively equivalent postoperative pain scores. In addition, multiple studies demonstrated that surgical sites involving the lip and nose were associated with higher average postoperative pain scores,[8,9,11] although other studies showed either no difference in postoperative pain scores based on anatomic location[3] or greater pain associated with other anatomic sites.[7,8,12] Even though the highest pain scores cited by Merritt and colleagues were reported in patients undergoing MMS on genital sites, it is difficult to conclude from these data that post-MMS wounds on the genitalia are, in fact, more commonly associated with pain than wounds on other anatomic sites because this conclusion was based on only 3 patients.

Based on the finding that high anxiety regarding pain can be associated with greater postoperative pain,[7] attempting to reduce preoperative and intraoperative anxiety by nonpharmacologic (eg, music) or pharmacologic (eg, zolpidem, diazepam) means may be a prudent strategy. Based on limited-quality level B evidence from a single prospective cohort study showing that pain anxiety can be associated with higher postoperative pain scores, the authors make a grade 2A recommendation for attempting to decrease pain anxiety related to dermatologic procedures.

No studies comparing nonpharmacologic interventions for postoperative analgesia, such as usage of icepacks, either in combination with pharmacologic interventions or as monotherapy, were found during the literature search. The investigators in some of the studies recommended that patients use icepacks postoperatively, but icepack usage was not tracked as a specific intervention in any of the studies included in this systematic review. Future research combining the use of icepacks with acetaminophen, ibuprofen, or a combination of the 2, may be helpful to determine whether any of the aforementioned combinations could either obviate or decrease the need for postoperative opioid prescriptions.

Most patients in the study by Sniezek and colleagues[9] thought that they had satisfactory postoperative pain control with acetaminophen alone, acetaminophen plus ibuprofen, or acetaminophen plus codeine. The combination of acetaminophen and ibuprofen led to better postoperative pain control after MMS without increasing the risk of postoperative bleeding compared with either acetaminophen alone or acetaminophen plus codeine. The finding that ibuprofen does not lead to an increased risk of postoperative bleeding matches the data published in a recent plastic surgery systematic review and meta-analysis.[13] Based on high-quality level A evidence from a double-blind randomized controlled trial, the authors give a grade 1 recommendation for using acetaminophen 1000 mg and ibuprofen 400 mg taken together immediately after surgery and every 4 hours for up to 4 doses to treat postoperative pain in the setting of MMS. However, care should be taken to not exceed the recommended maximum dose of 4000 mg of acetaminophen in a 24-hour period.

Because postoperative pain is greatest on the day of surgery and steadily decreases thereafter,[11,12] prescription medications for postoperative analgesia need only be given long enough to last a few days postoperatively. This guiding principle is especially true considering the fact that most of the patients who are prescribed opioids in the dermatologic setting either did not use them or only used 1 to a few of the pills prescribed.[11,12] Unfortunately, not enough data are available to make a recommendation about the specific number of days for which opioids should be prescribed because the studies that examined postoperative pain requirements varied in terms of the number of days in which postoperative pain scores were followed.[11,12]

One limitation in the available data is that none of the studies directly compared postoperative pain specifically related to nail procedures to postoperative pain experienced in other anatomic sites (eg, ear, nose). This limitation becomes especially important when considering the study by Topin-Ruiz and colleagues,[14] which showed that 8 out of 55 patients (15%) who underwent wide excision of the nail unit for subungual squamous cell carcinoma and full-thickness skin graft reconstruction reported experiencing severe pain days after surgery. Severe pain in this study was defined as a visual analog scale score greater than 7. Accordingly, average pain requirements for patients undergoing surgical procedures involving the nail unit may differ compared with those undergoing surgical procedures at other anatomic sites. The lack of available data may be due to the relative infrequency of subungual tumors treated by dermatologic surgeons compared with tumors involving other anatomic sites.

Another limitation of this systematic review is that original research articles pertaining to postoperative pain management for dermatologic procedures in patients younger than 18 years of age, pregnant women, and breastfeeding women were not available for analysis. Accordingly, the authors are unable to make evidence-based recommendations specifically for these patient populations. Anecdotally based recommendations published for these 3 patient populations are similar to those that have been made for nonpregnant, non-breastfeeding adults. Acetaminophen is often recommended as first-line therapy for mild postoperative pain in all patient populations, whereas small doses of opioids are recommended for moderate to severe pain. NSAIDs can also be used to control mild pain in the pediatric population, but aspirin should be avoided given the association of aspirin with the potentially fatal Reye syndrome in the pediatric population.[15,16]

SUMMARY

In summary, MMS and standard excision are procedures associated with relatively low postoperative pain. Attempts to reduce anxiety may decrease postoperative pain scores and, accordingly, present an opportunity for dermatologic surgeons to improve postoperative pain in a medication-free manner. The evidence clearly supports the use of acetaminophen and ibuprofen as first-line postoperative analgesia in dermatologic surgery. The authors are unable to make specific recommendations regarding when and for how long to prescribe opioids for postoperative pain given the lack of data. However, if opioids are to be given, the authors recommend prescribing a small quantity on the day of surgery based on the data showing that postoperative pain, although usually relatively low in the setting of dermatologic surgery, is typically at its peak immediately postoperatively and steadily decreases thereafter. In addition, the studies identified were highly variable with respect to which anatomic sites or reconstructions were most or least associated with postoperative pain, so it is difficult to provide evidence-based guidance on how dermatologic surgeons should approach pain control in a site and reconstruction-specific manner. Some evidence does suggest, however, that nail surgery may be more commonly associated with severe pain. Future research should further examine nonopioids or weaker opioids, whether as monotherapy or in combination, for the treatment of postoperative pain in dermatologic surgery and should provide clearer site and reconstruction-specific guidelines for the use of pain control following skin surgery.

REFERENCES

1. Legislatures NCoS. Prescribing policies: states confront opioid overdose epidemic. 2018. Available at: http://www.ncsl.org/research/health/prescribing-policies-states-confront-opioid-overdose-epidemic.aspx. Accessed August 11, 2018.
2. Harris K, Calder S, Larsen B, et al. Opioid prescribing patterns after Mohs micrographic surgery and standard excision: a survey of American Society for Dermatologic Surgery members and a chart review at a single institution. Dermatol Surg 2014; 40(8):906–11.
3. Harris K, Curtis J, Larsen B, et al. Opioid pain medication use after dermatologic surgery: a prospective observational study of 212 dermatologic surgery patients. JAMA Dermatol 2013;149(3):317–21.
4. Cao S, Karmouta R, Li DG, et al. Opioid prescribing patterns and complications in the dermatology medicare population. JAMA Dermatol 2018;154(3): 317–22.
5. Kreicher KL, Bordeaux JS. Addressing practice gaps in cutaneous surgery: advances in diagnosis and treatment. JAMA Facial Plast Surg 2017;19(2): 147–54.
6. Robinson JK, Dellavalle RP, Bigby M, et al. Systematic reviews: grading recommendations and evidence quality. Arch Dermatol 2008;144(1):97–9.
7. Chen AF, Landy DC, Kumetz E, et al. Prediction of postoperative pain after Mohs micrographic surgery with 2 validated pain anxiety scales. Dermatol Surg 2015;41(1):40–7.
8. Merritt BG, Lee NY, Brodland DG, et al. The safety of Mohs surgery: a prospective multicenter cohort study. J Am Acad Dermatol 2012;67(6):1302–9.
9. Sniezek PJ, Brodland DG, Zitelli JA. A randomized controlled trial comparing acetaminophen, acetaminophen and ibuprofen, and acetaminophen and codeine for postoperative pain relief after Mohs surgery and cutaneous reconstruction. Dermatol Surg 2011;37(7):1007–13.
10. Tschoeke N, Fisk S, Pellino T, et al. Patients' pain experience during and following the mohs' procedure. Dermatol Nurs 2010;22(6):11–7.
11. Firoz BF, Goldberg LH, Arnon O, et al. An analysis of pain and analgesia after Mohs micrographic surgery. J Am Acad Dermatol 2010;63(1):79–86.
12. Limthongkul B, Samie F, Humphreys TR. Assessment of postoperative pain after Mohs micrographic surgery. Dermatol Surg 2013;39(6):857–63.
13. Kelley BP, Bennett KG, Chung KC, et al. Ibuprofen may not increase bleeding risk in plastic surgery: a systematic review and meta-analysis. Plast Reconstr Surg 2016;137(4):1309–16.
14. Topin-Ruiz S, Surinach C, Dalle S, et al. Surgical treatment of subungual squamous cell carcinoma by wide excision of the nail unit and skin graft reconstruction: an evaluation of treatment efficiency and outcomes. JAMA Dermatol 2017;153(5):442–8.
15. Tyler KH. Dermatologic therapy in pregnancy. Clin Obstet Gynecol 2015;58(1):112–8.
16. Yates B, Whalen J, Makkar H. An age-based approach to dermatologic surgery: kids are not just little people. Clin Dermatol 2017;35(6):512–6.

Surgical Dressings and Novel Skin Substitutes

Eileen Axibal, MD, Mariah Brown, MD*

KEYWORDS

- Surgical wounds • Second intention • Wound care • Dressings • Skin substitutes • Skin cancer
- Dermatology • Mohs surgery

KEY POINTS

- An understanding of dressing goals and materials is necessary to optimize wound outcomes in dermatologic surgery.
- Conventional surgical dressings are best applied in a layered fashion.
- Second intention and poorly healing wounds may require the use of occlusive dressings or tissue-engineered skin substitutes.
- There are numerous skin substitute options and their utilization in dermatologic surgery is rising.

INTRODUCTION

Wounds from dermatologic surgery require meticulous care during the postoperative period. The management of acute wounds created by primary surgical incision sites and chronic wounds created by surgical sites that are healing by second intention or with slow progression are addressed in this review. Chronic wounds, such as the decubitus, neuropathic, vascular, inflammatory, and rheumatologic subtypes, are not covered, but many of the same wound care principles and techniques apply.

The concept of a surgical dressing is simple—a covering over a wound—but its importance and intricacy cannot be overstated. An ideal dressing provides pressure and hemostasis, protects the site from infection and foreign material, immobilizes surrounding tissues, cushions against mechanical trauma, provides a moist environment for healing, and wicks away blood and exudate.[1] In addition, an ideal surgical dressing should be simple to apply and maintain, nonallergenic, aesthetically pleasing, cost permissive, and easily stored.[2] Selection of the proper dressing is challenging given the wide range of wounds encountered in dermatologic surgery and the myriad dressing options available to clinicians. Although no perfect dressing exists, a thorough understanding of wound care goals and supplies allows for tailored decision making and optimal outcomes.

CONVENTIONAL SURGICAL DRESSINGS

Conventional surgical dressings are best applied in a layered fashion. The layers, from bottom to top, include ointment, contact layer, absorbent layer, contouring layer, and securing layer. Not all dressings require all components, and some materials may be useful for more than 1 layer.[1] Regardless of the specifics, the most important principles of a wound dressing are to keep the wound clean, moist, and covered.[3]

The ointment layer (**Fig. 1**) limits bacterial growth, provides hydration, and prevents the dressing from sticking to the wound. For routine dermatologic procedures, plain white petrolatum is preferred. A 2015 systematic review and meta-analysis did not show a statistically significant difference in incidence of postsurgical wound

Disclosure Statement: The authors have no commercial or financial conflicts of interest.

Mohs Micrographic Surgery and Cutaneous Oncology, Department of Dermatology, University of Colorado Hospital and School of Medicine, University of Colorado, 1665 Aurora Court, Mail Stop F703, Aurora, CO 80045, USA

* Corresponding author.

E-mail address: Mariah.Brown@ucdenver.edu

Dermatol Clin 37 (2019) 349–366
https://doi.org/10.1016/j.det.2019.03.005

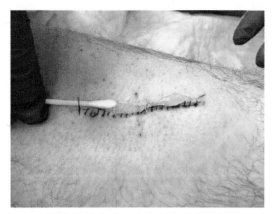

Fig. 1. Ointment layer of a conventional surgical dressing.

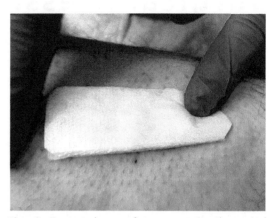

Fig. 2. Contact layer of a conventional surgical dressing.

infections between the use of topical antibiotics and petrolatum/paraffin for clean and clean-contaminated wounds.[4] There may be special circumstances in which a physician may deem the infection risk for a particular clean wound to be increased (ie, surgical site, poor personal hygiene, or contact with an individual with active infection), but there is no evidence in the literature to support the use of topical antibiotics in these cases.[5] Not only are topical antibiotics ineffective in decreasing wound infection but also they are associated with worse outcomes, such as skin edge necrosis and inflammatory chondritis.[6,7] Notably, topical antibiotics may cause allergic contact dermatitis (ACD); neomycin and bacitracin are the most common offenders, with ACD rates of 8% and 11%, respectively.[8,9] Contact allergens in commercial nonantibiotic ointments also can result in ACD. A 2013 study by Morales-Burgos and colleagues[10] showed that the rate of wound redness was higher for surgical wounds treated with Aquaphor Healing Ointment (52%) versus plain white petrolatum (12%), likely due to the allergenic ingredients lanolin and bisabolol. Lastly, topical antibiotics are contributing to emerging antibiotic resistance.[11] Despite being ineffective and posing a risk to patients, topical antibiotics continue to be used as infection prophylaxis; between 1993 and 2007, 212 million clean dermatologic procedures were performed and topical antibiotics were used in approximately 10.6 million (5.0%) of these cases.[5]

The contact layer (Fig. 2) touches the wound. It consists of a nonadherent material that allows exudate to pass through to the absorbent layer rather than adhere to the epithelium. The contact layer material should be chosen based on the type of wound dressed. Commonly used products include nonadherent pads (ie, Telfa, Cardinal Health, Dublin, OH, USA), impregnated gauze (eg,

Xeroform [Cardinal Health, Dublin, OH, USA], Vaseline Petrolatum Gauze [Petrolatum Gauze, Cardinal Health, Dublin, OH, USA], and ADAPTIC [Non-Adhering Dressing, Acelity L.P. Inc., San Antonio, TX, USA]), paraffin gauze (eg, Jelonet [Smith & Nephew, London, UK]), silicone net dressings (eg, Mepitel [Mölnlycke Health Care, Gothenburg, Sweden]), and gas-permeable film dressings (eg, Tegaderm [3M, Maplewood, MN, USA]). Some contact dressings have antibiotics or antiseptics embedded within them (eg, Bactigras [Smith & Nephew, London, UK] and Sofra-Tulle [Hoechst Marion Roussel Ltd., Mumbai, India]).[12]

The absorbent layer (Fig. 3) is placed on top of the contact layer and serves to wick and retain wound exudate, so that crust and necrotic material do not accumulate on the wound.[1] A landmark study by Winter and Scales in 1963[13] demonstrated that wounds with a thick scab, as a result of being uncovered and air dried, are slower to re-epithelialize because the regenerating epidermal cells need to migrate below the eschar until they

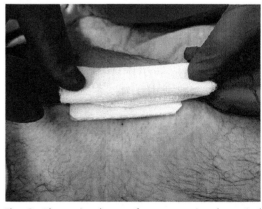

Fig. 3. Absorptive layer of a conventional surgical dressing.

reach a moist region conducive to survival.[14] Commonly used absorbent products include dry gauze pads and cotton balls. The materials can be made to be bulky or thin, depending on if pressure is required. In many cases, applying a well-padded and firmly adhesive pressure dressing and leaving it in place for 48 hours can greatly minimize bleeding complications.[15] A contour layer, if indicated, helps fill anatomic depression or support protruding structures, such as the ears and nose, so that the dressing is more secure. Dental rolls, gauze pads, and other materials may be used.

The final securing layer (**Fig. 4**) consists of tape or other wrapping materials, such as gauze rolls, tubular gauze, and elastic bandages. These materials serve to apply pressure and keep the underlying layers in place. Stretchable porous fabric and paper tape should be used in patients with fragile skin. Commonly used fabric tapes include Hypafix (BSN Medical, Hamburg, Germany), Medipore (3M, Maplewood, MN, USA), and Mefix (Mölnlycke Health Care, Gothenburg, Sweden). Hypafix uses a water-insoluble adhesive that is retained in the presence of moisture but can be removed easily with peanut or olive oil.[16] Paper tapes, such as Steri-Strips (3M, Maplewood, MN, USA) and Micropore (3M, Maplewood, MN, USA), often are placed over incision lines postoperatively and may constitute the entire dressing. They are latex-free and hypoallergenic and prevent stretching of the wound by reducing shear forces and tension on the wound edges.[17] They have the added benefit of preventing excessive soft tissue formation, thus reducing scar volume as well as keeping the wound moist and minimizing scab formation.[18] It is important to consider the potential for iatrogenic vascular insufficiency from circumferential securing bandages, particularly on the digits. With little manipulation, dressings may lift and roll distally up a digit and result in hypoxia and tissue necrosis. To prevent this tourniquet effect, digital dressings should also include the hand and wrist.[19]

When the dressing principles discussed previously, are followed, acute incisional wounds tend to progress in a sequenced fashion through the 4 major phases of wound healing: coagulation, inflammation, proliferation, and remodeling. When a wound becomes stalled in 1 of the stages of healing, it becomes a chronic wound.[20] In chronic wounds, elevated inflammatory cytokines, matrix metalloproteinases, and oxygen-free radicals result in destruction of extracellular matrix components and growth factors that are essential for healing.[21,22] Second intention surgical wounds that display minimal signs of healing after approximately 4 weeks also classify as chronic wounds, and they present challenges to surgeon and patient. Because the underlying tissue is exposed in second intention healing wounds, wound beds may be more susceptible to infection, pain, desiccation, and additional trauma. In the past, standard management of chronic wounds was with wet-to-dry gauze dressings; the problem lies in that these dressings become adherent to the wound bed once dry and result in reinjury, pain, and delayed wound healing on removal.[23] Gauze dressings do not support optimal healing and are more labor intensive to use than modern occlusive dressings and skin substitutes.[3,24]

OCCLUSIVE DRESSINGS

Occlusive dressings typically are divided into 5 major groups: films, foams, hydrogels, hydrocolloids, and alginates. Common trade names are listed in **Table 1**. Newer hydrofiber and hydroconductive dressings also are available. The designs of occlusive dressings are constantly changing, with the goal of improved and simplified care for a greater range of wounds. Composite dressings, which combine 2 or more types of semiocclusive dressings into 1 product, also are available. The goal of occlusive dressings is to prevent wound desiccation and maintain an optimal physiologic wound-healing environment. The decision of which type of occlusive dressing to use is guided based on the type of wound being managed. Although these materials often are used for chronic nonhealing wounds, there also is evidence for the use of occlusive dressings in acute postoperative surgical sites healing by second, and occasionally primary, intention (see **Table 1**).

Films

Film dressings are thin, flexible, transparent polyurethane or copolyester sheets with an acrylic self-adhesive backing. Oxygen, water vapor, and carbon

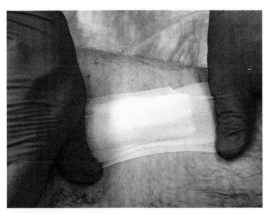

Fig. 4. Securing layer of a conventional surgical dressing.

Table 1
List of selected occlusive dressing materials

Type	Examples
Films	Tegaderm (3M, Maplewood, MN, USA)
	Mepore Film (Mölnlycke, Gothenburg, Sweden)
	Suresite (Medline Industries, Northfield, IL, USA)
	Kendall Polyskin II (Cardinal Health, Dublin, OH, USA)
	OPSITE (Smith & Nephew, London, UK)
	DermaView II (DermaRite Industries, North Bergen, NJ, USA)
	Silon-TSR (Bio Med Sciences, Allentown, PA, USA)
Foams	Mepilex and Lyofoam (Mölnlycke)
	ALLEVYN (Smith & Nephew)
	Kendall Foam (Cardinal Health)
	Biatain Foam (Coloplast, Humlebaek, Denmark)
	HydraFoam (DermaRite Industries, North Bergen, NJ, USA)
	Sof-Foam and Biopatch (Johnson & Johnson, New Brunswick, NJ, USA)
	PolyMem (Ferris Mfg. Corp, Fort Worth, TX, USA)
Hydrogels	AquaFlo (Cardinal Health, Dublin, OH, USA)
	Aquasite Hydrogel Sheet (Derma Sciences, Princeton, NJ, USA)
	Nu-Gel (Johnson & Johnson)
	Clearsite (ConMed, Utica, NY, USA)
	2nd Skin (Spenco, Waco, TX, USA)
	Vigilon (Bard, Murray Hill, NJ, USA)
Hydrocolloids	DuoDERM (Convatec, Deeside, UK)
	Exuderm (Medline, Northfield, IL, USA)
	N-Terface (Winfield Labs, Richardson, TX, USA)
	Comfeel (Coloplast, Humlebaek, Denmark)
	NU-DERM (KCI - An Acelity Company, San Antonio, TX, USA)
	REPLICARE (Smith & Nephew)
	Tegasorb (3M)

(continued on next page)

Table 1
(continued)

Type	Examples
Alginates	Algisite (Smith & Nephew)
	AlgiCell (Integra LifeSciences, Plainsboro, NJ, USA)
	Kaltostat (ConvaTec)
	Kalginate (DeRoyal, Powell, TN, USA)
	Melgisorb (Mölnlycke)
	Sorbsan (Aspen Medical Europe Limited, Ashby-de-la-Zouch, UK)

dioxide can permeate films, but bacteria and water cannot. Film dressings allow for a moist healing environment but do not have any absorptive capabilities, so they should not be used in wounds with excessive exudate or signs of infection.[25] In the postoperative setting, films may be used to cover primarily closed incisions, second intention surgical sites, and skin graft donor sites. They also may be used as a secondary dressing over other dressing materials. In 1991, Rubio[26] published a report of 3637 surgical incisions that were covered with a semiocclusive, transparent film dressing and found that, compared with conventional gauze dressings, the film dressing resulted in faster wound healing, decreased pain, and less scarring. No patient exhibited any symptoms of wound infection, and the dressing allowed for visual monitoring of the site. Because they are flexible, film dressings are easy to apply and they maximize patient range of motion.[27] Films can be left in place for up to 7 days but often need to be changed a few times per week.

Foams

Foam dressings are composed of an opaque polyurethane or silicone sponge-like polymer with a semiocclusive hydrophobic backing. They are permeable to both gases and water vapor and impermeable to fluid and bacteria. They are highly absorbent and provide cushion and thermal insulation. Foam dressings are indicated for moderate to heavy exudative wounds, granulating or slough-covered wounds, and graft donor sites.[25] They are too drying for wounds with little to no exudate. Two studies have demonstrated that foams are superior to gauze dressings in terms of pain reduction, nursing time, cost effectiveness, and patient satisfaction for second intention surgical wounds.[28,29] Foams can be either adhesive or nonadhesive, and a secondary dressing is required for the latter. The dressings should be changed once saturated with exudate; this can range from once daily to once or twice weekly.

Hydrogels

Hydrogel dressings are made of cross-linked starch polymers in 80% to 90% water base and are available as free-flowing gels, flexible sheets, and impregnated gauze. They are semitransparent and semipermeable to gases and fluid. Hydrogels donate fluid to dry wounds, promoting autolytic débridement, granulation, and re-epithelialization.[23] They have limited absorptive capacity due to their high water content and, as a result, should not be used in highly exudative or bleeding wounds. Hydrogels reduce the temperature of a wound bed by up to 5°C and, because of this cooling effect, can decrease perceived pain.[25] A 1993 study comparing the use of a hydrogel sheet dressing versus a hydrocolloid dressing on 8 full-thickness circular surgical wounds produced on the backs of micropigs showed a more rapid rate of closure and re-epithelialization with the hydrogel dressing.[30] Geronemus and Robins[31] also found that, in pigskin split-thickness wounds, 100% of hydrogel-treated wounds were healed by postoperative day 4 compared with 32% of open-air wounds. Hydrogels require a secondary dressing and should be changed approximately every 1 day to 3 days depending on the hydration status of the wound. Care must be taken to ensure the dressing changes are frequent enough to avoid maceration of the surrounding skin.[20]

Hydrocolloids

Hydrocolloid sheet dressings consist of an inner, self-adhesive layer composed of a hydrophilic polymer matrix with dispersed gelatin, pectin, and other substances; this material turns into a gel with absorption. The outer layer usually consists of polyurethane and protects the wound from bacteria, foreign debris, and shear forces.[25] Hydrocolloids also are available in pastes and powders. The dressing is semipermeable to water and gas vapors but impermeable to fluid and bacteria. Hydrocolloid dressings help promote a moist healing environment, autolytic débridement, angiogenesis, and granulation tissue formation. The ideal surgical wound is one with low to moderate exudate. In 2013, Nguyen and colleagues[32] published a technique of using hydrocolloid dressings on a Mohs surgery defect on the vertex scalp with exposed bone devoid of periosteum; the dressings allowed for the development of robust granulation tissue amenable to successful delayed full-thickness skin grafting. Hydrocolloids are waterproof and cushioned and do not require a secondary dressing, so they are convenient to use.[2] Hydrocolloids should be kept in place until drainage is noted beneath the dressing; this typically requires once-daily changes early in the treatment course, with a decrease to every 3 days to 7 days over time.

Alginates

Alginates are made up of soft, nonwoven alginic acid fibers, a cellulose-like polysaccharide derived from seaweed, covered in calcium and sodium salts. They are used most widely in sheet form, but ribbons and ropes also are manufactured and can be used to pack deeper wounds. When placed on a wound, sodium ions in the exudate are exchanged for calcium ions in the dressing, resulting in the formation of a hydrophilic gel.[33] Alginates are highly absorbent (15–20× their weight in fluid), nonadherent, and biodegradable.[27] They are the optimal dressing choice for highly exudative wounds. Because the calcium ions released from the dressing activate prothrombin in the clotting cascade, they also are helpful for hemostasis.[34] The entangled fibrous structure of the dressing contributes further to coagulation. Alginates have no hydration properties and thus should be avoided in dry wounds. They require a secondary dressing and should be changed up to weekly or until the gel loses its viscosity. Because they are soluble and can be removed by saline irrigation, alginate dressings changes are less painful. The yellow-brown color and malodorous smell of alginates may be falsely mistaken for infection.

HYDROFIBER AND HYDROCONDUCTIVE DRESSINGS

Hydrofiber dressings (Aquacel) are newly developed and consist of sodium carboxymethylcellulose prepared as fibers that form a band or plate. The hydrofibers are structurally and functionally similar to alginate fibers, turning into a gel once in contact with wound exudate.[35] The dressing is comfortable, easy to remove, and indicated for heavily exudative or infected wounds; the dressing can increase its weight up to 25-fold. Hydrofibers may be left in place for up to 3 days to 7 days or until saturated.[25]

Hydroconductive dressings (Drawtex) work via capillary, hydroconductive, and electrostatic action. The dressing uses 2 types of absorbent cross-action structures that facilitate the movement of large volumes of exudate, bacteria, and debris away from the wound bed into the dressing core. It provides a 90% reduction in bacterial numbers over a 24-hour period and can hold up to 8-times to 50-times its own weight, thus proving useful for highly exudative wounds.[25,36]

COMPARATIVE OUTCOMES BETWEEN CONVENTIONAL AND OCCLUSIVE DRESSINGS

Evidence comparing outcomes between gauze-based versus occlusive surgical wound healing comes mainly from the general surgery and wound care literature. For incisional wounds, although gauze dressings are not inferior with regard to cosmetic appearance or healing time, they require more frequent dressing changes and are less comfortable.[37,38] For second intention wounds, some studies report quicker healing times with occlusive dressings.[39,40] Other studies conclude that occlusive dressings do not lead to reduction in wound healing time or pain, and the decreased frequency of dressing change does not balance its higher cost.[41]

ANTIMICROBIAL DRESSINGS (SILVER, POLYHEXAMETHYLENE BIGUANIDE, IODINE, AND HONEY)

To prevent antibiotic resistance, dressings containing nonantibiotic antimicrobial compounds may be used for infected or high-risk wounds. Silver has strong and broad-spectrum antimicrobial characteristics. Silver cations exert antimicrobial activity by disruption of the cell wall, deactivation of cellular enzymes, and prevention of transcription by attaching to DNA.[42] In the past, the use of silver was limited due to its toxicity to humans, but, more recently, nanostructured silver particles with a high surface area (and therefore a higher area-to-volume ratio)

have been developed, which demonstrate greater efficacy against bacteria and less toxicity to humans.[43] A 2010 systematic review and meta-analysis showed that silver-impregnated dressings may improve short-term wounds and ulcers, but long-term data on complete wound healing are insufficient.[44] Polyhexamethylene biguanide (PHMB), a low-molecular-weight polymer with a structure related to chlorhexidine, also may be used in surgical dressings. A 2012 study by Eberlein and colleagues[45] compared the use of PHMB-containing biocellulose wound dressing against silver dressings in painful, critically colonized, and locally infected wounds and found that PHMB dressings were significantly faster and better at removing the bacterial load. It has been demonstrated, however, that soaking tie-over bolster dressings with PHMB solution in full-thickness skin grafting had no effect on postoperative bacterial loads and rather increased the risk of surgical site infection.[46] Iodine also is considered a broad-spectrum antimicrobial and is available in several dressing forms. Vermeulen and colleagues'[47] 2010 systematic review of iodine in wound care demonstrated that iodine did not lead to a reduction or prolongation of wound-healing time compared with other antiseptic wound dressings. Some of the individual trials, however, did show that iodine had significant superiority to paraffin dressings, zinc paste, silver sulfadiazine cream, and chlorhexidine dressings but was inferior to topical rifamycin dressings. Medical grade manuka honey from New Zealand and Australia is

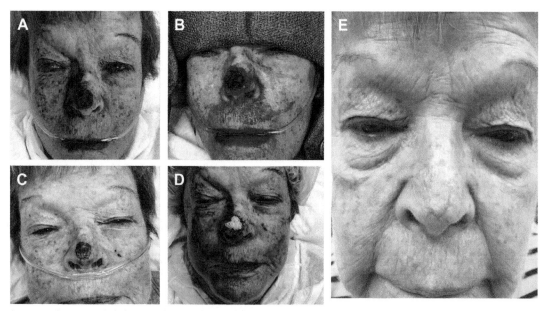

Fig. 5. Mohs surgical defect on the nasal tip (*A*). Bovine dermal regeneration template sutured into place (*B*). Three weeks later, before (*C*) and after (*D*) full-thickness skin graft placement. Three-month follow-up (*E*).

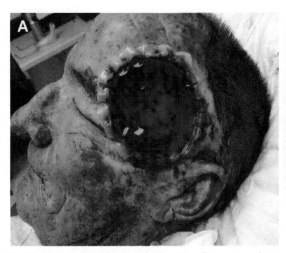 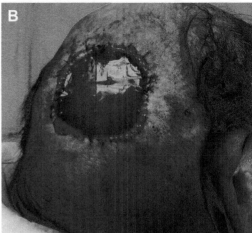

Fig. 6. Bovine dermal regeneration template sutured into large surgical defects on the left temple (*A*) and right occipital scalp (*B*).

believed to have antibacterial activity that can inhibit many bacterial species.[48] Manuka honey is available both as topical preparations (gel and paste) or impregnated into occlusive dressings (MEDIHONEY). Although there is evidence from different animal models that honey may accelerate healing compared with conventional dressings, the most recent Cochrane review in 2015 demonstrated only low-quality evidence showing that medical-grade honey heals infected postoperative wounds more quickly than antiseptics and gauze.[49,50] Nonmedical honey should not be used in wounds, because it may contain microbes and spores that can contaminate wounds.[2]

SKIN SUBSTITUTES

The advent of tissue-engineered skin substitutes has revolutionized the therapeutic potential for second intention and recalcitrant surgical wounds.[51] The goal of a skin substitute is to provide matrix materials, cells, and other key healing elements that are diminished in granulating or chronic wounds.[52,53] Unlike the other dressings, discussed previously, these materials are biodegradable and ultimately are replaced by a patient's own tissue. Skin substitutes are categorized into 3 types: epidermal, dermal, and composite (both epidermal and dermal). Dermal skin substitutes are divided further into acellular and cellular. The materials these grafts comprise may be biologic or synthetically manufactured; biologic skin substitutes are derived from a patient's own skin (autograft), another person's skin (allograft), or animals (xenograft).[54]

Epidermal Skin Substitutes

Epidermal autografts (EpiCel, EpiDex, and Laserskin) and allografts have been carried out by culturing keratinocytes from a patient's own skin and donor skin, respectively. The donor skin may be from cadavers, elective surgery patients, or neonatal foreskin (Celaderm).[55] Although they have been used to treat conditions, such as pyoderma gangrenosum, epidermolysis bullosa, severe second-degree burns, and chronic lower extremity ulcers, their use in postsurgical wounds is limited; this is because epidermal autografts take approximately 3 weeks to 4 weeks to cultivate, are extremely friable, and have a high risk of infection and poor graft take.[54,56–58]

Dermal Skin Substitutes

Dermal skin substitutes are of greater dermatologic relevance and can be divided into acellular and cellular products. Acellular dermal matrices comprise materials similar to the host extracellular matrix and function both as a barrier to fluid loss and contamination and as a template for dermal regeneration and angiogenesis.[53,59] They tend to be less expensive, be easier to produce and store, and incorporate better into the host tissue than

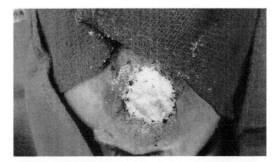

Fig. 7. Application of porcine urinary bladder matrix to a second intention Mohs surgical defect on the nasal supratip.

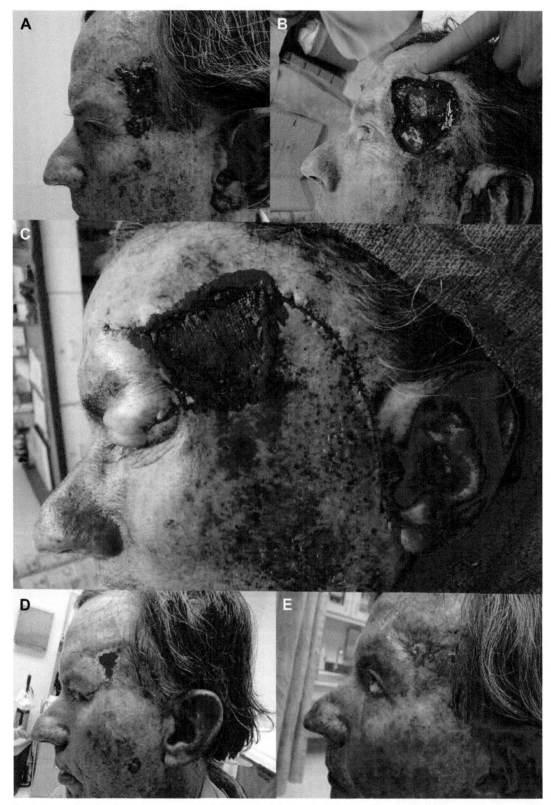

Fig. 8. Large basal cell carcinoma on the left temple (*A*). Surgical defect after Mohs micrographic surgery (*B*). Rotation flap with second intention and porcine xenograft sutured into place (*C*). Three-month follow-up (*D*). One-year follow-up, after small full-thickness skin graft placement (*E*).

cellular matrices due to their decreased antigenicity.[53,58,60] Cellular dermal matrices are composed of structural dermal scaffold as well as viable donor fibroblasts. These fibroblasts supply cytokines and growth factors required for wound healing.[58] The source of cells in these products are derived from human neonatal foreskin or maternofetal membranes. Both cellular and acellular grafts provide a barrier from the environment, protection against infection, and reduced wound pain.

Acellular dermal allografts (AlloDerm/Cymetra, AlloMax, DermaMatrix, GRAFTJACKET, FlexHD, and DermACELL) provide a scaffold into which host tissue integrates and revascularizes. They are believed to provide vascular linkage within 3 days of transplantation versus the 2 weeks to 3 weeks observed with xenografts.[58] These products have been used in patients with Mohs micrographic surgery defects as an alternative to granulation or as a bridge to split-thickness or full-thickness grafting.[61–64] Bovine (Integra and Matriderm) and porcine (Oasis, Cytal/MatriStem, and EZ Derm) acellular dermal xenografts have been used successfully in dermatologic surgery reconstruction. They are advantageous for deep wounds or those with bone, tendon, or cartilage exposure, allowing for pain reduction and dermal regeneration prior to definitive repair.[55,58] Examples of the application and outcomes of wounds treated with Integra, MatriStem, and EZ Derm can be seen in **Figs. 5–8**. Rogge and colleagues[65] published a series of 11 patients with calvarium-exposed scalp defects who underwent bovine xenograft placement and found that they had had increased rates of healing compared with second intention alone. Yang and Ochoa[66] demonstrated, by reviewing 225 porcine xenografts placed for Mohs and surgical excision defects, that they are safe and suitable methods to augment second intention healing and are applicable to many different sites and patient settings. Marzolf and colleagues'[67] retrospective review of

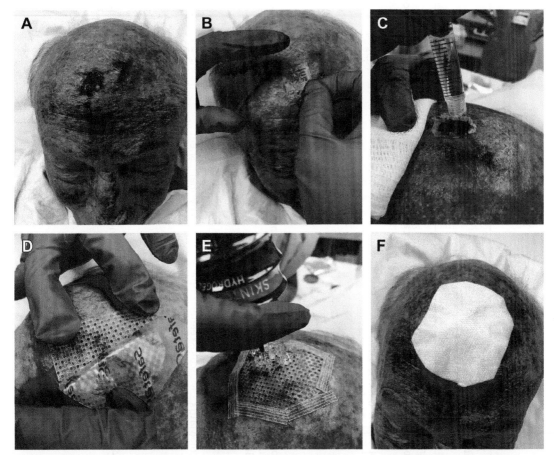

Fig. 9. Second intention wound of the midfrontal scalp (A). Application of dehydrated human amnion-chorion membrane (B). Hydration of the substitute with drops of sterile saline (C). Application of contact layer (D). Contact layer secured with paper tape and hydrated (E). Site covered with nonadherent pad and tape (F).

Table 2
Acellular dermal substitutes

Name	Manufacturer	Composition	Formulations	Storage	Application Instructions	Product Orientation
Allografts						
AlloDerm	Allergan	Dehydrated cadaveric human dermis	Sheet • AlloDerm Regenerative Tissue Matrix	Room temperature	1. Rehydrate in a 2-step bath, per instructions 2. Apply to surgical site with proper orientation	Basement membrane side: repels blood, pink when rinsed Dermal side: absorb blood, red when rinsed Meshed grafts have the letter "L" in the pattern; if you can read the letter, it is oriented properly
			Injectable particulate form • Cymetra Micronized AlloDerm	1°C–10°C	1. Rehydrate with lidocaine 2. Draw into syringe 3. Inject onto/into wound	
AlloMax Surgical Graft	C.R. Bard	Processed human dermal collagen	Sheet	Room temperature	1. Rehydrate ×5 minutes in sterile saline 2. Apply to surgical site with proper orientation 3. Suture into place	Basement membrane side: dotted, shiny, and has visible pores Dermal side: rough, with no visible pattern
DermaMatrix	Musculoskeletal Transplant Foundation/ Synthes	Donated human dermal collagen	Sheet	Room temperature	1. Rehydrate in 100 mL of saline or lactated ringers 2. Transplant onto the patient with proper orientation	Tissue notch should be on the upper left corner, facing left, when positioned correctly
GRAFTJACKET	Wright	Donated human dermis	Sheet	Room temperature	1. Rehydrate in a 5-step process, per instructions 2. Trim to dimensions 3. Apply to surgical site with proper orientation	Basement membrane side: dull, rough, buff-colored, repels blood Dermal side: Shiny, smooth, white, absorbs blood

FlexHD	Musculoskeletal Transplant Foundation	Donated human skin	Sheet	Room temperature	1. Soak in sterile solution 2. Trim to dimensions 3. Apply to surgical site with proper orientation; can be rolled or folded to desired thickness	Basement membrane side: more pigmentation, drop of blood rinsed off looks pink Dermal side: less pigmentation, drop of blood rinsed off looks red Tissue notch should be in the upper left-hand corner, facing left, when positioned correctly (epidermal side up)
DermACELL	LifeNet Health/ Stryker	Human dermis	Sheet	Room temperature	1. Immerse in sterile isotonic saline for at least 1 min, max of 4 h 2. Apply to surgical site, trim to dimensions PRN 3. Secure to wound bed/edges with suture, staples, liquid adhesive, or Steri-Strips	Basement membrane side: duller, smaller pores, repels blood Dermal side: lighter, larger pores, absorbs blood
Xenografts						
Bovine						
Integra	LifeSciences	Dermal Regeneration Template: cross-linked bovine tendon collagen and shark-derived chondroitin-6-sulfate ± disposable semipermeable silicone layer	Sheet • Bilayer matrix (Integra Dermal Regeneration Template) • Single-layer matrix (Integra Dermal Regeneration Template Single Layer) Flowable • Integra Flowable Wound Matrix	Room temperature	1. Soak in sterile saline until ready for application 2. Cut to size 3. Place collagen layer in contact with wound bed (silicone layer facing up, if using bilayer) 4. With single layer, can place an immediate split-thickness skin graft	The outer silicone layer has a black thread and should face up

(continued on next page)

Table 2
(continued)

Name	Manufacturer	Composition	Formulations	Storage	Application Instructions	Product Orientation
					5. Secure with surgical tapes or suture. With bilayer matrix, remove silicone layer 14–28 d later by peeling it back, can be replaced with a split-thickness skin graft	
MatriDerm (not available in United States)	MedSkin Solutions/ Dr Suwelack	Bovine collagen and elastin	Sheet • 1-mm thick • 2-mm thick	Room temperature	1. Apply onto wound bed, straight from pack 2. Rehydrate in the wound bed as needed with sterile saline 3. 1-mm thick: 1-step procedure with split-thickness skin graft placed same day 4. 2-mm thick: 2-step procedure with split-thickness skin graft placed 7 d later	N/A
Porcine						
OASIS	Smith & Nephew	Porcine small intestine submucosa	Sheet • One layer (OASIS Wound Matrix) • Three layers (OASIS ULTRA Matrix)	Room temperature	1. Cut to shape and apply onto wound bed 2. Secure with bandages (1 layer) or sutures/staples (3 layers) 3. Hydrate with sterile saline or hydrogel 4. Cover with dressing	N/A

Product	Company	Source	Form	Storage	Application	Notes

Cytal MatriStem	ACell	Porcine urinary bladder matrix	Sheet
			• Cytal Wound Matrix:
			  1-layer
			  2-layer
			  3-layer
			  6-layer
				Room temperature	1. Hydrate with room temperature saline for 2–45 min (1 layer and 2 layers), 5–60 min (3 layers and 6 layers)
					2. Cut sheet to desired size
					3. Apply to wound bed
					4. Cover with nonadherent dressing
						For 2-layer, 3-layer, and 6-layer devices: the tissue notch should be in the upper right-hand corner, facing right, when positioned correctly (epidermal side up)

			Particle • MatriStem MicroMatrix	Room temperature	1. Apply powder to wound bed, lightly covering entire wound; product can be poured directly from container or hydrated with sterile saline to make a paste 2. Cover with nonadherent dressing	N/A
EZ Derm	Mölnlycke	Aldehyde cross-linked porcine dermis	Sheet Comes perforated (meshed) and nonperforated	Room temperature	1. Apply either side of product to wound in a single layer 2. Surgically fix to wound 3. Leave in place until it sloughs naturally, trimming any nonadherent dry product as needed	N/A

Table 3
Cellular dermal substitutes

Name	Manufacturer	Composition	Formulation	Storage	Application Instructions	Product Orientation
Neonatal foreskin						
Dermagraft	Organogenesis	Cryopreserved human neonatal foreskin fibroblasts seeded onto a bioabsorbable polyglactin mesh		Frozen at −75°C	1. Thaw by submerging bag a warm water bath for no more than 3 min 2. Rinse per protocol 3. Cut to size of wound bed 4. Implant into débrided wound 5. Cover with nonadherent, moist dressing 6. Start dressing changes 72 h later	N/A
Maternal/fetal membranes						
EpiFix	MeMedx Group, Inc	Dehydrated human amnion/chorion membrane: single layer of epithelial cells, a basement membrane, and an avascular connective tissue matrix that contains extracellular matrix proteins, growth factors, and cytokines	Sheet Mesh	Room temperature for up to 5 y	7. Trim EpiFix to fit 8. Place on wound bed with proper orientation 9. Hydrate with sterile saline 10. Fix to wound (if applicable) with sutures or tape 11. Cover with nonadherent contact layer 12. Apply weekly until epithelialization is achieved	Orient the product onto the wound using the letter embossment "UP" as a guide, ensuring that the it reads from left to right
Grafix	Osiris Therapeutics	Cryopreserved placental membrane	Sheet	Frozen at −80°C for up to 2 y	1. Thaw product by submerging in water or saline for no more than 15 min 2. Remove from plastic backing and apply to wound bed 3. No fixation is needed 4. Apply a nonadherent, moist dressing 5. Apply weekly	N/A

128 cases of EZ Derm application at their institution revealed that the porcine xenografts were associated with minimal pain and low rates of infection (see **Figs. 5–8**).

Cellular dermal allografts can be derived from human neonatal foreskin (Dermagraft), human amniotic/chorionic membranes (EpiFix), and placental membrane (Grafix). Fibroblasts from these allografts synthesize proteins of the extracellular matrix to stimulate wound healing but also may cause an immunologic host response. Dermagraft has been successfully used for covering intraoral defects after excision of squamous cell carcinoma, resulting in complete closure of the wounds by day 11 with no evidence of fibrosis.[68] A 2014 report described patients with nonhealing postsurgical wounds that healed with the application of EpiFix dehydrated amniotic membrane material; the material was well tolerated and the wounds did not recur with long-term follow-up.[69] **Fig. 9** demonstrates the standard application of EpiFix.

Tables 2 and **3** detail many of the currently available dermal skin substitutes. The bulk of the research and approval of these products are with regard to breast reconstruction, burns, hernia surgery, and chronic venous, diabetic, and pressure ulcers. Because wound healing principles can be extrapolated across disciplines, the relative paucity of reports within the dermatology literature should not deter specialists from utilization of these skin substitutes (see **Tables 2** and **3**).

Composite Skin Substitutes

Composite grafts have both epidermal and dermal components, thus recreating natural tissue layers. Apligraf (Organogenesis) and OrCel (Forticell Bioscience) consist of both xenogenic (bovine type I collagen) and allogeneic (live human neonatal foreskin) components. StrataGraft (Mallinckrodt Pharmaceuticals) contains human dermal fibroblasts and a fully stratified, biologically active epidermis derived from near-diploid immortalized keratinocyte S (NIKS) cells—a pathogen-free, long-lived, consistent, human keratinocyte progenitor.[70] A 2002 prospective case series by Gohari and colleagues[71] evaluated the safety and efficacy of Apligraf versus second intention healing for full-thickness Mohs and excisional surgery defects. They found that, although healing time and symptoms were similar between the groups, those treated with Apligraf had more pliable, less vascular, and more cosmetically appealing scars.

Synthetic Skin Substitutes

Biobrane (Smith & Nephew) consists of an inner layer of nylon fabric mesh that allows fibrovascular ingrowth and an outer layer of silicone that serves as a vapor and bacterial barrier.[72] The dressing is temporary and should be removed once the underlying tissue has re-epithelialized, typically in 7 days to 14 days. It has been widely used in the treatment of burns and skin graft donor sites.[73] Within dermatology, it has been used for erosive skin diseases and cosmetic procedures. A 2014 case series by Gladsjo and colleagues[74] highlighted its effective use in temporary closures, delayed reconstructions, and secondary intention healing in Mohs surgery.

Collagen Dressings

Topical wound dressings composed of type I collagen scaffolding, such as Puracol Plus (Medline), Fibracol Plus (Systagenix), or BioPad (Angelini Pharma), primarily function to absorb wound exudate and prevent desiccation of the wound rather than provide bioactive components. The benefit of these materials over standard wound dressings is that, as the scaffold absorbs liquid, it protects the wound by forming a gel and sequesters damaging matrix metalloproteinases. These products, however, typically are replaced after only a few days and thus do not function as a typical scaffold to direct tissue repair.[75] One study showed that the use of Puracol Plus, a xenograft consisting of 100% pure native bovine-derived collagen in its native triple-helix formation, can be used successfully for reconstruction of dermatologic surgical scalp wounds extending to the calvarium.[65]

SUMMARY

To optimize outcomes of acute and chronic surgical dermatology wounds, a sound understanding of wound care materials and principles is necessary. Dressings are constantly undergoing innovation and investigation, and this review highlights the current landscape of wound management within dermatologic surgery.

REFERENCES

1. Winton GB, Salasche SJ. Wound dressings for dermatologic surgery. J Am Acad Dermatol 1985; 13(6):1026–44.
2. Broussard KC, Powers JG. Wound dressings: selecting the most appropriate type. Am J Clin Dermatol 2013;14(6):449–59.
3. Kannon GA, Garrett AB. Moist wound healing with occlusive dressings. A clinical review. Dermatol Surg 1995;21(7):583–90.
4. Saco M, Howe N, Nathoo R, et al. Topical antibiotic prophylaxis for prevention of surgical wound infections from

dermatologic procedures: a systematic review and meta-analysis. J Dermatolog Treat 2015;26(2):151–8.

5. Levender MM, Davis SA, Kwatra SG, et al. Use of topical antibiotics as prophylaxis in clean dermatologic procedures. J Am Acad Dermatol 2012;66(3):445–51.

6. Dixon AJ, Dixon MP, Dixon JB. Randomized clinical trial of the effect of applying ointment to surgical wounds before occlusive dressing. Br J Surg 2006;93(8):937–43.

7. Campbell RM, Perlis CS, Fisher E, et al. Gentamicin ointment versus petrolatum for management of auricular wounds. Dermatol Surg 2005;31(6):664–9.

8. Gehrig KA, Warshaw EM. Allergic contact dermatitis to topical antibiotics: epidemiology, responsible allergens, and management. J Am Acad Dermatol 2008;58(1):1–21.

9. Sheth VM, Weitzul S. Postoperative topical antimicrobial use. Dermatitis 2008;19(4):181–9.

10. Morales-Burgos A, Loosemore MP, Goldberg LH. Postoperative wound care after dermatologic procedures: a comparison of 2 commonly used petrolatum-based ointments. J Drugs Dermatol 2013;12(2):163–4.

11. Elston DM. Topical antibiotics in dermatology: emerging patterns of resistance. Dermatol Clin 2009;27(1):25–31.

12. Boateng J, Catanzano O. Advanced therapeutic dressings for effective wound healing–a review. J Pharm Sci 2015;104(11):3653–80.

13. Winter GD, Scales JT. Effect of air drying and dressings on the surface of a wound. Nature 1963;197:91–2.

14. Winter GD. Formation of the scab and the rate of epithelization of superficial wounds in the skin of the young domestic pig. Nature 1962;193:293–4.

15. Chen DL, Carlson EO, Fathi R, et al. Undermining and hemostasis. Dermatol Surg 2015;41(Suppl 10):S201–15.

16. Patel NG, Gore S, Shelley OP. Hypafix versus Mefix. J Plast Reconstr Aesthet Surg 2009;62(3):351.

17. Atkinson JA, McKenna KT, Barnett AG, et al. A randomized, controlled trial to determine the efficacy of paper tape in preventing hypertrophic scar formation in surgical incisions that traverse Langer's skin tension lines. Plast Reconstr Surg 2005;116(6):1648–56 [discussion: 1657–8].

18. Commander SJ, Chamata E, Cox J, et al. Update on postsurgical scar management. Semin Plast Surg 2016;30(3):122–8.

19. Hart RG, Wolff TW, O'Neill WL Jr. Preventing tourniquet effect when dressing finger wounds in children. Am J Emerg Med 2004;22(7):594–5.

20. Dabiri G, Damstetter E, Phillips T. Choosing a wound dressing based on common wound characteristics. Adv Wound Care (New Rochelle) 2016;5(1):32–41.

21. Bennett NT, Schultz GS. Growth factors and wound healing: biochemical properties of growth factors and their receptors. Am J Surg 1993;165(6):728–37.

22. Mast BA, Schultz GS. Interactions of cytokines, growth factors, and proteases in acute and chronic wounds. Wound Repair Regen 1996;4(4):411–20.

23. Dhivya S, Padma VV, Santhini E. Wound dressings - a review. Biomedicine (Taipei) 2015;5(4):22.

24. Ovington LG. Hanging wet-to-dry dressings out to dry. Home Healthc Nurse 2001;19(8):477–83 [quiz: 484].

25. Sood A, Granick MS, Tomaselli NL. Wound dressings and comparative effectiveness data. Adv wound care (New Rochelle) 2014;3:511–29.

26. Rubio PA. Use of semiocclusive, transparent film dressings for surgical wound protection: experience in 3637 cases. Int Surg 1991;76(4):253–4.

27. Landriscina A, Rosen J, Friedman AJ. Systematic approach to wound dressings. J Drugs Dermatol 2015;14(7):740–4.

28. Vermeulen H, Ubbink DT, Goossens A, et al. Systematic review of dressings and topical agents for surgical wounds healing by secondary intention. Br J Surg 2005;92(6):665–72.

29. Markl P, Prantl L, Schreml S, et al. Management of split-thickness donor sites with synthetic wound dressings: results of a comparative clinical study. Ann Plast Surg 2010;65(5):490–6.

30. Gokoo C, Burhop K. A comparative study of wound dressings on full-thickness wounds in micropigs. Decubitus 1993;6(5):42–3, 46, 48 passim.

31. Geronemus RG, Robins P. The effect of two new dressings on epidermal wound healing. J Dermatol Surg Oncol 1982;8(10):850–2.

32. Nguyen CV, Washington CV, Soon SL. Hydrocolloid dressings promote granulation tissue on exposed bone. Dermatol Surg 2013;39(1 Pt 1):123–5.

33. Thomas S. Alginate dressings in surgery and wound management–Part 1. J Wound Care 2000;9(2):56–60.

34. Lee KY, Mooney DJ. Alginate: properties and biomedical applications. Prog Polym Sci 2012;37(1):106–26.

35. Skorkowska-Telichowska K, Czemplik M, Kulma A, et al. The local treatment and available dressings designed for chronic wounds. J Am Acad Dermatol 2013;68(4):e117–26.

36. Edwards-Jones V, Vishnyakov V, Spruce P. Laboratory evaluation of Drawtex Hydroconductive dressing with LevaFiber technology. J Wound Care 2014;23(3):118, 120, 122-113 passim.

37. Shinohara T, Yamashita Y, Satoh K, et al. Prospective evaluation of occlusive hydrocolloid dressing versus conventional gauze dressing regarding the healing effect after abdominal operations: randomized controlled trial. Asian J Surg 2008;31(1):1–5.

38. Holm C, Petersen JS, Gronboek F, et al. Effects of occlusive and conventional gauze dressings on incisional healing after abdominal operations. Eur J Surg 1998;164(3):179–83.

39. Nemeth AJ, Eaglstein WH, Taylor JR, et al. Faster healing and less pain in skin biopsy sites treated with an occlusive dressing. Arch Dermatol 1991; 127(11):1679–83.

40. Bethell E. Why gauze dressings should not be the first choice to manage most acute surgical cavity wounds. J Wound Care 2003;12(6):237–9.

41. Ubbink DT, Vermeulen H, Goossens A, et al. Occlusive vs gauze dressings for local wound care in surgical patients: a randomized clinical trial. Arch Surg 2008;143(10):950–5.

42. Feng QL, Wu J, Chen GQ, et al. A mechanistic study of the antibacterial effect of silver ions on Escherichia coli and Staphylococcus aureus. J Biomed Mater Res 2000;52(4):662–8.

43. Rizzello L, Pompa PP. Nanosilver-based antibacterial drugs and devices: mechanisms, methodological drawbacks, and guidelines. Chem Soc Rev 2014;43(5):1501–18.

44. Carter MJ, Tingley-Kelley K, Warriner RA 3rd. Silver treatments and silver-impregnated dressings for the healing of leg wounds and ulcers: a systematic review and meta-analysis. J Am Acad Dermatol 2010;63(4):668–79.

45. Eberlein T, Haemmerle G, Signer M, et al. Comparison of PHMB-containing dressing and silver dressings in patients with critically colonised or locally infected wounds. J Wound Care 2012;21(1):12, 14-16, 18-20.

46. Saleh K, Sonesson A, Persson K, et al. Can dressings soaked with polyhexanide reduce bacterial loads in full-thickness skin grafting? A randomized controlled trial. J Am Acad Dermatol 2016;75(6): 1221–8.e4.

47. Vermeulen H, Westerbos SJ, Ubbink DT. Benefit and harm of iodine in wound care: a systematic review. J Hosp Infect 2010;76(3): 191–9.

48. Powers JG, Higham C, Broussard K, et al. Wound healing and treating wounds: chronic wound care and management. J Am Acad Dermatol 2016; 74(4):607–25 [quiz: 625–6].

49. Jull AB, Cullum N, Dumville JC, et al. Honey as a topical treatment for wounds. Cochrane Database Syst Rev 2015;(3):CD005083.

50. Jull AB, Rodgers A, Walker N. Honey as a topical treatment for wounds. Cochrane Database Syst Rev 2008;(4):CD005083.

51. Clark RA, Ghosh K, Tonnesen MG. Tissue engineering for cutaneous wounds. J Invest Dermatol 2007; 127(5):1018–29.

52. Morton LM, Phillips TJ. Wound healing and treating wounds: differential diagnosis and evaluation of chronic wounds. J Am Acad Dermatol 2016;74(4): 589–605 [quiz: 605–6].

53. Kallis PJ, Friedman AJ, Lev-Tov H. A guide to tissue-engineered skin substitutes. J Drugs Dermatol 2018; 17(1):57–64.

54. Junkins-Hopkins JM. Biologic dressings. J Am Acad Dermatol 2011;64(1):e5–7.

55. Cronin H, Goldstein G. Biologic skin substitutes and their applications in dermatology. Dermatol Surg 2013;39(1 Pt 1):30–4.

56. Limova M, Mauro T. Treatment of pyoderma gangrenosum with cultured keratinocyte autografts. J Dermatol Surg Oncol 1994;20(12): 833–6.

57. Wollina U, Konrad H, Fischer T. Recessive epidermolysis bullosa dystrophicans (Hallopeau-Siemens)–improvement of wound healing by autologous epidermal grafts on an esterified hyaluronic acid membrane. J Dermatol 2001;28(4): 217–20.

58. Foley E, Robinson A, Maloney M. Skin substitutes and dermatology: a review. Curr Dermatol Rep 2013;2:101–12.

59. Chern PL, Baum CL, Arpey CJ. Biologic dressings: current applications and limitations in dermatologic surgery. Dermatol Surg 2009;35(6):891–906.

60. Livesey SA, Herndon DN, Hollyoak MA, et al. Transplanted acellular allograft dermal matrix. Potential as a template for the reconstruction of viable dermis. Transplantation 1995;60(1):1–9.

61. Kontos AP, Qian Z, Urato NS, et al. AlloDerm grafting for large wounds after Mohs micrographic surgery. Dermatol Surg 2009;35(4):692–8.

62. Kolenik SA 3rd, Leffell DJ. The use of cryopreserved human skin allografts in wound healing following Mohs surgery. Dermatol Surg 1995;21(7):615–20.

63. Stebbins WG, Hanke CW, Petersen J. Human cadaveric dermal matrix for management of challenging surgical defects on the scalp. Dermatol Surg 2011;37(3):301–10.

64. Carucci JA, Kolenik SA 3rd, Leffell DJ. Human cadaveric allograft for repair of nasal defects after extirpation of Basal cell carcinoma by Mohs micrographic surgery. Dermatol Surg 2002;28(4): 340–3.

65. Rogge MN, Slutsky JB, Council ML, et al. Bovine collagen xenograft repair of extensive surgical scalp wounds with exposed calvarium in the elderly: increased rates of wound healing. Dermatol Surg 2015;41(7):794–802.

66. Yang YW, Ochoa SA. Use of porcine xenografts in dermatology surgery: the mayo clinic experience. Dermatol Surg 2016;42(8):985–91.

67. Marzolf S, Srivastava D, Nijhawan RI. Porcine xenografts for surgical defects: experience of a single center with 128 cases. J Am Acad Dermatol 2018; 78(5):1005–7.

68. Gath HJ, Hell B, Zarrinbal R, et al. Regeneration of intraoral defects after tumor resection with a bio-engineered human dermal replacement (Derma-graft). Plast Reconstr Surg 2002;109(3):889–93 [discussion: 894–5].

69. Sheikh ES, Fetterolf DE. Use of dehydrated human amniotic membrane allografts to promote healing in patients with refractory non healing wounds. Int Wound J 2014;11(6):711–7.

70. Centanni JM, Straseski JA, Wicks A, et al. Strata-Graft skin substitute is well-tolerated and is not acutely immunogenic in patients with traumatic wounds: results from a prospective, randomized, controlled dose escalation trial. Ann Surg 2011; 253(4):672–83.

71. Gohari S, Gambla C, Healey M, et al. Evaluation of tissue-engineered skin (human skin substitute) and secondary intention healing in the treatment of full thickness wounds after Mohs micrographic or exci-sional surgery. Dermatol Surg 2002;28(12):1107–14 [discussion: 1114].

72. Halim AS, Khoo TL, Mohd Yussof SJ. Biologic and synthetic skin substitutes: an overview. Indian J Plast Surg 2010;43(Suppl):S23–8.

73. Whitaker IS, Prowse S, Potokar TS. A critical evaluation of the use of Biobrane as a biologic skin substitute: a versatile tool for the plastic and reconstructive surgeon. Ann Plast Surg 2008;60(3): 333–7.

74. Gladsjo JA, Kim SS, Jiang SI. Review of the use of a semisynthetic bilaminar skin substitute in derma-tology and a case series report of its utility in Mohs surgery. J Drugs Dermatol 2014;13(5):537–41.

75. Turner NJ, Badylak SF. The use of biologic scaffolds in the treatment of chronic nonhealing wounds. Adv Wound Care (New Rochelle) 2015;4(8):490–500.

Patient-Centered Care in Dermatologic Surgery
Practical Strategies to Improve the Patient Experience and Visit Satisfaction

Michael P. Lee, BS*,[1], Shannon W. Zullo, MS[1],
Joseph F. Sobanko, MD, Jeremy R. Etzkorn, MD

KEYWORDS

- Mohs • Dermatologic surgery • Patient experience • Patient satisfaction • Best practices
- Patient-centered care

KEY POINTS

- Most of the skin cancer treatment procedures are performed by dermatologists who have a responsibility to deliver the highest quality of care.
- Understanding and addressing specific patient values and concerns sets the stage for patient-centered care, empowering patient autonomy and allowing for shared medical decision-making.
- Effective physician communication with thorough explanations of the surgical process can set realistic patient expectations, increased treatment compliance, and improved treatment outcomes.
- Anxiolytics, adequate pain management with proper local anesthetic injection technique, and appropriate patient-staff interactions can improve the intraoperative experience.
- Surgical patients experience elevated concerns for postoperative scarring and appearance changes. Strategies should be implemented to identify and help those at risk.

INTRODUCTION

With an aging population and an increasing incidence of skin cancer, the demand for surgical services is growing. Medicare data show that dermatologists perform the vast majority of surgical procedures for skin cancer excision and cutaneous reconstruction.[1] Therefore, dermatologists have a responsibility to properly manage and accommodate this patient population through delivery of the highest quality of care.

Barriers to providing optimal care arise throughout the surgical experience, from initial scheduling to postoperative follow-up. Occasionally, physicians and patients may prioritize aspects of care in different ways.[2] For example, patients may prioritize a positive patient-physician relationship through clear communication, as opposed to greater skill level of the surgeon, when reporting satisfaction with their surgical care.[3,4]

Limited high-quality research exists on improving the patient experience during dermatologic surgery. This review aims to provide practical and actionable information on methods to positively affect the patient experience.

PREOPERATIVE CARE AND CONSULTATION

The preoperative period can be challenging to navigate. Health care system and insurance hurdles offer resistance to smooth scheduling, which increases patient waiting time and may negatively

Disclosure Statement: Authors have no conflict of interest to disclose.
Department of Dermatology, University of Pennsylvania, 3400 Civic Center Boulevard, Suite 1-330S, Philadelphia, PA 19104, USA
[1] Co-first authors.
* Corresponding author.
E-mail address: michael.lee3@uphs.upenn.edu

Dermatol Clin 37 (2019) 367–374
https://doi.org/10.1016/j.det.2019.03.006

affect preconsultation satisfaction. Streamlining the process for new patient onboarding through implementation of checklists and standardized procedures can help decrease scheduling wait time and improve office flow. In the authors' practice, several strategies have been implemented to prepare patients for Mohs micrographic surgery (MMS) and minimize the impediments to patient scheduling. These strategies include the following: (1) using a standardized referral system that includes obtaining biopsy pathology reports and previous treatment history; (2) requesting biopsy photos to objectively confirm the anatomic site. Patient biopsy selfie photos can prove helpful in instances where photos are not taken by a referring provider[5]; and (3) instituting an evaluation system and checklist (**Table 1**) to predict the duration required to treat a tumor with MMS in order to improve surgical flow and reduce patient wait times. Practices may consider implementing similar assessment strategies to improve practice efficiency. One such scoring system is performed by allocating numerical values to tumor characteristics such as biopsy size, recurrence, and pathologic aggressiveness.[6] High-scoring tumors are correlated with increased surgical time[6] (**Table 2**).

Recent studies have investigated methods to improve practice efficiency and patient satisfaction during the surgical consultation. Most patients, especially those with a prior history of MMS or excision and larger tumor size, prefer a consultation on the day of surgery.[7] Attributes of patients preferring separate day visits include lower educational level, less experience with the health care system, and a previous history of surgical complications.[7] Same-day consultation as MMS reduces patient travel, time, and costs associated with treatment. Patients may also recall less than half of the information provided to them by their physician and use of video modules may improve education and satisfaction.[8] New and experienced patients were receptive to educational videos and agreed they were helpful in understanding Mohs surgery.[8] Furthermore, patients preferred high-definition video modules supplemented during the informed consent over provider information alone, resulting in increased patient comprehension and clinic efficiency.[9]

Preoperative telephone calls and shared medical appointments are 2 additional methods that have been investigated to improve patient satisfaction. Although preoperative educational

Table 1 New patient onboarding considerations and checklist	
Scheduling	Referral documentation: ☐ Pathology report ☐ Biopsy photos ☐ Tumor treatment history ☐ Estimated tumor size (dime, nickel, etc.): _____ ☐ Patient skin cancer history ☐ Pertinent medical history Complex tumor type: (case limit per day per surgeon) ☐ Melanoma ☐ Merkel cell carcinoma ☐ Invasive SCC ☐ Other: _____
Interdepartmental collaboration	Invasive tumor requiring collaboration: ☐ Sentinel lymph node biopsy ☐ Reconstruction Department: ☐ Plastic surgery ☐ Hematology/Oncology ☐ Urology ☐ Oculoplastic ☐ Radiation oncology ☐ Other: _____ Imaging: ☐ CT scan ☐ MRI ☐ PET
Surgical considerations	Requires additional surgical time due to anticipated: ☐ Anatomic complexity of tumor ☐ Advanced reconstruction Requires additional pathology processing time: ☐ Excision size/number of pieces ☐ Immunostaining
Physician recommendations	Scheduling timeline: ☐ Any invasive or locally advanced tumor (2–4 wk) ☐ Melanoma (<4 wk) ☐ SCC (4–8 wk) ☐ BCC next available unless ☐ critical anatomic location Requires surgical review and planning: ☐ Tumor board review ☐ Pathology review Recommendations for scheduling: ☐ Schedule as planned ☐ Requires preoperative consultation

Abbreviations: BCC, basal cell carcinoma; CT, computed tomography.

Table 2
Summary of recommendations in the preoperative setting

Preoperative Setting	Recommendation	Level of Evidence	Grade
Site identification	Biopsy site photo/patient selfie photos	2B	B
Scheduling	WAR triaging system for visit time	2C	C
	Shared medical appointments	2C	C
Patient education	Traditional or narrative educational videos	2B	B
Informed consent	Supplemental high-definition video modules	2C	C
Shared decision-making	Understanding patient priorities—local recurrence	2C	C
	Perceived involvement in treatment choices	2B	B
	Clear communication addressing expectations and concerns	1A	A

Key Points: Developing and implementing systematic approaches to new patient onboarding in preparation for MMS can lead to increased practice efficiency; effective physician communication with thorough explanations of disease prognosis and surgical process can set realistic patient expectations; understanding and addressing specific patient values and concerns sets the stage for patient-centered care, empowering patient autonomy, and allowing for shared medical decision-making; identifying patients at high risk for increased anxiety and allocating more time to focus on concerns may prove beneficial.

telephone calls do not seem to reduce anxiety or improve satisfaction,[10] shared medical appointments for initial consultation resulted in high patient satisfaction.[11] This group visit format allowed patients to receive valuable information regarding their disease and upcoming treatment while benefiting from the added questions and dialogue of their peers. However, implementation of this strategy may be logistically challenging.

More than half of preoperative Mohs patients report independently researching information about their upcoming MMS procedure but information quality available to patients can vary markedly.[12] Academic and professional society Websites tend to provide the most detailed, accurate information.[10] However, online MMS resources are often written at a reading level too difficult for most patients to comprehend.[13] Given the variability of information available online, it is important to gauge patient understanding and expectations to improve preoperative counseling.

In addition to education, identifying what patients value can improve shared decision-making and increase care quality.[14] A recent conjoint analysis demonstrated that patients preferentially selected surgical methods according to lowest rate of recurrence rather than other potential influences such as cost, travel, and surgical logistics.[14] Additional factors influencing patient preference included out-of-pocket costs and the need for

multiple visits requiring increased time commitment.[14] A second study identified similar patient priorities: high cure rate, preference for a skin cancer specialist, and not beginning reconstruction until their cancer was fully removed.[15] Understanding the importance of a patient's values can set the groundwork for providing patient-centered care and shared decision-making.

Effective physician-patient communication increases patient engagement and active participation in their care.[16] Active dialogue with patients regarding their disease, prognosis, and treatment can provide patients with a sense of autonomy, which can positively affect their perception of their overall treatment.[16] Effective communication aligns patient expectations with likely outcomes. For instance, patient expectations of excision size and scar length frequently do not align with their surgeon's estimate[17] and targeted preoperative counseling may help bridge this gap. Successful communication is also highly correlated with a patient's odds of adhering to physician recommendations and improved treatment outcomes.[18]

Recognition of elevated levels of anxiety and decreased quality of life in the preoperative period can help tailor counseling and improve the patient experience.[19,20] More than half of patients undergoing MMS have concerns regarding anticipated postsurgical changes to their appearance.[20] Most patients identified their surgeon as the appropriate person with whom best to discuss these concerns.[20] Younger age and female gender were risk factors for reduced preoperative quality of life.[19,20] Increased awareness of these at-risk patient populations can assist surgeons to effectively target patient concerns during a visit.

INTRAOPERATIVE CARE

Dermatologic surgery is a unique outpatient experience in which patients are awake and aware of the surroundings. Staff interaction with patients and their families affects patients' perceptions of the surgery. Strategies should be in place to anticipate patient concerns and minimize elements that may negatively affect the patient experience.

Anxiolytics in Dermatologic Surgery

Patients experience surgery from a different perspective than the physician. Multiple factors such as an unfamiliar environment, fear of pain, and unnerving thoughts of negative outcomes contribute to patient anxiety. Feelings of unease may not only negatively affect the patient experience but can also affect other physiologic properties increasing risks of complications.

Anxiolytic medications have been shown to be a safe and effective therapy for anxious patients, providing reduced alertness and amnesia.[21] Midazolam, compared with placebo, significantly reduces anxiety during MMS.[21] This effect is more pronounced in very anxious patients interested in anxiety-reducing treatment.[21] Although no clinically significant complications were associated with midazolam administration, patients may experience a mild drop in systolic blood pressure, which may confer some protection against bleeding-related complications.[21,22]

Midazolam has a rapid onset of action and short effect duration making it particularly suitable for short procedures. Alternatively, anxiolytic medications including lorazepam and diazepam have also been used effectively. Midazolam achieves peak concentration at 1 hour and has a mean half-life of 4 hours. The intermediate acting anxiolytic, lorazepam, is commonly used in the clinic and demonstrates a peak concentration at about 2 hours and half-life of 15 hours. Diazepam exerts longer-acting effects due to its half-life of 40 hours. These medications can be safely administered with proper clinical supervision during the procedure and by ensuring patients are discharged with a reliable chaperone.

Intraoperative Pain Management

Proper pain management for the awake patient is paramount. Procedural pain negatively influences patient perception and satisfaction with treatment.[23] It is a common practice to assess a patient for pain in the inpatient setting, but there is not a universal pain assessment strategy for dermatologic surgery. Approximately one-third3 of Mohs patients report procedural pain, many of whom experience moderate or severe pain.[22] Risk factors for pain include 3 or more intraoperative stages for tumor clearance or sensitive anatomic sites such as nose and periorbital skin.[24] MMS patients rarely report pain unless directly asked, as many expect to experience pain.[24] Implementing standardized protocols of intraoperative pain assessment, especially for procedures with long wait times, may reveal opportunities for practice improvement.

Local anesthetics possess low pH properties and can induce discomfort. Traditional strategies to mitigate injection pain include warming the solution, buffering with sodium bicarbonate, and cooling the skin.[25] The needle should be inserted perpendicular to the skin to minimize nerve irritation and the anesthetic administered slowly with needle advancement to ensure adequate infiltration.[25] Recently, use of a vibrating kinetic anesthetic device during lidocaine injections significantly reduced pain scores during injection, and patients preferred its use over control.[26] Adjunctive long-acting bupivacaine to lidocaine can also decrease the need for repeated local anesthetic injection and reduces intraoperative pain during long wait times.[27]

Additional Strategies to Improve Patient Comfort

Music intervention may reduce patient anxiety and pain when played before, during, or after surgery.[28] Music supplementation allows patients to focus their attention on a more soothing and pleasurable state. Specific to the MMS experience, patients demonstrated significantly reduced anxiety levels through personalized music choice during surgery.[29] An even more prominent reduction in anxiety was seen in patients undergoing MMS for the first time.[29] These findings were not duplicated when the selected music was not patient driven.[30]

Virtual reality may also reduce anxiety for patients undergoing skin cancer surgery.[31] Salivary cortisol levels decreased when patients were distracted from the surroundings and immersed in a relaxing environment.[31] As with music therapy, personalized, self-selected scenes or themes can improve the patient experience. These strategies may be beneficial for patients who continue to experience anxiety during surgery despite administration of anxiolytic medication or for those who prefer not to take medication.

The environment in the procedure and waiting rooms should be effectively managed with compassionate dialogue and calming interactions. Discussions between the surgeon and other staff members during a procedure may evoke anxiety in the patient through vivid imagery. Standard terms such as "cauterize" or "skin hook" may induce unnecessary anxiety. Replacing commonly used technical terms during surgery with nonverbal hand signals may be useful.[32] In the authors' experience, substituting more graphic and stress-inducing terminology such as "skin hook" with "dermal elevator" has kept patients at ease and improved their perception of the procedure.

MMS patients inherently spend a significant amount of time in the waiting room between stages and reconstruction. Altering the perception of wait times with proactive, unsolicited information delivery can improve patient satisfaction.[33] Frequent updates with explanations of long delays and providing food, beverages, and waiting-room entertainment increase engagement, positively affecting patient perception of wait time and overall experience (**Table 3**).

POSTOPERATIVE CARE

The period following dermatologic surgery represents an important opportunity to enhance a patient's perception of the overall experience. Patient concerns and priorities, including pain, physical appearance, and return to daily activities, evolve during the postoperative phase. Patient counseling should strive to anticipate issues and prepare patients for the postoperative experience. Open lines of communication and access to adequate postoperative visits permit physicians to address patient concerns in a timely fashion.

Counseling and Pain Assessment

In the authors' clinic, extensive time is spent on counseling patients for expectations in the immediate postoperative period. Before leaving clinic, staff members provide patients and family members with comprehensive verbal and written information on anticipated issues including swelling, bleeding, and pain and when to expect them. Wound care supplies are given to patients to ensure they are fully equipped to manage their wounds.

Although postoperative pain after dermatologic surgery is typically short lived and of low intensity, it is frequently a significant concern for patients. Patients experience their highest pain scores on the day of skin surgery, which significantly subside by postoperative day 4.[34] Most patients require only nonnarcotic pain medications.[34] Wound reconstruction type is correlated with pain level, with flaps and grafts associated with higher pain scores and requiring narcotic prescriptions more frequently than linear closures.[34] Patient anxiety is another pain risk factor. Patients with elevated anxiety scores may experience greater postoperative pain after MMS.[35] It may be worthwhile to identify these individuals with instruments such as the Pain Catastrophizing Scale or Pain Anxiety Symptoms Scale in order to target appropriate counseling and management.

Follow-Up Calls and Visits

Telephone calls after surgery serve as an important tool to gather information about potential complications and to address patient concerns. Same day, follow-up telephone calls after MMS result in higher satisfaction scores.[36] Patients

---

Table 3
Summary of recommendations in the intraoperative setting

Intraoperative Setting	Recommendation	Level of Evidence	Grade
Anxiety	Use of midazolam/anxiolytic medication	1B	A
	Personalized music therapy	1C	B
	Use of virtual reality	2B	B
Pain	Standardized pain assessment	3B	C
	Use of vibrating kinetic anesthetic device with analgesic techniques	2B	B
	Bupivacaine as adjunct to lidocaine	2B	B
Graphic terminology	Replace with hand signals or substitute terms	5	D
Waiting area	Provide shorter perception of wait time by keeping patients engaged	2C	C

Key Points: Dermatologic surgery is a unique surgical setting in which patients are awake and aware of their surroundings; consider anxiolytics, adequate pain management with proper local anesthetic injection, and appropriate patient and staff interactions; the perception of wait time may influence overall patient satisfaction more than actual wait time.

Table 4
Summary of recommendations in the postoperative setting

Postoperative Setting	Recommendation	Level of Evidence	Grade
Pain	Address common postoperative pain patterns	2C	C
	Identify highly anxious patients who are at risk	2C	C
Follow-up	Same day telephone calls by staff member	2B	B
	Follow-up visit within 4 wk	3B	C
Early scar revision	585-nm pulsed dye laser	2B	B
	Safe treatments to improve patient perception	2B	B

Key Points: Important setting for continued physician communication and follow-up to address concerns, align expectations, and optimize overall experience; period of increased patient concern for scarring and appearance changes, appropriate management should be targeted at those with increased risk of postoperative dissatisfaction including scar revision to improve cosmetic outcomes.

appreciate the personalized care, whether the surgeon or another health care provider makes the call.[36]

In the authors' clinic, patients can access staff by telephone and an online communication portal that facilitates sharing of surgical site photos and medical concerns. On postoperative day 1, office staff actively reach out to patients via telephone call to elicit and address any concerns. In addition, surgeons provide their personal phone numbers for after-hours or emergency concerns. Simply having the surgeon's phone number for emergencies provides comfort to patients and allows the surgeon to address patient concerns and complications in an expeditious fashion. Through these steps, the authors strive to eliminate any uncertainty or confusion following surgery and enhance the patient experience.

Postoperative follow-up visits are another tool in addressing patient concerns and expectations. Eighty-nine percent of patients from a dermatologic surgery practice considered postoperative follow-up important, with 55% of these patients opting for a follow-up visit within 4 weeks.[37] The major reason to request follow-up was to ensure wounds were healing correctly.[37]

Impact of Surgery on Patient Quality of Life

Patient quality of life (QOL) domains evolve differently after MMS. One to two weeks after surgery, patient anxiety about skin cancer is reduced but concerns about physical appearance persist.[19] Patient-centered outcomes such as physical appearance should be carefully addressed throughout the perioperative period. Scarring and disfigurement are highly relevant outcome measures to patients who have the potential to detract

from patient QOL.[38] Elevated anxiety about disfigurement may impair one's ability to cope effectively with outcomes after surgery.[39] There is also frequent disagreement between physicians and patients in scar assessments.[17] Because of commonly discordant perceptions of surgery outcomes between patients and physicians, it may be beneficial to longitudinally measure patient-reported outcomes using validated QOL instruments, such as skin cancer index. This may allow surgeons to identify at-risk patients and intervene in targeted ways.

It is important to set patient expectations during the preoperative period regarding scar evolution and anticipated timeline. However, many patients prefer to expedite cosmetic improvement. Early pulsed dye laser (PDL) is an effective and safe treatment to improve surgical scar appearance.[40] After 3 treatments with 585-nm PDL, a significant difference was seen with scar vascularity and pliability.[40] Early postoperative intervention with fractional CO_2 laser also produces patient-reported scar improvement, despite limited objective improvements.[41] Early intervention with lasers seems safe and helps to quell patient concerns during a high-risk period for patient psychological distress (**Table 4**).

SUMMARY

Numerous barriers to improving the patient experience exist throughout the perioperative period. Increased awareness and acknowledgment of these factors allows surgeons to take practical steps toward overcoming common impediments. Preoperatively implementing strategies that streamline patient scheduling, increase health literacy, and elicit patient preferences may decrease patient anxiety and improve shared decision making. Addressing intraoperative anxiety and pain with delicate communication, anxiolytics, strategic anesthetic injections, and distractions such as music can improve the overall experience. Proactive patient counseling of anticipated issues and outcomes, wound care instructions, and pain management improve the postoperative experience. Additionally, open lines of postoperative communication with practice staff and surgeons reassure patients and increase treatment compliance. Lastly, continued evaluation of patient appearance related concerns throughout the perioperative period helps to define patient expectations and anticipate issues.

REFERENCES

1. Kantor J. Dermatologists perform more reconstructive surgery in the Medicare population than any other specialist group: a cross-sectional individual-level analysis of Medicare volume and specialist type in cutaneous and reconstructive surgery. J Am Acad Dermatol 2018;78(1):171–3.e1.

2. Harun NA, Finlay AY, Salek MS, et al. Appropriate and inappropriate influences on outpatient discharge decision making in dermatology: a prospective qualitative study. Br J Dermatol 2015;173(3):720–30.

3. Fiala TG. What do patients want? Technical quality versus functional quality: a literature review for plastic surgeons. Aesthet Surg J 2012;32(6):751–9.

4. Golda N, Beeson S, Kohli N, et al. Recommendations for improving the patient experience in specialty encounters. J Am Acad Dermatol 2018;78(4):653–9.

5. Highsmith JT, Weinstein DA, Highsmith MJ, et al. BIOPSY 1-2-3 in dermatologic surgery: improving smartphone use to avoid wrong-site surgery. Technol Innov 2016;18(2–3):203–6.

6. Rivera AE, Webb JM, Cleaver LJ. The Webb and Rivera (WAR) score: a preoperative Mohs surgery assessment tool. Arch Dermatol 2012;148(2):206–10.

7. Sharon VR, Armstrong AW, Jim On SC, et al. Separate- versus same-day preoperative consultation in dermatologic surgery: a patient-centered investigation in an academic practice. Dermatol Surg 2013;39(2):240–7.

8. Newsom E, Lee E, Rossi A, et al. Modernizing the Mohs surgery consultation: instituting a video module for improved patient education and satisfaction. Dermatol Surg 2018;44(6):778–84.

9. Migden M, Chavez-Frazier A, Nguyen T. The use of high definition video modules for delivery of informed consent and wound care education in the Mohs Surgery Unit. Semin Cutan Med Surg 2008;27(1):89–93.

10. Sobanko JF, Da Silva D, Chiesa Fuxench ZC, et al. Preoperative telephone consultation does not decrease patient anxiety before Mohs micrographic surgery. J Am Acad Dermatol 2017;76(3):519–26.

11. Knackstedt TJ, Samie FH. Shared medical appointments for the preoperative consultation visit of Mohs micrographic surgery. J Am Acad Dermatol 2015;72(2):340–4.

12. Miller CJ, Neuhaus IM, Sobanko JF, et al. Accuracy and completeness of patient information in organic World-Wide Web search for Mohs surgery: a prospective cross-sectional multirater study using consensus criteria. Dermatol Surg 2013;39(11):1654–61.

13. Vargas CR, DePry J, Lee BT, et al. The readability of online patient information about Mohs micrographic surgery. Dermatol Surg 2016;42(10):1135–41.

14. Etzkorn JR, Tuttle SD, Lim I, et al. Patients prioritize local recurrence risk over other attributes for surgical treatment of facial melanomas-Results of a stated preference survey and choice-based conjoint analysis. J Am Acad Dermatol 2018;79(2):210–9.e3.

15. Chuang GS, Leach BC, Wheless L, et al. Preoperative expectations and values of patients undergoing Mohs micrographic surgery. Dermatol Surg 2011;37(3):311–9.

16. Martinez KA, Resnicow K, Williams GC, et al. Does physician communication style impact patient report of decision quality for breast cancer treatment? Patient Educ Couns 2016;99(12):1947–54.

17. Zhang J, Miller CJ, O'Malley V, et al. Patient and physician assessment of surgical scars: a systematic review. JAMA Facial Plast Surg 2018;20(4):314–23.

18. Zolnierek KB, Dimatteo MR. Physician communication and patient adherence to treatment: a meta-analysis. Med Care 2009;47(8):826–34.

19. Zhang J, Miller CJ, O'Malley V, et al. Patient quality of life fluctuates before and after Mohs micrographic surgery: a longitudinal assessment of the patient experience. J Am Acad Dermatol 2018;78(6):1060–7.

20. Pearl RL, Shao K, Shin TM, et al. Acute appearance concerns in patients undergoing mohs surgery: a single-institution cross-sectional study. Dermatol Surg 2018;44(10):1349–51.

21. Ravitskiy L, Phillips PK, Roenigk RK, et al. The use of oral midazolam for perioperative anxiolysis of healthy patients undergoing Mohs surgery: conclusions from randomized controlled and prospective studies. J Am Acad Dermatol 2011;64(2):310–22.

22. Jayasekera PSA, Kai A, Lawrence CM. Preoperative hypertension increases intraoperative bleeding in patients undergoing Mohs micrographic surgery. J Am Acad Dermatol 2019;80(2):562–4.

23. Glass JS, Hardy CL, Meeks NM, et al. Acute pain management in dermatology: risk assessment and

treatment. J Am Acad Dermatol 2015;73(4):543–60 [quiz: 561–2].

24. Connolly KL, Nehal KS, Dusza SW, et al. Assessment of intraoperative pain during Mohs micrographic surgery (MMS): An opportunity for improved patient care. J Am Acad Dermatol 2016;75(3):590–4.

25. Mustoe TA, Buck DW 2nd, Lalonde DH. The safe management of anesthesia, sedation, and pain in plastic surgery. Plast Reconstr Surg 2010;126(4):165e–76e.

26. Fix WC, Chiesa-Fuxench ZC, Shin T, et al. Use of a vibrating kinetic anesthesia device (KAD) reduces the pain of lidocaine injections: a randomized split-body trial. J Am Acad Dermatol 2019;80(1):58–9.

27. Chen P, Smith H, Vinciullo C. Bupivacaine as an adjunct to lidocaine in Mohs micrographic surgery: a prospective randomized controlled trial. Dermatol Surg 2018;44(5):607–10.

28. Kuhlmann AYR, de Rooij A, Kroese LF, et al. Meta-analysis evaluating music interventions for anxiety and pain in surgery. Br J Surg 2018;105(7):773–83.

29. Vachiramon V, Sobanko JF, Rattanaumpawan P, et al. Music reduces patient anxiety during Mohs surgery: an open-label randomized controlled trial. Dermatol Surg 2013;39(2):298–305.

30. Alam M, Roongpisuthipong W, Kim NA, et al. Utility of recorded guided imagery and relaxing music in reducing patient pain and anxiety, and surgeon anxiety, during cutaneous surgical procedures: a single-blinded randomized controlled trial. J Am Acad Dermatol 2016;75(3):585–9.

31. Ganry L, Hersant B, Sidahmed-Mezi M, et al. Using virtual reality to control preoperative anxiety in ambulatory surgery patients: a pilot study in maxillofacial and plastic surgery. J Stomatol Oral Maxillofac Surg 2018;119(4):257–61.

32. Fulchiero GJ, Vujevich JJ, Goldberg LH. Nonverbal hand signals: a tool for increasing patient comfort during dermatologic surgery. Dermatol Surg 2009;35(5):856–7.

33. Thompson DA, Yarnold PR, Williams DR, et al. Effects of actual waiting time, perceived waiting time, information delivery, and expressive quality on patient satisfaction in the emergency department. Ann Emerg Med 1996;28(6):657–65.

34. Firoz BF, Goldberg LH, Arnon O, et al. An analysis of pain and analgesia after Mohs micrographic surgery. J Am Acad Dermatol 2010;63(1):79–86.

35. Chen AF, Landy DC, Kumetz E, et al. Prediction of postoperative pain after Mohs micrographic surgery with 2 validated pain anxiety scales. Dermatol Surg 2015;41(1):40–7.

36. Hafiji J, Salmon P, Hussain W. Patient satisfaction with post-operative telephone calls after Mohs micrographic surgery: a New Zealand and U.K. experience. Br J Dermatol 2012;167(3):570–4.

37. Sharon VR, Armstrong AW, Jim-On S, et al. Post-operative preferences in cutaneous surgery: a patient-centered investigation from an academic dermatologic surgery practice. Dermatol Surg 2013;39(5):773–8.

38. Etzkorn JR, Gharavi NM, Carr DR, et al. Examining the Relevance to Patients of Complications in the American College of Mohs Surgery Registry: results of a delphi consensus process. Dermatol Surg 2018;44(6):763–7.

39. Sobanko JF, Sarwer DB, Zvargulis Z, et al. Importance of physical appearance in patients with skin cancer. Dermatol Surg 2015;41(2):183–8.

40. Nouri K, Jimenez GP, Harrison-Balestra C, et al. 585-nm pulsed dye laser in the treatment of surgical scars starting on the suture removal day. Dermatol Surg 2003;29(1):65–73 [discussion: 73].

41. Sobanko JF, Vachiramon V, Rattanaumpawan P, et al. Early postoperative single treatment ablative fractional lasing of Mohs micrographic surgery facial scars: a split-scar, evaluator-blinded study. Lasers Surg Med 2015;47(1):1–5.

Surgical and Noninvasive Modalities for Scar Revision

Rachel E. Ward, MD[a,1], Lindsay R. Sklar, MD[b],
Daniel B. Eisen, MD[b],*

KEYWORDS

- Scar revision • Noninvasive • Surgery • Laser • Dermabrasion • Silicone gel sheeting • Subcision
- TCA CROSS

KEY POINTS

- Every surgeon needs to revise an unsatisfactory outcome at some point. Knowledge of available revision techniques helps in choosing the correct methodology.
- Modalities include surgical revision, topical treatments, and mechanical and energy-based techniques.
- Appropriate patient selection and revision technique are important to optimize patient satisfaction and outcome.

INTRODUCTION

Treatments to improve the function, texture, contour, and color of the skin have been around since at least the sixteenth century. Several modalities exist for the treatment of suboptimal scars. These include the use of silicone gel sheets, resurfacing with electrosurgical instruments (electrobrasion), manual or mechanical dermabrasion, chemical peels, subcutaneous incisionless surgery (subcision), intralesional steroid injection, laser, and, lastly, excisional modalities and/or surgical rearrangement of skin. Thorough understanding of the benefits and potential complications of each of these techniques helps physicians individualize care for their patients with suboptimal surgical scars. Herein is a discussion of these scar revision modalities as well as the advantages and disadvantages of each (**Table 1**).

DERMABRASION

Dermabrasion is one of the oldest and most widely studied techniques for scar resurfacing. This procedure improves scar contour and color match with the surrounding skin through use of either sterile sandpaper for manual dermabrasion (dermasanding) or diamond fraise (or wire brush) for mechanical dermabrasion. Both approaches have a common outcome of promoting dermal fibroplasia as a means for scar improvement (**Fig. 1**).[1] The target depth of dermabrasion typically is the papillary dermis.[2]

The most cost-effective way to dermabrade is with sterile commercial-grade sandpaper wrapped around a cylindrical object. Most surgeons begin dermabrasion with a medium-to-fine grit sandpaper until the papillary or superficial reticular dermis is reached.[2–4] Another option is to use a sterile cautery scratch pad folded on itself.[5]

Disclosure Statement: The authors have nothing to disclose.
[a] Department of Dermatology, Wayne State University School of Medicine, Detroit, MI, USA; [b] Department of Dermatology, University of California Davis Medical System, 3301 C Street, #1400, Sacramento, CA 95816, USA
[1] Present address: 18100 Oakwood Boulevard, Suite 300, Dearborn, MI 48124.
* Corresponding author.
E-mail address: deisen123@gmail.com

Dermatol Clin 37 (2019) 375–386
https://doi.org/10.1016/j.det.2019.03.007

Table 1
Modalities for scar revision

Revision Modality	Advantages	Disadvantages	Indications
Dermabrasion	Ease of use Cost efficient	Risk of scarring Risk of blood-borne pathogen transmission (with mechanical dermabrasion)	Scars that are uneven, bumpy, have color or contour irregularity
Electrobrasion	Ease of use Cost efficient No need to purchase additional equipment	Nonuniform response to treatment	Scars that are uneven, bumpy, have color or contour irregularity
Re-excision	Relatively quick procedure	Invasive Patient hesitation for further surgical intervention	Small to moderately sized undesirable scars (hypertrophic, atrophic, depressed, widened)
Serial excision	Ability to use adjacent skin from similar cosmetic subunit	Widening of scar if closed under too much tension Lengthy procedure Patient must return for numerous procedures	Large undesirable scars (hypertrophic, atrophic, depressed, widened)
Z-plasty	Lengthening of scar Reorientation of scar (often to be parallel to RSTLs and perpendicular to free margins)	Zigzag scar may be more noticeable than linear scar	Ectropion, eclabium, skin webbing Misoriented smaller scars
Silicone gel	Ease of use Cost efficient Painless	Nonuniform response to treatment	Generalized scar improvement Erythema
Intralesional corticosteroid and massage	Quick procedure Cost effective	Nonuniform response to treatment Need for repeated injections Painful	Trapdoor deformity Keloid/hypertrophic scar
Subcision	Ease of use Cost efficient	Nonuniform response to treatment Risk of redepression of scars Risk of needlestick injury to surgeon Possible postoperative hypertrophic scarring	Small, depressed scars
TCA CROSS	Ease of use Cost efficient	Risk of hyperpigmentation, especially in darker skin types Risk of postoperative hypertrophic scarring	Small, depressed scars Uneven, bumpy scars
Lasers			
Nonablative fractional	Less downtime and less discomfort than fully ablative lasers	Cost of treatment Discomfort Less significant results compared with ablative lasers Erythema and edema	Depressed, uneven, or lumpy scars

(continued on next page)

Table 1 (continued)			
Revision Modality	Advantages	Disadvantages	Indications
Fully ablative	Significant results	Cost of treatment Risk of scarring Prolonged downtime and edema Persistent erythema Keloid formation Permanent dyschromia	Depressed, uneven, or lumpy scars
PDL	Well tolerated	Possible postoperative purpura	Erythema

Alternatively, there are various motorized derm-abrasion units that can be purchased to employ mechanical dermabrasion.[2] These units typically are fitted with diamond fraises or wire brushes of varying shape, grit, and width. The authors prefer to avoid the mechanical option for all but very large scars. The time required to set up the device, the need for special protective equipment during the procedure, and the propensity for gauze to become entangled on the fraise are all disadvantages of mechanical dermabrasion.

The surgeon uses a manual or mechanical dermabrasion modality, traversing the designated area in a back-and-forth manner until diffuse punctate bleeding is appreciated. This bleeding designates that the upper papillary dermis has been reached. After completion of the procedure, profuse bleeding is typical. The authors cover the

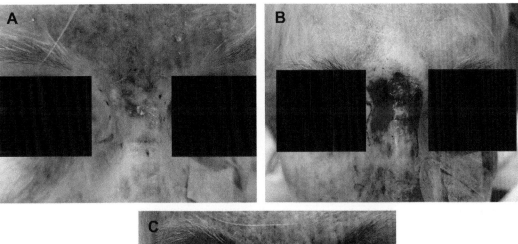

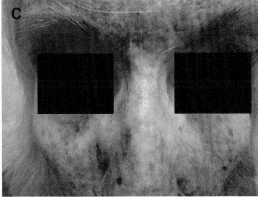

Fig. 1. Electrobrasion and dermabrasion. (A) Patient with nasal root and glabella graft exhibiting textural and color mismatch with surrounding skin. She was treated with dermabrasion on the left half of the wound and elec-trobrasion on the right half as part of an institutional review board–approved clinical trial. (B) Immediately after electrobrasion and dermabrasion. (C) Two months after treatment, both sides have improved.

abraded site with lidocaine and epinephrine–soaked gauze until bleeding stops. Complete re-epithelialization usually occurs in 7 days to 10 days.

Previous studies have compared dermabrasion with laser modalities. In 1 study, the ablative non-fractionated pulsed CO_2 laser was comparable in outcome to dermabrasion.[6] A randomized controlled split-scar trial comparing fractionated CO_2 laser resurfacing to diamond fraise dermabrasion on postsurgical scars on the face showed similar outcomes, with the laser-treated scars having less erythema and edema than those treated with dermabrasion.[7]

There are several advantages to dermabrasion. Dermabrasion can be used in any outpatient setting, and the cost of treatment is low, especially in comparison to laser treatment. One of the main disadvantages to dermabrasion is risk of further scarring if the surgeon abrades tissue too deeply.[2] With mechanical dermabrasion, there also is an increased theoretic risk of transmission of blood-borne pathogens.[2] Additionally, dermabrasion in darker skin types increases the risk for persistent dyschromia.[3]

ELECTROBRASION AND ELECTROABLATION

The term, *electrobrasion*, was first introduced in 2010 as a method of achieving similar results to dermabrasion using a hyfrecator to superficially ablate the skin.[8]

A standard electrosurgical unit is used to superficially ablate the scar and several millimeters of surrounding tissue. The depth of treatment can be controlled by adjusting the power of the tool, time of contact with tissue, and distance between the electrosurgical tool and the skin surface. The authors typically use low-power settings (5–10 W).

A randomized, double-blind trial comparing the effectiveness of electrobrasion to manual dermabrasion with sterile sandpaper showed that both modalities improved scar appearance, and there was no statistical difference between outcomes.[9] The authors concluded that electrobrasion was an acceptable, cost-effective alternative to dermabrasion that also decreased postprocedure bleeding time.

Electroablation is the use of an electrosurgical instrument with an epilating needle to drill small holes in protuberant tissue.[8,10] Similar to fractionated ablative lasers, the treatment causes immediate tissue contraction. The authors find this technique useful for treating protuberant grafts, flaps with trapdoor deformities, or standing cones (**Fig. 2**). Disadvantages of this technique are the potential risk of scarring from overtreatment and the need for an electrosurgical instrument and epilating needles.

RE-EXCISION

The least technically demanding modality of invasive scar revision is a fusiform or curvilinear re-excision. This typically is used for small to moderately sized scars that have become depressed, hypertrophic, or widened after the initial surgery. Re-excision should be performed on scars that have had at least 6 months to mature.[11]

One of the most important principles in re-excision is scar placement. Ideally, the final scar should run parallel to resting skin tension lines (RSTLs) and perpendicular to free margins. The ellipse is drawn around the margins of the scar, and the surrounding skin is widely undermined (**Fig. 3**). Suturing techniques, such as set-back suturing for subcutaneous sutures, vertical mattress or running subcuticular sutures for cuticular suture placement, and the running horizontal mattress suture can improve cosmetic outcomes.[12–14]

An advantage of elliptical re-excision is that it is a relatively simple procedure. A disadvantage of re-excision is that the resultant scar always is longer than the original, and many patients are unwilling to undergo the procedure again after a poor outcome from the original excision.

SERIAL EXCISION

At times, scars are too large or inelastic to allow for revision in 1 stage. Serial excision allows for a staged procedure wherein normal adjacent skin is recruited to replace a functionally or cosmetically flawed scar. Serial excision relies on the principle of mechanical tissue creep, where microfragmentation of elastic fibers, dehydration of the affected tissue, and collagen fiber rearrangement allow for stretching of the tissue beyond its original capabilities.[15] Biological tissue creep then follows with synthesis of new collagen and elastin fibers and neovascularization.[15]

For scarred skin, it has been suggested that serial incisions should be made at the periphery of the scar.[16] The authors of this article prefer a central incision for simplicity's sake, because there is no evidence that other techniques result in better outcomes.

One advantage of serial excision is that the adjacent skin typically is from a similar cosmetic subunit, so it has the best color and texture match to the target area. This is especially advantageous for scalp scars, whereby adjacent hair-bearing

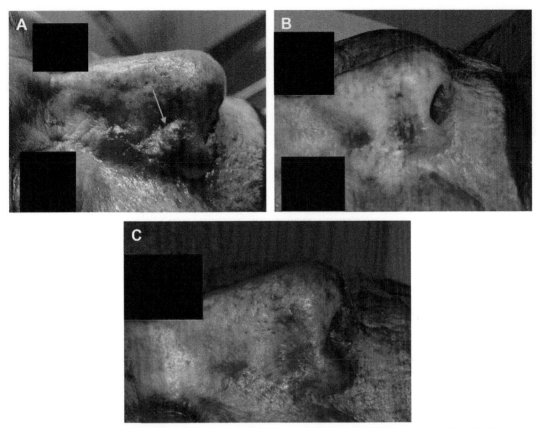

Fig. 2. Electroablation. (*A*) Trapdoor deformity resulting from tunneled cheek interpolation flap. (*B*) Flap immediately after electroablation. (*C*) Four-month follow-up.

skin can be advanced to replace alopecic scars.[17] A disadvantage of serial excision is that the patient must return for more than 1-staged procedures.

Z-PLASTY

A Z-plasty is used to lengthen and reorient contracted scars. Although this technique can be used in nearly any location, the most common areas of use are the canthi, oral commissures, and alar bases.[11] Advantages of Z-plasties include redirecting scars to be parallel to the RSTLs, lengthening scars, and redistributing tension (which is especially important to correct ectropion, eclabium, and skin webs). Additionally, some investigators suggest the zigzag configuration may allow the final scar to be less visible.[18] They posit that breaking a long scar into multiple smaller sub-units, through the Z-plasty technique, makes the scar less visible. A recent national survey study found, however, significantly more patients preferred linear scars to the same scar in a zigzag confirmation.[18] Although there is doubt as to whether the zigzag configuration of Z-plasties improves aesthetic outcomes over linear closures, it

is clear that it has significant benefit for scar webs, eclabium, ectropion, or misoriented scars.

Many variations on the Z-plasty have been described, including altering the angle size, limb length, and number of flaps.[19] As the limb angle increases, so does the final length of the scar; 30° angles increase the final scar length by 25%, 45° angles increase the final scar length by 50%, and 60° angles lengthen the final scar length by 75%.[20] The most commonly used angle is 60°. For longer scars, often a surgeon must use multiple adjacent and consecutive smaller Z-plasties rather than 1 large Z-plasty to preserve surrounding tissue, redistribute tension over a greater area, and allow the final scar to be less visible (**Fig. 4**).[12] Although Z-plasties predictably increase scar length, the overall lengthening may vary significantly patient to patient, depending on several factors, including the nature of the scar, age, and location, among other variables.

SILICONE GEL

Silicones are made up of polymerized siloxanes, or polysiloxanes, which are chains of alternating

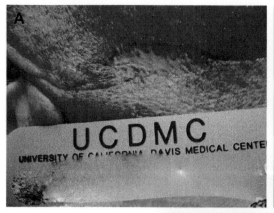
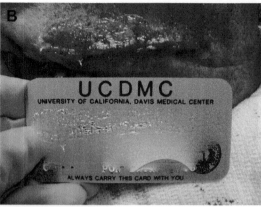
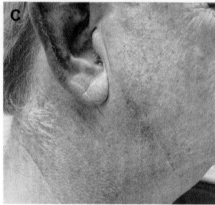

Fig. 3. Re-excision. (*A*) Patient with a widened scar with prominent track marks. (*B*) Scar excised and sutured. Note the excised tissue is, by necessity, longer than the original scar. This is something that needs to be explained to the patient prior to the procedure. (*C*) Result at 3 months.

silicone and oxygen atoms combined with other elements. The most common polysiloxane is polydimethylsiloxane, which is used in medical-grade silicone products, including silicone gel and sheeting. Silicone-based products are used most often in patients who have, or are at high-risk for the development of, hypertrophic or keloidal scarring. It has been postulated that these products act via occlusion and hydration of the stratum corneum rather than by direct action of the silicone element itself.[21] These materials have been shown to improve color, thickness, and elasticity of scars.[22]

Guidelines are lacking regarding the optimal timing of onset and duration of treatment with silicone-based products. Some studies have shown promising results when the sheet is applied for at least 4 hours daily with a duration of use of at least 3 months.[22] Some sources recommend starting treatment when the scar is less than 3 months old. Other studies, however, have shown efficacy for scars older than 12 months.[22]

Numerous randomized controlled and split-scar trials have shown superior results in scar appearance when using silicone gel or sheeting as directly compared with control and onion extract use,[23,24] although some investigators have criticized the quality of these trials. Despite these concerns, many sources consider silicone-based products the gold standard of noninvasive modalities for scar prevention and treatment.[25]

Silicone-containing products are easy to use, painless, and have minimal, if any, side effects. Another advantage is that the sheeting can be washed and reused for up to 4 weeks to 8 weeks, which decreases the overall cost of treatment.[22] The disadvantages of this treatment include the nonuniform response to treatment.

INTRALESIONAL CORTICOSTEROIDS AND MASSAGE THERAPY

Intralesional corticosteroids typically are used in the treatment of trapdoor deformities, hypertrophic scarring, and keloidal scarring (**Fig. 5**). Corticosteroids have numerous effects on bulky scars,

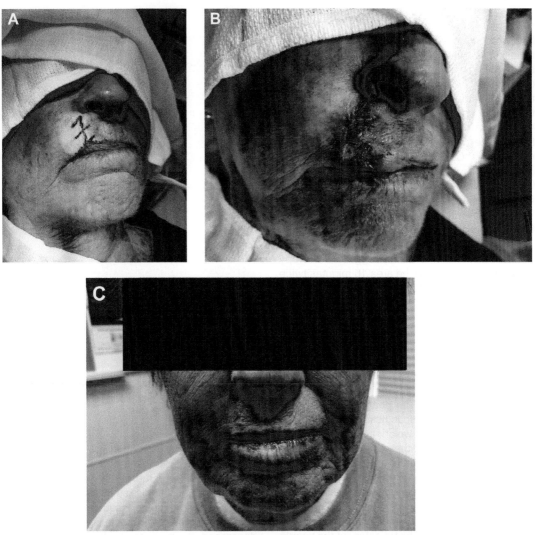

Fig. 4. Z-plasty. (A) Patient with eclabium and planned Z-plasty revision. (B) Sutured flaps. (C). Result at 5 months with resolution of eclabium.

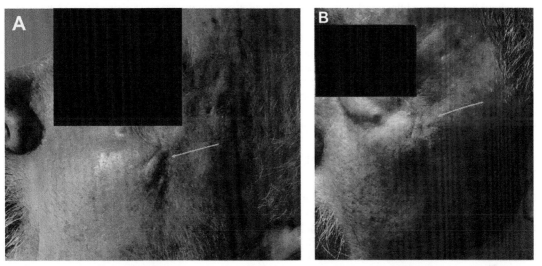

Fig. 5. Kenalog. (A) Rhombic flap with prominent trapdoor scarring. (B). Two months after injection of 0.2-mL of 40-mg/mL triamcinolone acetonide.

including decreasing inflammatory mediators, inhibiting keratinocyte and fibroblast proliferation, and reducing nourishment to scar tissues via vasoconstriction.[26] Triamcinolone acetonide 0.1% is the steroid of choice for many physicians and typically is used in dilutions from 10 mg/mL to 40 mg/mL. Injections are repeated at 2-week to 8-week intervals or until the desired endpoint is reached.[27,28] Corticosteroids may cause atrophy of the dermis and subcutaneous fat, which can lead to depigmentation, telangiectasias, and surface irregularities.

The use of scar massage therapy can be beneficial in improving, and possibly preventing, the development of hypertrophic scarring, although scientific data are weak.[29] Suggested therapy ranges from massaging the area 10 minutes twice daily to 30 minutes 3 times daily to 30 minutes 3 times per week.[29]

SUBCISION

Subcision[30] is an alternative to surgery and mainly is used in the treatment of bound-down or tethered scars, such as the rolling and depressed scars seen in acne scarring. The goal is to both break up the dense, fibrous scar tissue and stimulate new collagen growth, which act in concert to elevate the concavity of the scar.

To perform the procedure, the surgeon inserts a hypodermic needle (the authors recommend a Nokor needle (**Fig. 6**) (Nokor needle, Becton, Dickinson and Company, New Jersey), which contains a flat cutting tip) into the dermis underlying the scar at a shallow angle, with the trajectory of the needle running parallel to the epidermal surface. The needle then is inserted repeatedly in a fanning motion throughout the entirety of the scar.

Subcision typically is well tolerated, inexpensive, and easy to perform in an outpatient setting. The main disadvantages are the varied response to treatment and the risk of redepression of scars, which can occur up to 10 days postprocedure.[31] Other disadvantages include risks of permanent hyperpigmentation, hypertrophic scarring, and needlestick injury for surgeons.[32]

TRICHLOROACETIC ACID AND CHEMICAL RECONSTRUCTION OF SKIN SCARS

Chemical peeling of the skin has been used for decades due to its ability to exfoliate the skin and stimulate collagen growth and remodeling. The chemical reconstruction of skin scars (CROSS) technique was first described by Lee and colleagues[33] in 2002, whereby varying concentrations of trichloroacetic acid (TCA) were focally

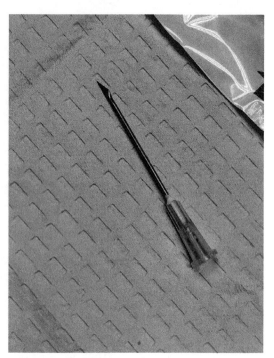

Fig. 6. Nokor needle. The presence of a flat cutting tip facilitates easy subcision of scars. The needle is inserted at the edge of the depressed scar and fanned underneath the area.

applied at the base of atrophic acne scars, with the result of elevating the base of the scar. Since then, comparative studies have shown similar results using other acids, such as phenolic acid,[34] as well as to fractionated resurfacing. The CROSS technique has been most effective for deep, depressed scars, such as those seen in acne scarring.

For this technique, a tapered wooden applicator is dipped in the TCA solution and carefully applied to the base of the depressed scar. The endpoint is a white frost-like appearance to the scar (**Fig. 7**), which can be achieved with a low volume of acid. This procedure can be repeated every 2 weeks to 4 weeks until a desired appearance is reached.

TCA CROSS is an inexpensive and quick procedure to complete. Caution must be used when treating darker skin types due to the risk of permanent dyschromia.[35] There also is a risk of hypertrophic scar development, especially with higher concentrations of acid.[36]

LASERS

Ablative lasers, including the 10,600-nm CO_2 laser and the 2940-Er:YAG laser, have been used in the treatment of hypertrophic and atrophic scars. The goal is to destroy the fragmented

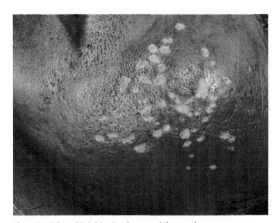

Fig. 7. TCA CROSS. Patient with sunken acne scars; 100% TCA was applied with a toothpick after first performing a test site 2 months earlier. This is advisable with patients with darker skin types. The toothpick is dipped in the acid and ground into the bottom of the scar until a white discoloration becomes apparent. The same procedure can be performed for sunken surgical scars.

collagen, which comprises the majority of the scar, and promote new collagen growth. Use of ablative lasers, especially nonfractional ablative lasers, is limited by adverse side effects, such as prolonged downtime, edema, persistent erythema, keloidal scar formation, and temporary or permanent dyschromia. These side effects are lessened by using a nonablative laser, especially a nonablative fractional laser. Nonablative lasers also induce extracellular matrix remodeling but to a lesser degree than ablative lasers.[37] Especially for atrophic scarring, such as acne scarring, the nonablative lasers achieve inferior results compared with ablative lasers.[38]

Fractionated photothermolysis, which can be used with both ablative and nonablative lasers, has transformed the ability for surgeons to treat hypertrophic and atrophic scars while avoiding many of the adverse effects of nonfractionated lasers (Fig. 8). The principle behind this technology is to create microthermal zones throughout the treatment area, which allows for quicker healing and reepithelization from the neighboring islands of untreated skin.[39] Although underpowered, a randomized controlled split-face trial comparing the efficacy and safety of the ablative fractional CO_2 laser to the nonablative fractional 1550-nm Er:glass laser showed superior results using the ablative fractional CO_2 laser.[37] A study comparing the ablative fractional 2940-nm Er:YAG laser to the ablative fractional 10,600-nm CO_2 laser showed a greater improvement in the pliability of scars when using the fractional CO_2 laser.[39] Tidwell and colleagues[40] conducted a randomized controlled split-scar study comparing the fractionated Er:YAG laser to the fully ablative (nonfractionated) Er:YAG laser, which showed statistically significant superior results in both physician and patient assessment scores with the fractionated Er:YAG laser. One study showed efficacy in the treatment of hypopigmented scars with use of the fractionated 1550-nm erbium-doped laser in combination with topical prostaglandin analog (bimatoprost) and tretinoin or pimecrolimus.[41]

For the ablative and nonablative laser treatments, each treatment area should be cleansed thoroughly with topical alcohol or acetone in the preoperative setting. Use of a topical or local anesthetic or nerve block can be used to mitigate discomfort during these procedures. Intraoperative use of a forced air-cooling device, wet gauze, or ice packs also can be used to further decrease

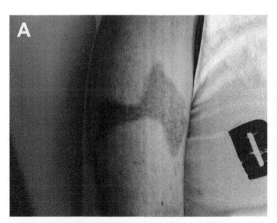
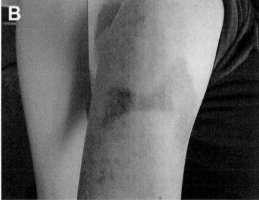

Fig. 8. Fractionated photothermolysis. (A) Hyperpigmented scar resulting from water burn. (B) Two-month follow-up after 3 fractionated 1540-nm erbium-doped fiber treatments. A test site was performed prior to treatment of the entire scar due to patient's dark skin type, something that is always recommended.

patient discomfort. No definitive guidelines have been established for the use of topical or oral antibiotics postoperatively. Some investigators recommend the use of oral anti-inflammatory medications postoperatively to reduce pain and swelling, and prophylactic and postoperative use of antiviral agents is recommended in patients with a history of herpes labialis infections. Sunscreen use is recommended postoperatively, and it is recommended patients avoid sun exposure during the healing process to avoid potential dyschromia.[42]

The 585-nm and 595-nm pulsed dye lasers (PDLs) work on the principle of selective thermolysis, wherein oxyhemoglobin within the vasculature is targeted and destroyed, thus causing localized thrombosis, vasculitis, and tissue remodeling. This collectively acts to decrease the vascular appearance, height, and volume of scars. The efficacy of PDL lasers is well studied, with numerous split-scar studies comparing PDLs to untreated scars, showing significant improvement in pigmentation, vascularity, pliability, and height in the PDL-treated halves.[43] A split-scar study comparing PDL to the ablative fractional 10,600-nm CO_2 laser showed superior results in the decrease in vascularity and improvement in pigmentation using the PDL laser, whereas the CO_2 laser showed superior results in increasing pliability and decreasing thickness.[44] A study comparing the nonablative fractional 1550-nm Er:YAG laser to PDL showed superior results using the Er:YAG laser on postoperative scars.[45] PDL treatment typically is well tolerated with minimal discomfort. The main side effect of PDL treatment is postoperative purpura. Studies have shown, however, comparable improvements in scar appearance using nonpurpuric PDL settings.[46] In addition, studies have shown synergistic effects when PDL is used in combination with ablative fractional CO_2 lasers.[47]

RECOMMENDED APPROACH TO SCAR TREATMENT

Patient expectations and concerns should be the primary drivers of all scar revision treatments. A patient with an unsightly scar who is happy with the outcome probably needs no further treatment. For everyone else, it is important to determine which features about the scar bother the patients, because they may not be the same as those of concern to the surgeon.

A safe, universal recommendation for most patients is the use of silicone gel sheets. Many patients are interested in doing some form of scar treatment, even before they return for follow-up. Providing them with a recommendation prevents the use of other unproved or potentially deleterious treatments that patients may find on their own. Similarly, patients with excellent surgical outcomes who are unsatisfied and have high risk-to-benefit ratios for other treatments can be safely recommended to try this treatment.

For patients with small focally depressed scars, subcision, TCA CROSS, or fractionated laser can be useful, quick, and low risk. Although a full discussion is outside the constraints of this current discussion, anecdotal evidence also has shown success using normal saline and various types of fillers for atrophic scars.[48,49] Especially for rolling and boxcar scars, microneedling has shown success in increasing collagen, dermal thickness, and elastic fibers.[50]

Scars with significant erythema or prominent surrounding telangiectasia treatment can be treated with a vascular laser, silicone gel sheets, and reassurance that the erythema is likely to resolve with time. Hypopigmented scars potentially are improved with the use of a fractionated laser with the addition of topical prostaglandin analog and tretinoin or pimecrolimus.

For widened scars, excision or serial excision often results in excellent outcomes, despite the occurrence of a suboptimal outcome after the original wound repair.

Trapdoor defects or hypertrophic scars should be treated aggressively with intralesional steroids. Occasionally, electroablation or surgical debulking may be necessary where intralesional treatments fail to accomplish the desired outcome.

For lumpy, topographically uneven scars or skin grafts, dermabrasion, electrobrasion, TCA peels, or CO_2 laser resurfacing can produce excellent outcomes.

Ectropion, eclabium, or skin webs often can be addressed with Z-plasty. Similarly, scars not oriented in RSTLs can be redirected via this technique.

SUMMARY

There are many modalities for scar revision, including silicone gel or sheeting, electrosurgery, dermabrasion, chemical peels, subcision, lasers, and surgical excision. Patient characteristics and desires dictate which technique will provide the optimal outcome. The variety of available scar revision techniques broadens the depth of the dermatologic surgeon's capability to create a more cosmetically appealing scar and, therefore, aids in increasing patient satisfaction.

REFERENCES

1. Harmon CB, Zelickson BD, Roenigk RK, et al. Dermabrasive scar revision. Immunohistochemical and ultrastructural evaluation. Dermatol Surg 1995; 21(6):503–8.
2. Cerrati EW, Thomas JR. Scar revision and recontouring Post-Mohs surgery. Facial Plast Surg Clin North Am 2017;25(3):463–71.
3. Smith JE. Dermabrasion. Facial Plast Surg 2014; 30(1):35–9.
4. Ardeshirpour F, Shaye DA, Hilger PA. Improving posttraumatic facial scars. Otolaryngol Clin North Am 2013;46(5):867–81.
5. Kidwell MJ, Arpey CJ, Messingham MJ. A comparison of histologic effectiveness and ultrastructural properties of the electrocautery scratch pad to sandpaper for manual dermabrasion. Dermatol Surg 2008;34(9):1194–9.
6. Nehal KS, Levine VJ, Ross B, et al. Comparison of high-energy pulsed carbon dioxide laser resurfacing and dermabrasion in the revision of surgical scars. Dermatol Surg 1998;24(6):647–50.
7. Christophel JJ, Elm C, Endrizzi BT, et al. A randomized controlled trial of fractional laser therapy and dermabrasion for scar resurfacing. Dermatol Surg 2012;38(4):595–602.
8. Campbell TM, Eisen DB. Electrobrasion–an alternative to dermabrasion. Dermatol Surg 2010;36(11): 1739–42.
9. Kleinerman R, Armstrong AW, Ibrahimi OA, et al. Electrobrasion vs. manual dermabrasion: a randomized, double-blind, comparative effectiveness trial. Br J Dermatol 2014;171(1):124–9.
10. Campbell T, Eisen DB. Fractionated electroblation - using electro surgery for cutaneous redundancies and bulky flaps. Dermatol Online J 2010; 16(6):10.
11. Horswell BB. Scar modification. Techniques for revision and camouflage. Atlas Oral Maxillofac Surg Clin North Am 1998;6(2):55–72.
12. Lee KK, Mehrany K, Swanson NA. Surgical revision. Dermatol Clin 2005;23(1):141–50, vii.
13. Kantor J. The set-back buried dermal suture: an alternative to the buried vertical mattress for layered wound closure. J Am Acad Dermatol 2010;62(2): 351–3.
14. Wang AS, Kleinerman R, Armstrong AW, et al. Setback versus buried vertical mattress suturing: results of a randomized blinded trial. J Am Acad Dermatol 2015;72(4):674–80.
15. Mostafapour SP, Murakami CS. Tissue expansion and serial excision in scar revision. Facial Plast Surg 2001;17(4):245–52.
16. Quaba O, Shoaib T, Durrani AJ, et al. A user's guide for serial excision. J Plast Reconstr Aesthet Surg 2008;61(6):712–5.
17. Liotta DR, Costantino PD, Hiltzik DH. Revising large scars. Facial Plast Surg 2012;28(5):492–6.
18. Ratnarathorn M, Petukhova TA, Armstrong AW, et al. Perceptions of aesthetic outcome of linear vs multiple Z-plasty scars in a national survey. JAMA Facial Plast Surg 2016;18(4):263–7.
19. Furnas DW, Fischer GW. The Z-plasty: biomechanics and mathematics. Br J Plast Surg 1971; 24(2):144–60.
20. Kadakia S, Ducic Y, Jategaonkar A, et al. Scar revision: surgical and nonsurgical options. Facial Plast Surg 2017;33(6):621–6.
21. Liu A, Moy RL, Ozog DM. Current methods employed in the prevention and minimization of surgical scars. Dermatol Surg 2011;37(12):1740–6.
22. Westra I, Pham H, Niessen FB. Topical Silicone sheet application in the treatment of hypertrophic scars and keloids. J Clin Aesthet Dermatol 2016; 9(10):28–35.
23. Chan KY, Lau CL, Adeeb SM, et al. A randomized, placebo-controlled, double-blind, prospective clinical trial of silicone gel in prevention of hypertrophic scar development in median sternotomy wound. Plast Reconstr Surg 2005;116(4):1013–20 [discussion: 1021–2].
24. Cruz-Korchin NI. Effectiveness of silicone sheets in the prevention of hypertrophic breast scars. Ann Plast Surg 1996;37(4):345–8.
25. Meaume S, Le Pillouer-Prost A, Richert B, et al. Management of scars: updated practical guidelines and use of silicones. Eur J Dermatol 2014;24(4):435–43.
26. Morelli Coppola M, Salzillo R, Segreto F, et al. Triamcinolone acetonide intralesional injection for the treatment of keloid scars: patient selection and perspectives. Clin Cosmet Investig Dermatol 2018;11: 387–96.
27. Rahban SR, Garner WL. Fibroproliferative scars. Clin Plast Surg 2003;30(1):77–89.
28. Thomas JR, Somenek M. Scar revision review. Arch Facial Plast Surg 2012;14(3):162–74.
29. Shin TM, Bordeaux JS. The role of massage in scar management: a literature review. Dermatol Surg 2012;38(3):414–23.
30. Orentreich D, Orentreich N. Acne scar revision update. Dermatol Clin 1987;5(2):359–68.
31. Konda S, Potter K, Ren VZ, et al. Techniques for optimizing surgical scars, part 1: wound healing and depressed/atrophic scars. Skinmed 2017;15(4): 271–6.
32. Barikbin B, Akbari Z, Yousefi M, et al. Blunt blade subcision: an evolution in the treatment of atrophic acne scars. Dermatol Surg 2017;43(Suppl 1):S57–s63.
33. Lee JB, Chung WG, Kwahck H, et al. Focal treatment of acne scars with trichloroacetic acid: chemical reconstruction of skin scars method. Dermatol Surg 2002;28(11):1017–21 [discussion: 1021].

34. Dalpizzol M, Weber MB, Mattiazzi AP, et al. Comparative study of the use of trichloroacetic acid and phenolic acid in the treatment of atrophic-type acne scars. Dermatol Surg 2016;42(3):377–83.

35. Roberts WE. Chemical peeling in ethnic/dark skin. Dermatol Ther 2004;17(2):196–205.

36. Nguyen T, Rooney J. Trichloroacetic acid peels. Dermatol Ther 2000;13(2):173–82.

37. Cho SB, Lee SJ, Cho S, et al. Non-ablative 1550-nm erbium-glass and ablative 10 600-nm carbon dioxide fractional lasers for acne scars: a randomized split-face study with blinded response evaluation. J Eur Acad Dermatol Venereol 2010;24(8):921–5.

38. Balaraman B, Geddes ER, Friedman PM. Best reconstructive techniques: improving the final scar. Dermatol Surg 2015;41(Suppl 10):S265–75.

39. Choi JE, Oh GN, Kim JY, et al. Ablative fractional laser treatment for hypertrophic scars: comparison between Er:YAG and CO2 fractional lasers. J Dermatolog Treat 2014;25(4):299–303.

40. Tidwell WJ, Owen CE, Kulp-Shorten C, et al. Fractionated Er:YAG laser versus fully ablative Er:YAG laser for scar revision: results of a split scar, double blinded, prospective trial. Lasers Surg Med 2016; 48(9):837–43.

41. Massaki AB, Fabi SG, Fitzpatrick R. Repigmentation of hypopigmented scars using an erbium-doped 1,550-nm fractionated laser and topical bimatoprost. Dermatol Surg 2012;38(7 Pt 1):995–1001.

42. Gold MH, McGuire M, Mustoe TA, et al. Updated international clinical recommendations on scar management: part 2–algorithms for scar prevention and treatment. Dermatol Surg 2014;40(8):825–31.

43. Alster TS, Williams CM. Treatment of keloid sternotomy scars with 585 nm flashlamp-pumped pulsed-dye laser. Lancet 1995;345(8959):1198–200.

44. Kim DH, Ryu HJ, Choi JE, et al. A comparison of the scar prevention effect between carbon dioxide fractional laser and pulsed dye laser in surgical scars. Dermatol Surg 2014;40(9):973–8.

45. Tierney E, Mahmoud BH, Srivastava D, et al. Treatment of surgical scars with nonablative fractional laser versus pulsed dye laser: a randomized controlled trial. Dermatol Surg 2009;35(8):1172–80.

46. Gladsjo JA, Jiang SI. Treatment of surgical scars using a 595-nm pulsed dye laser using purpuric and nonpurpuric parameters: a comparative study. Dermatol Surg 2014;40(2):118–26.

47. Cohen JL, Geronemus R. Safety and efficacy evaluation of pulsed dye laser treatment, CO2 ablative fractional resurfacing, and combined treatment for surgical scar clearance. J Drugs Dermatol 2016; 15(11):1315–9.

48. Wollina U, Goldman A. Fillers for the improvement in acne scars. Clin Cosmet Investig Dermatol 2015;8: 493–9.

49. Bagherani N, Smoller BR. Introduction of a novel therapeutic option for atrophic acne scars: saline injection therapy. Glob Dermatol 2015;2(6):225–7.

50. Hou A, Cohen B, Haimovic A, et al. Microneedling: a comprehensive review. Dermatol Surg 2017;43(3): 321–39.

Pearls for Dermatologic Surgery in Pediatric Patients

Nnenna G. Agim, MD[a],*, Kishan M. Shah, BA[b]

KEYWORDS

- Pediatric • Caregiver • Anesthesia • Surgery • Pearls • Dermatology • Distraction

KEY POINTS

- Surgical treatment of pediatric patients requires consideration for developmental stages.
- Caregivers can play important roles when executing a procedure in a pediatric patient.
- Distraction techniques lower anxiety, improving overall satisfaction with pediatric surgical procedures.

Children under 18 years, and young adults between 18 and 25 years, with developmental delay or similar disabilities may be seen in the dermatologic surgery setting for diagnostic or therapeutic procedures. **Box 1** highlights several indications for pediatric surgical procedures. Lesions with impact on psychosocial development are considered to be those lesions, such as a visible birthmark, for which a child is bullied, adversely affecting the child's social development and psyche. Generally, any procedure that can be performed in an adult can be executed in a child. The indication to perform surgery is based on the diagnosis as assessed by the surgeon and the family's preference. When in doubt, a referral can always be made to Pediatric Dermatology, Pediatric Plastic Surgery, or Dermatologic Surgery (see **Box 1**).

Typical Diagnoses Requiring Surgical Intervention in Children

It is prudent to commit a patient and their family to surgery only when indicated and safe. As such, managing expectations and preprocedural investigation such as imaging may be required.

Midline lesions, aplasia cutis, dermal sinuses, and subungual exostoses are a selection of lesions for which imaging may alter the decision to proceed in the outpatient dermatologic surgery setting.[1–4]

As with adults, the most common procedures performed in the pediatric population include skin biopsies, excision and closure, destruction of benign neoplasia, intralesional injections, chemical peels, pulsed dye laser treatment, and nail avulsion with or without matrixectomy.

Excision may be necessary for both benign and malignant neoplasms such as nevus sebaceus, melanocytic nevi, dermoid cysts, macronodular juvenile xanthogranulomas (>2 cm), and pilomatricomas, which are the most commonly excised lesions.[5] Shave, punch, snip, and incisional biopsies may be needed for inflammatory, infectious, or neoplastic phenomena.[6] Destruction of verrucae, molluscum, and milia are a common occurrence in the typical pediatric dermatologic practice. Intralesional injection of hypertrophic scars, keloids, alopecia areata, and suppurative hidradenitis occurs more frequently in teenage patients.

Disclosure Statement: The authors have nothing to disclose.
[a] Pediatric Dermatology, University of Texas Southwestern, Dallas, TX, USA; [b] Indiana University School of Medicine, Indianapolis, IN, USA
* Corresponding author.
E-mail address: nnenna.agim@childrens.com

Dermatol Clin 37 (2019) 387–395
https://doi.org/10.1016/j.det.2019.03.008
0733-8635/19/

Box 1
Indications for pediatric dermatologic surgery

When is a pediatric surgical procedure indicated?

- Lesions representing significant health risk
- Lesions with potential for disfigurement
- Lesions with active symptoms
- Lesions with impact on psychosocial development
- Lesions best removed early for superior cosmetic outcome

Box 2
Indications for subspecialty referral

- Plastic surgery
  - Larger excisions, specialized ablative lasers
- Ophthalmology
  - Deep periocular, scleral, or corneal neoplasms
- Otorhinolaryngology
  - Extensive cervical and preauricular dermal sinuses, oral mucosal vascular lesions
- Neurosurgery
  - Midline and scalp sinuses or neoplasia
- Orthopedic surgery
  - Limb asymmetry, deep/circumferential lesions
- Urology
  - Perianal sinuses, distortion of genitalia

In this population, chemical peels with trichloroacetic acid $\pm$ CROSS technique for scarring and botulinum toxin injection for hyperhidrosis may be indicated.[7] Vascular laser treatment of capillary malformations, infantile hemangiomas, rosacea, spider, and neonatal lupus-associated telangiectasia, is also possible. Although requiring multiple sessions, early intervention greatly improves long-term outcomes.[8,9] Keratinaceous, inflammatory, and acneiform epidermal nevi, angiokeratoma, and lymphangioma circumscriptum may benefit from ablative laser therapy.

Nail detachment, biopsy, and/or matrixectomy may be necessary for congenital malalignment of the great toenail, subungual verrucae/exostosis, longitudinal melanonychia, onychomatricomas, and onychocryptosis. The type and frequency of these procedures performed will vary by surgeon. For some diagnoses, it is best to refer to another specialty (**Box 2**).

Approaching the Pediatric Patient

On determining that a procedure is indicated, enlisting the participants is the next step. Approaching this population differs from typical negotiations with an adult patient capable of independent consent. Addressing the needs of pediatric patients involves coordinating with their parents or caregivers while considering the unique aspect of childhood.

Following the first series of immunizations, most children develop an aversion to medical professionals and see them as "the one who gives shots." This translates into anxiety, which is sometimes triggered by visualizing the physician's office building. In this case, minimizing the inherent tension in a patient requiring a procedure is the overarching goal.

Consider a child's developmental stage when planning and executing any given procedure.[10] The Bayley Scales of Infant Development initially published in 1969 by Nancey Bayley, and restandardized to the Bayley-III in 2006, is an example of a tool for reference.[11] Assessment is aimed at children of 16 days to 42 months corrected age, the caveat being that each child progresses through development at their unique rate. Although the Bayley Scales of Infant Development is primarily administered by a trained professional over 45 to 60 minutes to identify the need for early childhood intervention, the concepts therein can be distilled to inform expectations for behavior at any given age, however brief the encounter. Also available are the American Academy of Pediatrics guidelines for developmental surveillance for ages 3 through 21 years.[12] Key considerations from these resources are summarized in **Table 1**.

For any given procedure, the players include the child, the parent/caregiver/family, and the treating medical team. Each possesses a role in making the best possible experience for the patient. Assuming that there is no need to include any foreign language or speech/hearing deficit interpreter during the visit, we will begin by discussing the family's role.

Properly Identify/Verify Primary Caregiver

- Individuals accompanying the patient are not always parents
- Parents may not always be responsible for consent
- Always verify who is responsible for consent of the procedure

Table 1
Developmental stage effects on surgical approach

Patient's Age Range	Expected Behavior	Possible Accommodations
Neonate (0–4 wk)	Crying with adverse/unfamiliar stimuli	Reassurance from physician and caregiver(s); swaddle
Infant (2–12 mo)	Crying with adverse/unfamiliar stimuli	Reassurance from physician and caregiver(s); swaddle
Toddler (12–36 mo)	Active resistance of restriction	Consider sedation if high anxiety; secure all limbs to minimize injury[a] or involve caregiver in positioning[b]
Early childhood (4–7 y)	Variable anxiety, underdeveloped understanding of procedure	Consider sedation if high anxiety; secure all limbs to minimize injury or involve caregiver in positioning
Late childhood (8–10 y)	Variable anxiety, open to negotiation	Consider sedation if anxiety is high; explain procedure, clearly offer reward
Preteen (11–13 y)	Variable anxiety, communicates needs clearly	Obtain assent, address questions directly, reassure, offer personalized comfort measures[c]
Teenage (over 13 y)	May demonstrates angst, indifference, withdrawal, resistance to or minimization of discomfort	Obtain assent, address questions directly, reassure, offer personalized comfort measures[c]

[a] Swaddling technique using sheet or thin blanket pictured below; pillowcase only if arms need to be secured.
[b] Positions of comfort as described and pictured in following segment.
[c] Choice of auditory, visual or environmental stimuli using tablets, screens, other devices.
 Data from Maccow G. Bayley Scales of Infant and Toddler Development. 3rd ed. San Antonio, TX: Pearson Education, Inc; 2008.

Because the consent of an adult caregiver is required before performing a procedure on a child, it is essential to establish who has the legal right to give such permission. An assumption could be made that the adult with whom the child presents is the parent with full rights, but simple questioning may reveal that this is not the case. Ideally, intake personnel establish the relationship between adult and child, but often an assumption is also made at this level and entered erroneously in the medical record. It is our duty as physicians to verify and ensure the child's safety. It is not unusual to encounter a child accompanied by a noncustodial parent, grandparent, birth parent's partner, older sibling, uncle, aunt, foster, or adoptive family, or with older teenagers, or a significant other. If a child is not emancipated, especially where written consent is indicated, the patient's legal guardian must give consent after appropriate counseling. When not present, they can be reached by telephone and a witnessed delegation of the duty to the accompanying adult may be documented. Informed consent must be obtained from the properly identified adult caregiver and clearly documented in the child's medical record.

Assess Degree of Engagement in Procedure

- Identify if there is an adult that the patient seeks for comfort
- Understand the comfort level of the adult with the procedure

If more than 1 adult is present with the patient, assess who controls the situation. With whom is the child more comfortable? Who do they seek out for comfort? Which adult can tolerate witnessing the procedure? Does the adult want to participate in comforting or encouraging the child, or would they be best served by sitting at a distance or outside the room? It is ideal to make sure everyone is on the same page and directing each activity toward a united goal. A guardian's presence has been shown to result in higher satisfaction with procedures and outcomes.[13] In addition, the presence of a caregiver has no effect on complications from procedures.[13] If a parent is squeamish, give them the option to stay behind curtain rather than leave room, allowing their participation through verbal encouragement. This can avoid an occasion in which the adult caregiver faints during the procedure creating a new patient encounter.

Address Anxiety in Caregivers

Although step-by-step understanding of a procedure in adult patients may alleviate anxiety, preprocedural anxiety in pediatric dermatologic procedures is multifactorial. A child's anxiety may be heightened because of the guardian's anxiety about the procedure. It is therefore useful to evaluate and treat the two as a unit.[14] Guardian anxiety has been shown to be directly correlated to the size of the lesion, and indirectly correlated to the age of the patient.[15] It is vital to implicitly address the caregiver's questions and concerns, as this allows for a greater understanding between the patient, caregiver, physician, and staff. It may also provide insight into the child's anxieties that he or she may have revealed to a guardian before the visit.

Address Anxiety in Children

A recent Cochrane review established that psychological methods including hypnosis and distraction were effective in decreasing preprocedural anxiety in children.[16] Distraction diverts attention from painful stimuli, and is most effective in children younger than 7 years old.[17] The use of smart devices, including iPhones, DVD players, and handheld gaming devices, can additionally distract patients form anticipating pain.[18] Anxiolytic treatment of pediatric patients with a combination of oral benzodiazepines and inhaled nitrous oxide, with appropriate preparedness should complications occur, have been shown to be a useful and safe adjuvant for surgical procedures.[19,20] The administration of oral benzodiazepines is not common practice for pediatric dermatologists. Institutional policies guide use of such drugs; for example, in our institution, anesthesiologists recommend dose, and administer these medications before procedures. Overall, as mentioned earlier, there will then be an unavoidable degree of fear in the preprocedural period. Therefore, it is best to control other aspects of the procedure including pain, surgery-related distress, the relationship between the surgical team, child and caregivers, for overall satisfaction.[21]

Encourage the Engaged Caregiver's Active Role

- Patients can be held during procedures
- Allow the adult and patient's input
- Engaging in conversation can reduce anxiety
- Set boundaries on recording procedures
- Use smart devices

If positioning for the procedure allows, the patient can be placed in their comforting adult caregiver's arms in any of the positions described below (**Box 3**).

Positions of Comfort

To prevent falls and injury to the patient or staff, while providing the familiar environment of a hug, positions of comfort and other forms of limb security can help improve procedure efficiency (see **Box 3**).

For procedures performed under general anesthesia, encourage parent and child interaction until the start of procedure. Pair duration with position (prone, supine, lateral), using gel bars/donuts to cushion pressure point. Safety straps and arm boards further customize security. Most surgical centers/outpatient operating rooms have a streamlined process for the tool assembly line. The tool assembly line refers to the tray with all items arranged in order of typical use for the assistant to pass to the surgeon.

Explain the positioning to the parent and child and practice before the actual procedure. Give opportunity for questions and options for an alternative arrangement. Keep a conversation going about the procedure and other aspects of the patient's life throughout, creating a reassuring setting and calming distraction. Older children sometimes ask to watch the procedure, which is at the physician's discretion. It is not unreasonable to have a clear policy regarding video recording. Patients or their caregivers may ask permission to, or spontaneously film on their smart devices, so this issue must addressing to avoid conflict. A smart device may be used to deploy distraction in the form or music, video, or games, none of which may be permitted to simultaneously film the procedure.

Stage the Treatment Room

To reduce anxiety, carefully select each team member's location in the room and the position of the tray relative to the treatment site (**Fig. 1**).

Consider what the child sees: a child-friendly examination room with a comfortable/steady examination table, chairs, and neutral or themed décor.

Box 3 Positions of comfort
Straddle position (arms, legs)
Side sitting (arms, legs, back)
Front to back (arms, face, trunk)
Superhero pillowcase ("cape")
Burrito

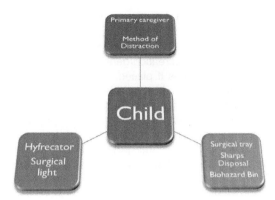

Fig. 1. Surgical room layout.

Avoid bright lights initially, keep the surgical tray and any sharps out of full view. Boredom can amplify anxiety, so keep the child occupied from arrival until the procedure. Possible distraction methods include activity/coloring books, music, movies, and wall-mounted play stations.[18,22]

Consider what the child hears: friendly staff, friendly physician or other provider, no loud sounds (tools clanging on tray); primary caregiver's voice reassuring. Given limitations in receptive and expressive communication, approach the child with succinct, direct phrases. Limit negotiation but avoid use of words that can threaten bodily injury or trigger anxiety. For example, instead of saying "I will inject your skin with local anesthetic then cut out the lesion," one might couch the same information as: "I will place some medication under your skin to help it go to sleep; once it is asleep, the 'bad spot' will be removed."

Consider what the child needs: "position of comfort," entrapment of active limbs, additional staff for security, topical anesthesia, bathroom break

- Assess placement of tools and rewards
- Keep sharps and irritants out of reach
- Secure the patient on the examination table

OLDER CHILDREN

Grade school-aged children and teenagers are usually adept at self-care, self-direction, self-regulation, emotional communication, and purposeful engagement. As such, involve them in the decision to proceed and consent throughout the procedure. Assess their level of interest, explain the procedure with more detail if they are interested, offer encouragement, and allow selection of a distraction technique. During the procedure, acknowledge expected discomfort, request feedback, and emphasize the timeline/progress if desired. For example, some children will want a

countdown before injections, while others prefer and clearly communicate the desire for a swift direct approach.

Topical Anesthesia

A eutectic mixture of lidocaine and prilocaine (EMLA) should be avoided in infants because of the risk of methemoglobinemia. EMLA is generally safe after age 1, regardless of prematurity and birthweight. Apart from this age group, application of a specified amount of EMLA, lidocaine (2%, 4%, or 5%), with or without occlusion, can initiate pain relief before the procedure. The area of application generally should not exceed 5 × 5 cm. The ideal time of application is between 60 and 15 minutes before the procedure, because, if applied too early or too late, it has no effect on perceived pain.

Local Anesthesia

Local anesthesia is a fundamental part of cutaneous surgery, widely used in adult and pediatric surgery. The injection of a local anesthetic is often the most painful and memorable part of the procedure for pediatric patients.[23] Vibratory tools, such as Buzzy (**Fig. 2**), allow for recruitment of pressure sensing nerves as does a generous pinch or depression on adjacent skin. This is a US Food and Drug Administration–approved neuromodulation method, which reduces the pain of an injection.

Smart devices or classic toys and games can also be used as distraction techniques. Reading a story book, blowing bubbles, a puppet show or magic tricks can divert the patient's attention from the painful procedure long enough to infiltrate

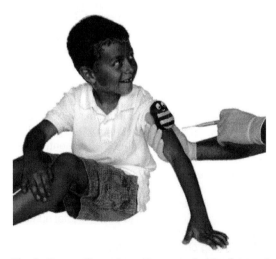

Fig. 2. Buzzy. (*From* https://www.pediatricsafety.net/2011/07/buzzy/ (Buzzy, Atlanta, Georgia).)

the skin with lidocaine or Marcaine. Lidocaine is not usually buffered in pediatric patients. Regulations on in-office compounding may preclude use of the buffered mixture. Marcaine is sometimes used to offer longer-lasting postsurgical anesthesia. Ultimately, the choice is left to the surgeon's preference. The needle and syringe should be kept out of the line of sight, further reducing anxiety. Where available, child life specialists can help with the distraction techniques.

General Anesthesia

- Most modern medications do not carry grave sequelae
- Pediatric anesthesiologists are an asset
- Estimated risk for major adverse event per American Society of Anesthesia = 1:20,000

When indicated, procedures estimated to take 60 minutes or less can be safely performed under general anesthesia. The frequency of major adverse events including nausea/vomiting, bradycardia, postintubation croup, malignant hyperthermia, cardiac arrest, respiratory failure, and death have been studied. The estimated risk is 0.0005% in facilities with pediatric anesthesiologists. Age cutoff is defined by comfort of the anesthesiologists in the institution. Most dermatologic surgeries last less than an hour. We start at age 6 months. Studies have shown safety down to 2 months.[24] Concerns relating to long-term intellectual disability relate to much longer procedures. For example, 6 pulsed dye laser treatments during which a child is exposed to general anesthesia for less than 10 minutes per session may not even approach this threshold. Privileges in a facility with pediatric anesthesiologists are indispensable for this arrangement, given the attributed 300-fold risk reduction in this situation.[24]

Establish the Surgical Team's Role(s)

The information contained in this article can be distilled for training support staff; their contribution to the overarching game plan will likewise minimize pain and anxiety. Assign team member roles before entering the room and introduce personnel to the family. Indicate whether the resident, if present, or attending will lead execution of procedure. If you host medical students, they can also help by engaging the patient and family in pleasant conversation. However, depending on the family's preference, you may need to limit the total number of staff in the room.

Depending on practice culture, nurses or medical assistants can apply topical anesthesia, supervise the surgical tray, and educate the family regarding wound care instructions. Postprocedure, emphasis should be placed on physical activity restrictions, avoiding immersion of wounds in water during recreation/general grooming, and duration of sutures if placed. Specific written instructions should be provided, especially for school and sporting commitments. Proper use of sunscreen and silicone dressing for optimizing scars may also be reviewed.

Expectations for the postoperative course, including the development of temporary edema, erythema, pruritus, and postanesthesia pain, along with ameliorating measures should be outlined unequivocally. A call to check on family within 48 hours can reaffirm provided instructions and prevent complications. Recommend in-office suture removal for complicated repairs; simple interrupted and running sutures can be removed by a local pediatrician or physician extender if the patient lives at a distance. To minimize postprocedural anxiety when a specimen is sent to pathology, also consider timely/thoughtful communication of results.

Tools

Because children generally have supple skin and exhibit rapid wound healing, they require a shorter duration for suture removal, usually 5 to 7 days. Depending on body location, a smaller-caliber suture may be needed. Prepubertal children do not have thick sebaceous skin on the face and trunk, also allowing use of smaller-caliber suture. Smaller-caliber sutures are also used for delicate areas to minimize scars. Under the age of 10, suture removal on scalp and trunk is recommended at 7 days. When placing sutures, space should be allowed for swelling to minimize track marks.

Tools that can enhance the procedure include use of a #15C blade for more precision in small spaces and delicate areas. For lesions on the oral mucosa, a chalazion clamp can help secure the treatment area and provide a measure of hemostasis.[25,26] A white eyeliner pencil may be useful for delineating capillary malformations in the operating suite.[27] Raney clips can be used for scalp surgery.[28]

Techniques

There are several different suturing techniques that may be used for pediatric dermatology procedures. First, purse string closure (**Fig. 3**) may be considered for excisions on the scalp, back, mid cheek, and abdomen. Purse string closure has been successfully used in patients from 4 months to 17 years for lesions less than 4 cm, especially if facial. A second procedure to convert the circular scar to a linear one may be necessary

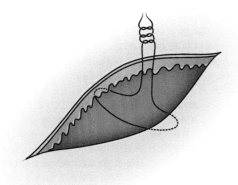

Fig. 3. Pursestring sutures in the upper dermis. (*Adapted from* Wagner AM. Slick suturing for impatient patients. *Pediatr Dermatol.* 1998;15(1):62-64; with permission.)

for older patients or larger lesions.[29] This usually has a reasonable cosmetic outcome and can minimize scar length.[30] Running subcuticular sutures allows prolonged approximation of suture line, and reduces subcuticular dissolvable suture spitting in active children (**Fig. 4**). Although the type of suture used is up to the surgeon discretion, we use clear polypropolene.[31] Individual horizontal mattress sutures can help closure of tight spaces. These may include, but are not limited to, perinasal, periocular, and periauricular lesions[32,33] (see **Figs. 3** and **4**).

Executing the Procedure

With the entire team and family's engagement, safe comfortable positioning and audible reassurance, the procedure may begin. The aim includes

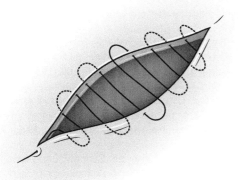

Fig. 4. Running subcuticular suture. (*Adapted from* Wagner AM. Slick suturing for impatient patients. *Pediatr Dermatol.* 1998;15(1):62-64; with permission.)

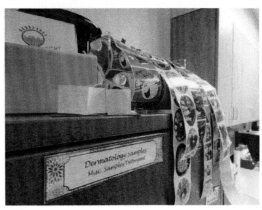

Fig. 5. Reward sticker rolls.

carrying out a coordinated, efficient procedure with a swift return to the preprocedural state.

To minimize interruptions, all instruments necessary should be in the room, and a negotiated reward should be easily accessible and/or visible to the patient. Younger patients readily accept stickers (**Fig. 5**) and small inexpensive plastic toys (**Fig. 6**) or books, in addition to congratulations on their bravery. To maintain a low-anxiety environment, the following are recommended:

- Soiled/bloody gauze pieces should be discarded discretely as soon as generated
- Sharp instruments should remain on the surgical tray when not in use and out of the line of sight
- Dropped instruments should be left of the floor without accompanying alarming exclamations
- If the bed or table is raised, it should be lowered before the patient gets up to avoid falls
- Dispose of all sharps before leaving the treatment room

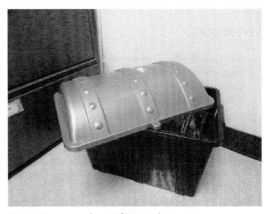

Fig. 6. Treasure chest of rewards.

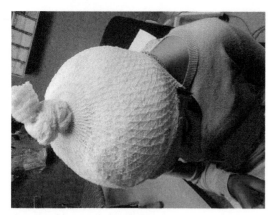

Fig. 7. Baklava style head dressing.

- Maintain conversation and request feedback throughout
- Congratulate parent and child participation in the procedure
- Review restrictions and wound care instructions verbally
- For younger children, provide tangible reward for effort

If necessary, once the procedure is complete, a secure dressing should be applied. Because children are generally physically active and may not fully understand restrictions, a simple wound dressing may come undone with vigorous physical activity. Any dressing should be planned with security against this fact. Strategies include using short adhesive strips over sutures, reusable stretch bandage wraps on limbs, and a balaklava style head dressing (**Fig. 7**) for the scalp. Running subcuticular sutures may offer more security in areas of frequent movement, minimizing scar spread. If a clear polypropolene or a similar nonabsorbable suture is used, these sutures can be left in for 2 weeks, offering a discrete scaffold for scar formation (see **Figs. 5–7**).

REFERENCES

1. Yan C, Low DW. A rare presentation of a dermoid cyst with draining sinus in a child: case report and literature review. Pediatr Dermatol 2016;33(4): e244–8.
2. Hsu JW, Tom WL. Omphalomesenteric duct remnants: umbilical versus umbilical cord lesions. Pediatr Dermatol 2011;28(4):404–7.
3. Kargl S, Silye R, Pumberger W. Sinus sternoclavicularis: a congenital cervical sinus. Pediatr Dermatol 2015;32(2):240–3.
4. Gokdemir G, Ekmen S, Gungor S, et al. Perianal rhabdomyosarcoma: report of a case in an infant and review of the literature. Pediatr Dermatol 2013; 30(1):97–9.
5. Bowen CD, Roberts JE, Dominguez AR, et al. Large, exophytic mass on the scalp of a newborn. Solitary infantile myofibroma. Pediatr Dermatol 2015;32(2): 281–2.
6. Brockman RM, Humphrey SR, Moe DC, et al. Mimickers of infantile hemangiomas. Pediatr Dermatol 2017;34(3):331–6.
7. Gelbard CM, Epstein H, Hebert A. Primary pediatric hyperhidrosis: a review of current treatment options. Pediatr Dermatol 2008;25(6):591–8.
8. Hochman M, Adams DM, Reeves TD. Current knowledge and management of vascular anomalies, II: malformations. Arch Facial Plast Surg 2011;13(6): 425–33.
9. Hochman M, Adams DM, Reeves TD. Current knowledge and management of vascular anomalies: I. Hemangiomas. Arch Facial Plast Surg 2011;13(3): 145–51.
10. Sharp M, DeMauro SB. Counterbalanced comparison of the BSID-II and Bayley-III at eighteen to twenty-two months corrected age. J Dev Behav Pediatr 2017;38(5):322–9.
11. Maccow G. Bayley scales of infant and toddler development. 3rd edition. San Antonio (TX): Pearson Education, Inc; 2008.
12. Committee on Practice and Ambulatory Medicine, Bright Futures Periodicity Schedule Workgroup. 2017 recommendations for preventive pediatric health care. Pediatrics 2017;139(4) [pii:e20170254].
13. Piira T, Sugiura T, Champion GD, et al. The role of parental presence in the context of children's medical procedures: a systematic review. Child Care Health Dev 2005;31(2):233–43.
14. Baxter L. Common office procedures and analgesia considerations. Pediatr Clin North Am 2013;60(5): 1163–83.
15. Hoetzenecker W, Guenova E, Krug M, et al. Parental anxiety and concern for children undergoing dermatological surgery. J Dermatolog Treat 2014;25(5): 367–70.
16. Taddio A, McMurtry CM. Psychological interventions for needle-related procedural pain and distress in children and adolescents. Paediatr Child Health 2015;20(4):195–6.
17. Kleiber C, Harper DC. Effects of distraction on children's pain and distress during medical procedures: a meta-analysis. Nurs Res 1999;48(1): 44–9.
18. Burk CJ, Benjamin LT, Connelly EA. Distraction anesthesia for pediatric dermatology procedures. Pediatr Dermatol 2007;24(4):419–20.
19. Otley CC, Nguyen TH, Phillips PK. Anxiolysis with oral midazolam in pediatric patients undergoing dermatologic surgical procedures. J Am Acad Dermatol 2001;45(1):105–8.

20. Otley CC, Nguyen TH. Conscious sedation of pediatric patients with combination oral benzodiazepines and inhaled nitrous oxide. Dermatol Surg 2000;26(11):1041–4.

21. El Hachem M, Carnevale C, Diociaiuti A, et al. Local anesthesia in pediatric dermatologic surgery: evaluation of a patient-centered approach. Pediatr Dermatol 2018;35(1):112–6.

22. Salvaggio HL, Zaenglein AL. "Magic goggles": a distraction technique for pediatric dermatology procedures. Pediatr Dermatol 2012;29(3):387–8.

23. Yates B, Whalen J, Makkar H. An age-based approach to dermatologic surgery: kids are not just little people. Clin Dermatol 2017;35(6):512–6.

24. Juern AM, Cassidy LD, Lyon VB. More evidence confirming the safety of general anesthesia in pediatric dermatologic surgery. Pediatr Dermatol 2010; 27(4):355–60.

25. Bodner L, Manor E, Joshua BZ, et al. Oral mucoceles in children–analysis of 56 new cases. Pediatr Dermatol 2015;32(5):647–50.

26. Pagliarello C, Paradisi A. Using ringed scissor handles to dry the operative field. Pediatr Dermatol 2010;27(1):115–6.

27. O'Regan GM, Benjamin LT. Delineating capillary malformations in the operating suite using white eyeliner pencil. Pediatr Dermatol 2011;28(6):746–7.

28. Williams JV, Bickel KD, Cunningham BB. Raney clips: excision of vascular lesions on the scalp made (ridiculously) simple. Pediatr Dermatol 2000; 17(3):238–9.

29. Mulliken JB, Rogers GF, Marler JJ. Circular excision of hemangioma and purse-string closure: the smallest possible scar. Plast Reconstr Surg 2002;109(5): 1544–54 [discussion: 1555].

30. Baraldini V, Coletti M, Cigognetti F, et al. Haemostatic squeezing and purse-string sutures: optimising surgical techniques for early excision of critical infantile haemangiomas. J Pediatr Surg 2007;42(2): 381–5.

31. Wagner AM. Slick suturing for impatient patients. Pediatr Dermatol 1998;15(1):62–4.

32. Bellet JS, Wagner AM. Difficult-to-control bleeding. Pediatr Dermatol 2009;26(5):559–62.

33. Wagner AM, Listina K. The ultimate dressing: no mess, no fuss, no phone calls. Pediatr Dermatol 1999;16(1):62–4.

Moving?

Make sure your subscription moves with you!

To notify us of your new address, find your **Clinics Account Number** (located on your mailing label above your name), and contact customer service at:

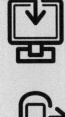

Email: journalscustomerservice-usa@elsevier.com

800-654-2452 (subscribers in the U.S. & Canada)
314-447-8871 (subscribers outside of the U.S. & Canada)

Fax number: 314-447-8029

Elsevier Health Sciences Division
Subscription Customer Service
3251 Riverport Lane
Maryland Heights, MO 63043

*To ensure uninterrupted delivery of your subscription, please notify us at least 4 weeks in advance of move.

Printed and bound by CPI Group (UK) Ltd, Croydon, CR0 4YY

03/10/2024

01040374-0020